Ethics in Health Care

S.A. Pera & S. van Tonder
(Editors)

WIRRAL EDUCATION CENTRE
JUTA
LIBRARY
0151 604 7291

First published 1996 as Ethics in Nursing Practice
Reprinted 1997
Reprinted 2002

Ethics in Health Care second edition 2005

©Juta & Co. Ltd PO Box 1473 Landsowne, 7779

ISBN 0 7021 66790

Editor: Louis van Schaik
Proofreader: Adrienne Pretorius
Cover design: WaterBerry Designs
Index by: Cecily van Gend
Typeset by Lebone Publishing Services
Printed and bound by Distinct Holdings Pty Ltd

Table of Contents

Page

Preface... iv

List of contributors vi

Part 1 Perspectives on health-care ethics

Chapter

1   The moral and ethical foundation of nursing 3
2   The caring ethic in nursing 11

Part 2 Perspectives on ethical theory, principles and decision-making in health care

3   Ethical theory and decision-making in nursing and health care 27
4   Ethical principles and rules in moral decision-making and
     professional-patient relationships 46

Part 3 Perspectives on rights and relationships in health-care practice

5   Human rights and legal liability in nursing practice 59
6   Ethical concerns in relationships between nurses, patients, family
     members and members of the health-care team 70
7   Ethical concerns in relationships between nurses, their employing
     authorities and trade unions 82
8   The rights of patients and nurses in health care 97

Part 4 Perspectives on ethical issues in health-care practice

9   Nursing and health-care issues from the beginning of life to adolescence 111
10   Nursing and health-care issues from the beginning of adulthood to the
     end of life 124
11   Management ethics 140
12   Ethics in research 147

Part 5 Perspectives on transcultural issues in health-care practice

13   Dealing with cultural differences 167
14   Religious and cultural forces in transcultural nursing 175

Part 6 Perspectives on the application of ethical theory in health-care

15   Ethical principles in caring for HIV/AIDS patients 201

References 221

Index 236

Preface

Since the appearance of this book in 1996, nurses in southern Africa have been faced by an increasing number of ethical dilemmas. While the new millennium has brought about many advances in our society, numerous problems remain in the provision of health care. Ethical issues in particular currently receive attention in the mass media in the form of legal decisions and reports.

The exploding AIDS crisis in Africa, the right to abortion, the plight of homeless and displaced persons, the escalation in child abuse, the status of live-in partners and the elderly, all of these raise crucial ethical questions. In the field of nursing practice, nurses have to provide care for increasing numbers of patients. At the same time, costs are being reduced in many hospitals and health-care centres in South Africa by cutting down on the number of nurses.

Confronted by staff shortages, nurses under very difficult conditions try to keep the interests of the patient foremost by providing a caring, qualitative nursing environment. Acting justly, challenging evolving policies and practices, promoting ethical conduct, cultural competence and a research ethic: these are just some of the challenges facing the nurse today.

We have thoroughly revised this edition and have added new material, while continuing to discuss ethical issues from the perspective of nursing. The structure of the book has been modified to accommodate the needs of diverse students in South Africa. All chapters have been updated and expanded to include new material and four new chapters have been added. The chapters have been reorganised into six parts and each chapter provides outcomes and critical thinking activities to expand the understanding of the content and to encourage reflection and dialogue. The index at the end of the book provides a quick reference-tool.

Part One presents perspectives on nursing ethics and caring. The two chapters deal with the moral and ethical foundation of nursing and the caring ethic in nursing. The new chapter on caring redefines nursing ethics as the ethic of caring, which is the hallmark of professional nursing.

Part Two contains two chapters, which deal with perspectives on ethical theory, ethical principles and decision-making in nursing and health care.

Part Three focuses on rights and relationships in nursing practice and consists of four chapters. The content deals with human rights and legal liability, and with problems in relationships between nurses, patients, families and doctors. Ethical concerns in relation to employers and trade unions are also dealt with. Systematic understaffing and staff shortages have lead to job dissatisfaction and are creating moral distress amongst nurses. A disturbing trend in South Africa is that nurses are being held accountable for a failing system over which they have no control. The rights of patients and nurses are also addressed.

Part Four highlights moral dilemmas in the context of health-care practice and consists of four chapters. Issues relating to nursing care from the beginning to the end of life are dealt with. The effects of the HIV/AIDS epidemic in South Africa are highlighted throughout. Two new chapters, which deal with current issues in the field of health care, have been added to this section. The issue of management ethics is addressed owing to a need to define boundaries for ethical behaviour. Rising costs, the increasing demand for quality care, the introduction of managed care and the possibility of fraud in relation to medical aid schemes give rise to the introduction of a new concept: organisational ethics. Nursing research and research in health sciences are gathering momentum in this country. Because the patient remains the nurse's primary concern, any involvement in research demands that the nurse extend the caring ethic into the realm of research to benefit the patient.

Part Five consists of two chapters that focus on transcultural issues in nursing practice. Religious and cultural factors, and problems of dealing with cultural differences, are addressed.

Part Six consists of one chapter, which deals with perspectives on the application of ethical theory in nursing practice. This chapter is entitled 'Ethical principles in caring for HIV/ AIDS patients' and in it both the bioethical and the public health perspectives on HIV/AIDS are addressed as well as the ethics of HIV testing, stigmatisation, tolerance, and research into HIV/AIDS related issues.

We are pleased that the response to this book has been such that we were asked to do a second edition. We want to thank all who contributed to this edition. Their specialised education, vast experience and deep understanding of the specific areas about which they write bring insight and understanding to issues confronting nurses today.

Once again we are indebted to Mrs Valerie Pretorius and wish to thank her for her overall secretarial assistance.

THE EDITORS

List of Contributors

S.A. Pera, B Cur (I et A) (Pretoria), M Cur (Pretoria), D Cur (UPE), DNE (Pretoria), RGN, RM, RT, RNA, RCN, Orth & Spinal N.
Professor Emeritus, Department of Nursing Science, UNISA, Pretoria.

S. van Tonder, B Cur (I et A) (Pretoria), Hons BA (Cur) (UNISA), M Cur (UNISA), D Cur (UPE), DNA (Pretoria), R Int, N, RGN, RM, RCN, RT, RNA Orth & Spinal N.
Professor Emeritus, Department of Nursing Science, UNISA, Pretoria.

T. Verschoor, B. Iur, LL.D. (Professor)
Vice-rector: Academic Operations, University of the Orange-Free State.

R.M. Jansen, B. Iur, LLM, LL.B, B. SocSc (Hons) Nursing, DNE.
Professor, Private Law, University of the Orange-Free State.

M.M. Groenewald, B.A. (Cur) (UNISA), MA (Nursing) (PU for CHE), RGN, RM, RCN, RT.
Lecturer, Department of Health Studies, UNISA, Pretoria.

M.J. Oosthuizen, B Cur (Pretoria), MA Cur (UNISA), HONS B.A. (Cur) (UNISA), D Litt et Phil (UNISA), DNE (Pretoria) RGN, RM, RT, RPN, RCN.
Lecturer, Department of Health Studies, UNISA, Pretoria.

D.M. van der Wal, RGN, BA. (Soc. Crim) UNISA, D. Litt et Phil (UNISA).
Senior Lecturer, Department of Health Studies, UNISA, Pretoria

N. Geyer, B Cur, M Cur (UP), RN, RM, RPN.
Deputy Director, Professional Matters, DENOSA.

T. Mngomezulu, BA Cur (UNISA), MPH (University of Dundee, Scotland), RN, RM.
Deputy Director, Industrial Relations, DENOSA.

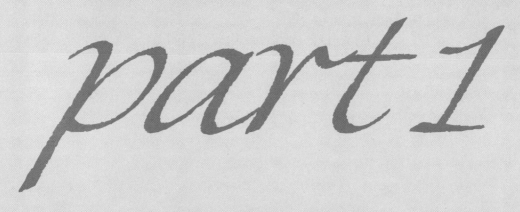

Perspectives on health-care ethics

You, the reader, whoever you are, are not a complete novice in ethics. You understand the meaning of 'good' and 'bad', 'right' and 'wrong', and you know that some actions are right while others are wrong and that some things are good while others are bad. These aspects are precisely what ethics as a subject of systematic study deals with

(Ewing 1995:1).

The moral and ethical foundation of nursing

Silvia Pera

Outcomes

Studying this chapter will enable you to:

- critically discuss the nursing profession's concern for ethics in nursing practice
- differentiate between ethics, morality and moral values
- outline the nature and scope of ethics
- describe the place of values in nursing practice
- distinguish between personal values and nursing values
- differentiate between values, attitudes and beliefs
- discuss the importance of values in providing guidelines for conduct in nursing practice.

Introduction

Nursing is a caring and inherently moral enterprise, and nursing practice is characterised by its long and noteworthy moral tradition. The nursing profession teaches its practitioners to advocate the well-being of patients and their families with compassion, commitment, confidence, competence and a deep sense of moral awareness. The primary task of caring for those in need is appropriate to the nursing profession because nursing practitioners have closer contact with patients and their families than practitioners of any other discipline. This unique position carries privileges and responsibilities that demand total commitment towards those who are ministered to and cared for. Nurses are taught to respect human life, to protect human dignity and to maintain a person-centred approach in nursing practice.

Ethics in nursing practice

The nursing profession's concern for ethics in nursing practice was expressed more than a century ago when the Nightingale Pledge was introduced as an oath for nurses completing their training. Fowler (1989:955) believes that nursing ethics is a social ethics because it is based on an enduring ideal of service, which is not confined to bedside nursing. Progress in society, in biomedical technology and in health care has brought about a greater awareness of ethical issues and the need for moral conduct. Moreover, nurses today practise their profession in multicultural societies where there is often a range of moral values which often differ. There has accordingly been a shift from a general moral consensus to the tolerance of diversity. In everyday practice, nurses come into contact with divergent moral beliefs. They often find themselves in situations where conflict exists between the value systems of patients, health-care institutions, and among other health professionals. Where these situations arise, nurses are required to make moral decisions, and they face the consequences of such decisions.

The aim of this text is to provide an overview of nursing ethics from the perspective of the authors and from the work of others. We believe that nurses in society should be guided by moral considerations and have knowledge of ethical views that support reasons for moral choices. The purpose of this chapter is to outline the discipline of ethics, define basic terms from a nursing perspective and explain the importance of values in nursing and health care.

The foundation of ethics

The ancient Greek philosopher Socrates (born 470 BC) is generally considered the founder of ethics in the Western tradition. Socrates was convinced that neither virtue nor ethical conduct is possible without an understanding of the meaning of ethical concepts (Husted & Husted 1995:5). The word 'ethics' derives from the Greek *ethikos*, while the word 'morals' derives from the Latin *moralis*. Both words relate to the customs, conventions or character peculiar to a given people. Although the concept of ethics still retains its original meaning, it has been extended to include the study of moral beliefs.

Ethics

The concept of ethics has several meanings. Sometimes it is used to refer to the practices or beliefs of a particular group of individuals, for example Christian ethics, medical ethics or nursing ethics. Sometimes it refers to the standards and behaviour expected of a group as described in the group's code of professional conduct. The concept is also used to refer to a philosophical method of enquiry, which enables us to understand the moral dimensions of human conduct. In this sense ethics is an activity, a particular method of enquiry that one undertakes to respond to particular questions about human welfare (Fry in Creasia & Parker 1991:149).

Ethics as a branch of philosophy is called moral philosophy and addresses issues of human conduct that are of great importance to nurses and other health professionals. Rumbold (1993:1) asserts that at its most fundamental, ethics is concerned with the meaning of words such as *right, wrong, good, bad, ought, duty*. Ethics explores the basis on which people, individually or collectively, decide whether actions are right or wrong, and whether something ought to be done, or whether they have the right to do something. Deloughery (1991:178-179) points out that etiquette is not an ethical issue because, while certain behaviour may violate social etiquette, such as chewing gum, using vulgar language or wearing unprofessional clothes, this type of behaviour is not unethical. However, a nurse or a doctor's violation of a patient's rights is rightly considered an ethical issue. Deloughery maintains that ethics is concerned with what people *ought to* attach value to and the reasons why conduct *ought to* be considered right or wrong, and not so much with what people do attach value to or consider right or wrong. Tschudin (1993:preface) maintains that ethics lies at the heart of nursing because nursing and caring are synonymous, and caring is inescapably an ethical issue. Ethics is thus a generic term for various ways of understanding and examining the moral life.

Morality

The term 'moral' tends to refer to the norms of conduct, which individuals and groups uphold and adhere to. The violation of a moral rule by an individual may, for example, elicit disapproval in the form of mistrust, hostility or ostracism by the group. Morals refer to what we should or should not do and, as Thompson & Thompson (1992:5) maintain, they embrace the 'oughts' and 'ought nots' of life. Good examples of moral principles are the Ten Commandments of Judaism and Christianity.

Norms about right and wrong human conduct are generally widely shared by members of a particular society. They form a stable social consensus and encompass standards of conduct, which include moral principles, rules, rights and virtues. Beauchamp and Childress refer to the notion of a *common morality* that all morally serious persons share. Likewise, most professions contain a professional morality with standards of conduct that are acknowledged by those in the profession who are serious about their moral responsibilities (Beauchamp & Childress 2001:3-5).

Moral values

Tschudin (1993:2) believes that values are closely related to the meaning of life. According to Steele (in Steele & Harmon 1983:1), a value is an affective disposition towards a person, an object or an idea and represents a way of life. Values relate to our identity and we find our values through specific experiences and from our association with other people.

Ethics and the law

Ethics is not synonymous with law, although Deloughery (1991:179) maintains that law and ethics sometimes overlap, for example when the law requires a nurse to provide a patient with sufficient information to enable the patient to make an informed decision on proposed treatment. At other times, judgements of law and ethics are dichotomous, for example when a distinction is made between taking a patient off a respirator and not putting the patient on a respirator in the first place. Deloughery maintains that ethicists would never make such a distinction.

The concepts of ethics and the law both serve as guides to action and both have social sanctions and functions. Laws are promulgated to maintain order in society and to establish minimum standards for social conduct. Ethics, on the other hand, may make a demand on an individual, which may conflict with or even violate the demands of the law. Ethics is regarded as higher than the law and often serves as a source of judgement of the law itself. At the level of everyday decision-making, disregard for the law may result in punishment, whereas disregard for ethical norms does not carry the same force (Fowler in Fowler & Levine-Ariff, 1987:26).

Wright (1987:xiii) warns against the temptation to consult the law when addressing ethical issues, particularly in the context of health care. He argues that, since legal decisions are made by individuals, judges and juries, such decisions are based on individual value judgements, which should be analysed in their own context and not merely accepted automatically.

Nursing ethics

Nursing ethics has evolved from philosophical schools of thought and has now become a specialised subject to meet the needs of the nursing profession. Deloughery (1991:178-

179) argues that nursing ethics is not synonymous with medical ethics, since nursing is a profession in its own right. Nursing ethics is concerned with specific moral problems that occur within the context of nursing practice.

Fowler (in Fowler & Levine-Ariff 1987:186) argues that nursing has a distinctive nursing ethics. Because nursing is a distinctive profession with its own distinctive concepts and caring function, it also has its own particular means of expression. She argues that, since nursing is not merely a branch of medical science, it is proper to discuss nursing ethics separately from medical ethics.

Caring and nursing ethics

Caring is the cornerstone of all nursing that is moral and centred on the well-being of patients. Caring is a commitment and entails respect for all persons (Bandman & Bandman 2002:13). Caring means that patients matter as persons. (This idea will be dealt with more fully in the next chapter.)

Bioethics or biomedical ethics

Bioethics is the study of the moral and social implications of techniques resulting from advances in the biological sciences. Bioethics has emerged partly because of the vulnerability of patients and the extremely intimate relationship between patients and health professionals, together with the undesirable degree of power, which health professionals hold over patients. Bioethics is especially important because humans are used as subjects of medical research and because of the growing threat of malpractice suits (Husted & Husted 1995:5-6). In practice, bioethics has come to be practically interchangeable with medical ethics or biomedical ethics (the ethics of health care) (Thompson & Thompson 1992:8).

Codes of ethics

Common guidelines, which are used by nurses for making ethical decisions, are contained in various codes or pledges. Like other professional codes of ethics, nursing codes contain rules and moral standards applicable to nursing conduct. While some codes address specific issues and are not confined to matters of etiquette or broad statements, most do not give guidance on conduct in specific situations. Nursing codes not only guide members of the profession but also serve as a declaration to the public they serve.

Established professions like the nursing profession tend to express explicitly the moral standards which guide their professional conduct. Professions consequently rely on the integrity of their members to carry out their work in the best interests of those whom they serve. In practice, then, while codes of ethics have limitations and cannot provide answers to day-to-day moral dilemmas, they do provide a framework of general rights, duties, values and policies that govern professional practice (Thompson, Melia & Boyd 1988:57-58).

The nature and scope of ethics

Ethics is a very specialised field of study, which deals with the dynamics of deciding what is right, and what is wrong. It can be approached from three different perspectives.

■ Descriptive ethics or the descriptive study of morality

Descriptive ethics consists of factual descriptions of conduct or moral beliefs that are often found in research studies undertaken by anthropologists, historians, sociologists and psychologists. In other words, descriptive ethics is merely concerned with stating what the actual beliefs of a person or group are. It does not pass moral judgements on conduct or beliefs; it merely describes what certain people believe to be right or wrong without judging these beliefs.

Fowler contends that while descriptive ethics can be applied to moral issues, it is not a formal branch of ethics. Descriptive ethics describes the values of a particular group of people or culture, that is, what they believe to be 'right' or 'wrong'. An example of descriptive ethics in nursing would be where a nursing educator or researcher would question a class of nurses on their views on abortion or euthanasia and then compile the results of the survey without making value judgements.

Nurses who study moral conduct also encounter descriptive ethics in the form of value clarification or in theories on moral development (Fowler in Fowler & Levine-Ariff 1987:27).

■ Analytical ethics or meta-ethics

The study of moral judgements is the domain of the professional ethicist. It is a field of study in which philosophers ask and attempt to answer questions about the meaning of words like 'right' and 'wrong' or 'good' and 'bad'. What, for example, does it mean to say that mercy killing is wrong (McConnell 1982:2)?

Meta-ethics is concerned with theories of ethics and analyses questions such as 'Why be good?' or 'What do we mean when we say a particular value is good or right?' Fowler (1989:956) believes that while the significance of such questions is not immediately apparent, they are important because they provide a critique on ethics.

According to Fry (in Creasia & Parker 1991:150), typical meta-ethical enquiries consider the connection between human conduct and morality or between ethical beliefs and the facts of the real world, and the relationship between the various theoretical principles of ethics and human conduct.

■ Normative ethics

A third way in which moral beliefs can be studied is normative ethics. Here the concern is not merely with what someone thinks is right but with what is in fact right. The focus is therefore on the justification of a particular moral belief. The study of ethics in the field of nursing and health care is primarily centred on normative ethics.

Normative ethics is generally divided into norms of value and norms of obligation. According to Fowler (1989:957) norms of value deal with what is 'good' or 'evil' in people. Early nursing ethics was concerned with virtue, within the domain of norms of value. The emphasis in nursing today has shifted from the moral character of nurses to the ethical duties and obligations of nurses. Norms of obligation are concerned with what is the 'right' or the 'wrong' thing to do. Ethical theories and principles specify what moral obligations are, and this will be dealt with in a subsequent chapter.

The place of values in nursing practice

Nurses constantly have to make ethical decisions about what should or ought to be done for a particular patient. Because nursing's primary goal is to provide the best care for each individual, a nurse needs to know herself, what she believes in and what she values.

This knowledge of self contributes to ethical decision-making and nursing practice. Nurses, however, are individuals with personal values, beliefs and attitudes. They should, therefore, never impose their own values on their patients, since patients are capable of making their own decisions based on all the relevant information (Thompson & Thompson 1992:75-76).

The foundation of professional nursing values

As previously explained, a value is a position taken and expressed through conduct, feelings, imagination and knowledge and is linked to a person's identity and way of life. According to Steele & Harmon (1983:1-2), there are two types of values, namely intrinsic values and extrinsic values. These values develop from association with other people, from life experiences, from the environment and from within the self. Intrinsic values relate to survival, such as the value of food, or to things we value for their own sake, such as truth, love, friendship or strength of character. Examples of extrinsic values are books, motorcars or the selection of a particular health-care facility.

Personal value systems differ from person to person. Nolan & Kirkpatrick (1982:17) maintain that our values are being challenged continuously by the worldviews of other people. Not only does a very broad range of values within Western civilisation confront us, but also by philosophies from the East and the Third World, which provide us with a whole range of new values to consider.

Values arise from cultural and ethnic backgrounds, family traditions, peer group ideas and practices, as well as political, educational and religious philosophies. In nursing, the most basic of all our professional values is that of caring. Unstal (in Fowler & Levine-Ariff 1987:138) maintains that caring is the springboard for the application of all other values inherent in the nurse-patient relationship. She firmly believes that this value, which is both a traditional and a contemporary one, is the cornerstone of the moral art of nursing.

The development of personal and professional values

Values are learned and, like other learned behaviour, take shape in early life and are influenced by early caregivers and the family. Gradually, as an individual grows and develops, formal learning, peer experiences and societal institutions shape values. When conduct becomes more autonomous, an individual's actions are influenced not only by personal values, but also by educational and religious philosophies with which the individual identifies. Values vary according to the importance an individual attaches to them. They can be both simple as well as complex, and they can help to explain similarities and differences between people (Lindberg, Hunter & Kruszewski 1990:296).

The difference between attitudes, beliefs and values

According to Steele & Harmon (1983:3-4) the major differences between these three concepts are:

An *attitude* is a feeling or disposition towards a person, an object or an idea, and includes cognitive, affective and behavioural components. Attitudes are generally assessed as 'positive' and 'negative' and, therefore, an evaluative process is involved.

A *belief*, on the other hand, represents personal confidence in the validity of some idea, person or object. The cognitive component is based on faith rather than on fact. Beliefs are true or false, correct or incorrect.

A *value* relates to modes of conduct and is expressed in terms of either right or wrong. Steele and Harmon argue that values help to determine reasons for people's actions and hold a key position in any decision-making process. Values, therefore, play a very important role in the lives of individuals and in the society to which they belong.

Fry (in Creasia & Parker 1991:188) maintains that values and beliefs function as screens of interpretation that provide evaluation criteria people use when they interact with the world around them. They also provide standards for relationships between people and essential elements of life.

The importance of values in providing guidelines for conduct in nursing practice

Nurses need to know and understand their own value systems, as this influences their relationships and the manner in which they practise professional nursing. Thompson & Thompson (1990:20) point out that nurses enter into a mutual agreement with their patients, namely to care for them with respect and dignity and to support their right to self-determination. A nurse may never abandon a patient, regardless of the health problem involved or whether the nurse disagrees with the patient on some issue - for example, abortion. Dissimilar values may contribute towards misunderstanding or serious conflict, and nurses need to find ways to accommodate these differences. This is essential for the sake of a patient's health care as well as for the nurse's personal and professional well-being. Knowing her/his own values is the first step in helping a nurse to identify, understand and learn strategies to accommodate differences (Lindberg, Hunter & Kruszewski 1990:298).

Wright (1987:7) believes that values influence ethical decision-making in three ways. Firstly, values frame the problem, that is, we see or fail to see a problem on the basis of the values we bring to a situation. Secondly, values provide alternatives for the resolution of a problem. Thirdly, values direct judgements. The way we judge and resolve a problem depends on the values we wish to uphold or promote. Wright warns that if the role of values in ethical decision-making is not recognised, important values will be overlooked when a decision is made.

Having clarity about one's values is essential for a meaningful life and is indispensable for self-knowledge. It also has a direct practical application in the case of a nurse whose response to the question 'Do I avoid terminally ill people?' might help her to deal with terminally ill patients.

Another application of value clarification is the ranking of specific values against each other where, for example a nurse has to choose between the possibility of a higher salary and job security when she decides whether or not to participate in strike action.

Steele & Harmon (1983:13) maintain that clarity about values should not be seen as a set of rules that interferes with conscientious decision-making. On the contrary, it helps the nurse establish, through her feelings and an analysis of her conduct, what choices to make when there are alternatives, and to identify whether or not these choices are rational choices or the result of previous conditioning.

Our values are part of a world we take for granted. But before we make ethical decisions, we need to be fully aware of what those values are. We need to remember that people do not always share the same perceptions or values. In particular, nurses and patients may have different perceptions and values. The nursing profession places a high premium on compassionate service to patients, on the competence of its practitioners, on conscientious decision-making, commitment to professional values and confidence in the professional role. These are only some of the values which ultimately influence society's view of the profession.

Concluding remarks

Nursing is an inherently moral enterprise and the nursing profession is only as strong as its commitment to its ethical obligations and values. Nursing codes of ethics have established high ideals and make many demands on nurses. Caring for patients is a profound activity and the driving force in the moral treatment of patients. The experience of genuinely caring for and about a patient confirms nursing potential in daily practice. Ethics as a mode of enquiry helps nurses to understand the moral dimensions of human conduct and to investigate matters of human concern.

Critical thinking activities
1. What is nursing ethics?
2. How does nursing ethics differ from biomedical ethics?
3. What are the three categories in the study of ethics?
4. Why is normative ethics considered of prime importance in the field of nursing and health care?
5. What is the difference between personal values and professional values?
6. Why are values important in providing guidelines for nursing conduct?

The caring ethic in nursing

Dirk van der Wal

Outcomes

Studying this chapter will enable you to:

- debate the semantics of the concept of caring
- list the essential attributes of caring
- conceptualise the phenomenon of caring
- discuss vulnerability as a fundamental principle of the caring ethic
- substantiate the claim that caring is an ethical principle
- critically discuss the individual as an ethical (and caring) agent
- appraise the self as an ethical agent
- give a broad outline of a learning program that would accommodate the development and maintenance of a caring and ethical concern in learners.

Introduction

It is often said that caring is the hallmark of the nursing profession. The notion of caring has indeed been the subject of much discussion in recent times, and one consequence of such discussion is that health professions have come to realise that ultimately, quality health care resides in caring. Caring thus becomes the essential indicator of quality health care and the capacity to care the defining attribute of the health-care professional. It can be argued, in fact, that caring is what makes us human, that it is an innate human attribute and not just a fragmented subject of interest and dispute among the health professions (Van der Wal 1996:320). It is the capacity for caring – and not mere technical proficiency in a particular profession – that secures the quality of ethical weight to that profession.

In the context of health services, the emphasis on caring has implications for our understanding of the notion of cure. Health care is not only about cure; indeed, where cure is an end in itself, caring is both a means to an end and an end in itself. Caring without cure is undoubtedly a worthwhile activity; however, cure without caring poses grave ethical questions. Cure without caring is a desolate and unfeeling experience for both the receiver and giver of health care.

When considering caring as an ethic in nursing and health care, the following issues are vitally important:

- the semantics involved in the concepts of *care* and *caring*
- the essential nature of the phenomenon of caring
- caring as an ethic

- care, caring and healing versus curing
- the individual as an ethical (and caring) agent
- teaching, learning and practising caring.

Caring as an ethical principle

Since the basic definition of the term ethic is a code or principle of behaviour whose aim is doing what is good and right, it is quite evident that caring is an ethic. Certainly, most nurses and other health professionals would agree that what they are doing entails care and, as such, is about doing what is good and right.

Caring certainly meets the four requirements for an ethical standard. According to Fry (1988:48), caring 1) is a principal value in guiding the action of nurses and other health professionals; 2) is a universal attitude that is appropriate across many contexts and cultures; 3) identifies specific behaviours that characterise excellence in human behaviour; and 4) is 'other-regarding'. We agree with Bevis (1981:49) that caring by its very nature can only be positive. Caring is the central ethic not only in nursing (Klimeck 1990:178) but also in other health-care services. One problem is that caring has not as yet been fully embraced by other health-care services, which tend to focus instead on the distinctive professional knowledge and skill that they have to offer.

Given the universality of caring across professions and disciplines, it is appropriate to speak of the caring sciences or caring professions. If indeed we intend to support the present Moral Regeneration Movement in South Africa (see MRM, 16-12-2004), there is no better way of doing so than by way of the caring professions.

Caring, curing and healing

According to Dunlop (1986: 662) the word *care* comes from the Old English *carina* meaning 'to trouble one', whereas *cure* comes from Latin via French, in which language it is one of the words for a priest. The different origins of the words *care* and *cure* suggest an original class difference: the higher orders cured while the lower orders cared. This distinction has found its way into modern health services in the sense that it is the male dominant field of medicine which cures, while care is relegated to women and thus to a female-dominated profession such as nursing. Benner (Stevenson and Tripp-Reimer 1990:5) asserts in this regard that caring is a word that, for some, calls to mind a form of oppression: 'the enslavement to unending, mindless, circular work that is consumed as soon as it is created'. This incriminates caring as an outmoded ideology. However, caring is far from being an outmoded ideology and, as Benner proceeds to point out, it in fact engenders pleasure in the midst of work: a sense that some things are worth doing and good in themselves. Caring is maligned only because it challenges the dominant technological cure paradigm. This paradigm, the so-called controlling paradigm, cannot, however, exist without the caring paradigm. Benner emphatically states that the control paradigm is an illusion carried on the back of caring (Benner in Stevenson and Tripp-Reimer 1990:6). If the control paradigm ever triumphs completely, cancelling out all caring ways of being, the consequence will be ecological and human disaster. The issue at hand is thus not so much a dispute between nursing and medicine. Within the health-care arena at large, it is a dispute about conflicting claims about the contributions of science and humanity. The valuing of science (procedure and cure) over humanity (caring, healing and cure) holds risks for all the health professions. Nonetheless, as Gadow (1988:5) points out, nurses feel the ethical differences between caring and curing more poignantly than any other professionals.

To comprehend the foundational difference between curing and caring (including healing), we need to understand the difference between the natural sciences and the human sciences. This is essentially the difference between two core elements: quantity/measurement and quality. In the continuing struggle of the nursing profession to free itself from being the handmaiden of medicine, Watson's (1985:10) summary of the essential differences between medicine and nursing and, therefore, between curing and caring, is useful (see Table 1).

Table 1

Traditional medical-natural science-human context	Emerging alternative nursing science and context for caring
Normative (norms set by science)	Ipsative
Reductionistic	Transactional
Mechanistic	Metaphysical and humanistic-contextual
Method-centred	Phenomena-centred
Neutrality of values	Value-laden; values acknowledged, clarified
Disease-centred (pathology-physiology), the physical body	Human response to illness and personal meanings of human condition
Ethics of 'science'	Humano-social ethics-morality
More quantitative	More qualitative
Absolutes, givens, laws	Relativism, probabilism
Human as object	Human as subject
Objective experiences	Subjective-intersubjective experiences
Facts	Experience, meaning
Nomothetic (relates to the generalised)	Idiographic (relates to the individually expressed life experience) and nomothetic
Concrete and observable things	Abstract things: may or may not be seen
Analytical	Dialectical, philosophical, metaphysical
Science as product	Science as creative process of discovery
Human = sum of parts (bio-psycho-socio-cultural-spiritual-being)	Human = mind-body-spirit gestalt of whole being (not only more than sum of parts, but different)
Physical materialistic	Existential-phenomenological-spiritual
'Real' is that which is measurable, observable, and knowable	'Real' is abstract, largely subjective as well as objective, but it may or may not ever be fully known, observable, measured; what is 'real' holds mystery and unknowns yet to be discovered

(Watson 1985:10)

In spite of the differences between caring and cure, no single profession can claim caring as its unique professional possession, especially not within the health care sector. Cure and caring are both seen as alternative forms of commitment to the patient. The distinction between the two forms of commitment is thus not so sharply made as to denote two distinct sets of character, but rather two distinct professions, namely medicine and nursing (or any other health-care profession). However, some professions, like nursing, are by their very nature, more attuned to caring. Certainly, nursing has given that from which other health professions can only benefit. It must be remembered that whereas cure is an end in itself, caring is both a means to an end and an end in itself. Where cure is no longer possible, caring prevails. Where cure serves science, caring always serves humanity; caring humanises the scientific business of cure. Where the process of curing might increase the patient's vulnerability, caring is always on the alert not to exploit vulnerability, but to nurture, protect and facilitate growth. If the ultimate aim of medicine is to cure, the ultimate aim of caring is to heal.

Experience with terminal conditions such as cancer, HIV/AIDS, aged fragility and the like, has led to the realisation that at some point in human life there is nothing that can alleviate human suffering. All that remains is the giving of oneself and being involved in the process of healing. Healing involves 'the process of bringing the parts of one's self together at a deep level of inner knowledge, resulting in an integrated, balanced whole with each part having equal importance and value' (Dozzy and Guzzetta 1995:6). In the professional field, healing is the exquisite blending of technology with caring and not just the curing of symptoms. For the health professional committed to caring, healing is a life-long journey in which engaging with the life of the client and attributing moments of meaning and insight amidst crisis, result in an understanding of the wholeness of human existence. Thus we seek harmony and balance through the expansion of our inner potential (Dozzy, Keegan, Guzzetta and Kolmeier 1995:xxvi). The essence of the process of healing, and by implication caring, is mindfulness; to see things as they are, without trying to change them. The point is to suspend one's reactions to disturbing emotions without rejecting the emotion itself. This allows one to look deeper into the moment. In this sense, mindfulness creates wise attention (Bennett-Goleman 2001:6-8) and wisdom.

Given the close relationship between caring and healing, with healing being the ultimate aim of caring, caring is clearly not a 'fall-back position' when cure becomes impossible (Gadow 1988:6). Caring and healing accompany the process of curing.

Caring

Caring: an innate human attribute

If one views caring as a professional attribute only, one can easily forget that it is part of the very essence of being human. This becomes apparent when one considers the origins of caring:

- Care is the human mode of being. The desire to care is human (Roach cited in Forrest 1989:816).
- Caring denotes a *primary mode of being* in the world, which is natural to us and of significance in our relationships to others. It might be argued that to care is part of one's concept of a whole person and that an uncaring person is, to some extent, crippled (Griffin 1983: 289).
- Caring is biologically programmed into human nature (Gaylin cited in Carper 1979: 14).
- Caring is founded on reverence for life, love of self and others, and a concern for improving the world. It is based on a dedication that motivates and energises the self and others towards mutual actualisation (Forsyth *et al* 1979: 165). This view is also reflected in the major religions of the world and, therefore, transcends cultural barriers.
- Caring is founded on two root elements, namely 1) the individual's longing to maintain, recapture or enhance his/her most caring and tender moments, and 2) the natural sympathy human beings feel for each another (Noddings cited in Dunlop 1986: 666).

Given prevailing social conditions and the general level of moral development and social responsibility of a large part of contemporary society, the second root-element appeals directly to the reinforcement of a global caring ethic and towards the improvement of basic living conditions of all peoples around the world. In this regard the Moral Regeneration Movement in South Africa merits our support. After all, the caring individuals we wish to attract to the caring professions are primarily nurtured by society. Furthermore, if this primary caring concern is not nurtured, the caring professions themselves will have to do this very difficult but extremely important job.

With the above in mind, Noddings states: 'Whatever I do in life, whomever I meet, I am first and always one-caring . . . I do not "assume roles" unless I become an actor. "Mother" is not a role; "teacher" is not a role' (Noddings 1984:145). By the same token, 'nurse' is not a role, neither is any other position taken in any other health-care professions a role.

Caring defined

There is an abundance of information on 'care' and 'caring'. In the nursing literature and the literature of moral philosophy the semantics of the term 'caring' are important. Although care and caring are often used synonymously, care sometimes implies a procedure and a scientific orientation that is lacking in the innate human attributes of concern and empathy. Be that as it may, two nodes of meaning crystallise, namely feelings/emotions and doing/action. Table 2 contains a summary of some of the words linked to the emotional component of caring, the so-called qualitative indicators of caring.

In the action/doing component of caring both the implementation of professional knowledge via procedure, skill and technology, as well as lay caring actions, are indicated. A major challenge in caring in the health care professions is to strike a balance between emotions and action within a caring relationship. To treat caring only as a verb (that is, as an action, procedure or technique) sets aside certain other senses of the word such as caring as a virtue or quality of human character (Gaut 1979: 79). Griffin (1983: 289) is in no doubt that it is the emotional element of the caring activity, which motivates and energises nursing action, thus enabling one to call it caring. However, caring for someone is not so much a matter of doing something as doing it at the right time in the right place, when needs are felt and communicated (Pribram cited in Gendron 1990:280). Caring involves more than just carrying out nursing procedures. True caring is based on an attitude of nurturing, of helping one another grow (Lindberg, Hunter, and Kruszewski 1990:5), of ' . . . stepping out of one's personal frame of reference into the other's, . . . [to] care is to act not by fixed rule but by affection and regard' (Noddings cited in Dunlop 1986: 667). This implies that caring excludes all forms of neglect, oppression, possessiveness and the cultivation of dependence and co-dependence. Caring does, however, include growth and the optimalisation of potential, without leaving the patient or client to his or her own devices. In this regard Watson (1985:54) points out that human care 'consists of transpersonal human to human attempts to protect, enhance, and preserve humanity by helping a person find meaning in illness, suffering, pain, and existence; to help another gain self-knowledge, control, and self-healing in which a sense of inner harmony is restored regardless of the external circumstances'. One way of achieving these objectives might be by implementing the principles of Viktor Frankl's existential therapy or logotherapy.

Table 2

Words associated with the term caring				
Acceptance	Confidence	Guidance	Meaningfulness	Self-develop-
Accommodation	Confidentiality	Healing	Mercifulness	ment
Accompaniment	Consideration	Helping	Mindfulness	Self-generating
Acknowledgement	Contact	Holism	Non-authoritarian	Self-healing
Action	Connectedness	Honesty	Non-manipulative	Self-maintain-
Advocacy	Conviction	Hope	Non-maleficence	ing
Affection	Covenant	Humaneness	Non-possess-	Service
Association	Democracy	Human mode	iveness	Serious attention
Attitude	Devotion	of being	Non-threatening	Sincerity
Appreciation	Discipline	Human right	Nurturing	Situation-specific
Authenticity	Doing	Interest	Oneness	Skills
Autonomy	Effort	Inviting	Participation	Spontaneity
Availability	End in itself	Individualism	Personal barriers	Supervision
Balance	Empathy	Interaction	Presence	Support
Being there	Empowerment	Innovative	Protection	Sympathy
Benevolence	Fairness	Involvement	Rational	Therapeutic
Calling	Faith	Justice	Reciprocity	Transaction
Caution	Feeling	Knowledge	Relational	Trust
Commitment	Fidelity	'Life-force'	Respect	Unbiased
Communication	Flexibility	Listening	Responsibility	Unity
Compassion	Freedom	Love	Secrecy	Universality
Competence	Giving of self	Maturity	Security	Warmth
Concern	Growth	Meaning	Self-actualisation	Way of life
		attribution	Self-care	Willingness
				Will

The essential structure of caring can be further explained by plotting its emotional and active components on a matrix. In this way we get a better idea of the different variants of caring (see Figure 1).

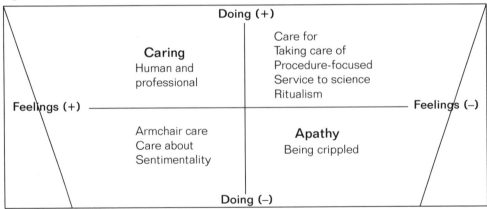

Fig 1 Variants of 'caring'

Note that the word 'caring' in the caption to Figure 1 is placed in inverted commas. This is to indicate that 'variants' of caring are not 'true' caring. At most, these can be labelled 'pseudo-caring'. Caring implies action and, in this sense, the complete opposite of caring is *apathy*, or 'being crippled' according to Griffin (1983: 289). The worse of the two remaining 'variants' of caring is perhaps 'armchair' caring. Here the individual professes but is not committed to caring. This is a kind of sentimental caring where 'caring' concern' is not put into action. The fourth quadrant in Figure 1 covers a situation in which action is not accompanied by any positive human emotion towards the object of care. For example, in many an emergency situation in health care the impression might be created that it is more about doing and less about caring, that caring is in the service of science rather than of humanity. Another example might be where the individuals who benefit from the health professionals' actions are not in immediate contact with the professional; for instance, in the case of officials who monitor the quality of food, air, drinking water, environmental safety, and the like.

Whatever the case, in the end it is only the individual carer who can tell whether his or her actions are conducted out of 'caring'.

In summary, caring:
- is not merely the present continuous form of the verb 'to care' but is a collective noun denoting a whole range of ethical, moral and religious concepts and principles
- is based on knowledge, skills, experience and values, is culturally situated and is ultimately about doing what is right and good
- is an ethic in itself; it is ethical behaviour par excellence
- humanises science and technical procedure
- determines the quality of the connectedness (intentionality) between subject and object
- brings about true job satisfaction (Van der Wal 2000)
- accompanies curing and oversees healing.

The reader might argue at this point that caring is unattainable. The fact is, so is absolute clinical sterility. But even if we cannot attain complete clinical sterility, we can strive towards it. In the case of caring, the ideal caregiver would be an individual who could integrate humane attitudes and emotions with scientific knowledge and technological skill in nursing and health care. In such an individual caring would manifest itself as the essence of being and the fulfilment of his/her relationship to others and the whole of creation.

The individual as an ethical agent

Many books on ethics teach isolated ethical principles, theories and concepts. Some courses and texts involve learners by analysing ethical situations, and identifying and resolving ethical dilemmas. However, very few deal with the philosophical underpinnings of ethics and, more specifically, a model of the individual. It is often mistakenly assumed that a purely theoretical understanding of ethics is sufficient for the nurturing of ethical, caring behaviour. However, for a course in ethics to have any positive result, it needs to:
- conceive of the individual (nurse or other health-care professional) as being able and wanting to act ethically
- conceive of the individual as the locus of social responsibility
- uncover what needs to be nurtured within the individual so that he/she can become an ethical and caring agent.

Essentially, such a model of the individual entails an inter-relationship of the individual's conscience, his/her will orientation, and the meaning he/she finds in life and how this inter-relationship affects the individual's ability to connect with others. Here we enter the realm of human spirituality; 'that part of the person that is most deeply concerned with feelings, with the need for meaning in life, with convictions, belief systems, values, dreams, interpersonal relationships, relationship to God, and so forth' (Dugan 1988:109). Spirituality, in this sense, 'has to do with depth value, relatedness, heart, and personal substance' and is not 'an object of religious belief or . . . something to do with immortality' (Moore cited in Goddard 1995:809). In this view, spirituality engages all the elements needed for caring.

Figure 2 gives a diagrammatic representation of the relationship between the components of a model of an ethical and caring agent (Van der Wal 2000:487).

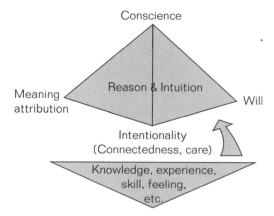

Fig 2 The basic component necessary for grounding the individual as an ethical agent

Intentionality

One may well ask: 'What kind of person is the caring professional ?' The answer to this question resides primarily in the so-called subject/object relationship, that is the relationship between the knowing mind and that which is known and can be known; in short, intentionality.

Intentionality is not used in the same sense as 'having good intentions' As Watson (1999:119) indicates: 'The term *intentionality*, within the mind-body field, is a more technical, philosophical term meaning "being directed towards a mental object"' (Watson 1999:119). At this point we need to explain that 'mental object' includes all human experiences and thoughts; whatever we experience we do so because we make 'mental' meaning of it – we interpret it. Watson cites Schiltz (1996:31) who defines intentionality thus: 'Philosophically, it is consciousness about something or some content of consciousness, such as belief, volition, expectation, attention, action, and even the unconscious.' Intentionality sits at an *interface* [our emphasis] between the subject and the object (Schiltz 1996:31), the subject being the thinking mind and the object anything (tangible or intangible, including norms and values) at which our thinking is directed. Intentionality is akin to what Benner and Wrubel (Moccia 1990:212) in their definition of caring call "connectedness" and "having something matter." Intentionality is all about being aware. In essence this awareness is value neutral and has infinite potential. It is as such neither good nor bad, neither right nor wrong. This is where caring comes into play. Caring, in its most fundamental form, represents a way of life, a sustained positive orientation (Bevis 1981:49). It is the determinant of the quality of the subject-object relationship, of our intentionality. As Benner and Wrubel (Moccia 1990:212) put it, caring ' . . . fuses thoughts, feelings, and action; it fuses knowing and being and so is primary to our existence . . . it creates possibility . . . connection and concern . . . sharing of help, allowing one to give and allowing another to receive'.

Will

Will is defined as either an altruistic humanistic or theistic orientation of the individual. Associated concepts are those of willingness, commitment, conviction, devotion, confidence, compassion and effort.

Will implies that the individual has the freedom to exercise choice. In those situations where choice can be exercised, it is up to the individual to choose whether to live up to or reject the caring ethic. Without freedom of choice, there can be no accountability or responsibility.

Kekes' concept of the 'informed will' well describes what we understand by the will. According to Kekes (1986:75; 89-90):

- The will is directed by feelings and intellect.
- The will is self-directed and is not manipulated. It is not imposed on an individual by some external power, but stems from character and circumstances.
- The exercise of will is not only to maintain one's life, but also to realise one's visions of the good life. However, what one wills can be limited by one's embodiment and by social factors (Kekes 1986: 89-90).

Conscience

The word 'conscience' is derived from the Latin words *con* and *scientia* and literally means 'knowledge with' or shared knowledge (Peterson 1982:8). This gives to conscience a social tone and, indeed, the term is often qualified in the literature as 'social conscience' as a reminder of its origins in social norms. Conscience is also regarded as the moral aspect of personality, a hypothetical part of the individual that judges behaviour according to the person's moral values. Conscience thus has a cognitive aspect, namely knowledge of, and insight into, the rules and values the individual adheres to; an affective side, namely feelings of obligation, shame, guilt and pride; and a conative aspect, namely decisions regarding future behaviour (Gouws *et al* 1979:105). The term usually refers to thoughts, feelings and actions involving human valuing and judgement (Peterson 1982:3).

Conscience is a summons to one's own 'potentiality-of-being' (Heidegger, as translated by Stambough 1996:256). Although the content and of conscience and will derive from the same sources, they are not necessarily always aligned. Conscience is indubitably ethical; it is the 'gatekeeper', and often appeals against our expectations and even against our will. 'The call comes "from me" and yet "over me"' (Stambough 1996:254). When it does call in this way, we have a personal ethical dilemma (Van der Wal 2000:504). The resolution of a conscience/will disagreement calls for rational consideration. If it is not resolved, we will end up not acting according to our convictions or our true and authentic ethical selves. Our actions then become merely ritualistic. In this regard, Frankl (Massey 1991:32) points out that tradition and conventional values do not constrain human behaviour as they once did. Authenticity sometimes requires that the individual disregard standards of social conscience for the sake of insight brought about by common sense (Massey 1991:32). Common sense in this instance includes sense created by scientific, professional and ethical knowledge.

The dialogue between conscience and will confirms certain fundamental ethical attributes of the individual as an ethical and caring agent, namely accountability, responsibility, autonomy and reason. These are fundamental to all ethical concepts. Table 3 (taken from Van der Wal 2000: 506) summarises the outcome of the dialogue between conscience and will.

Table 3

The relationship between conscience and will and its implications for ethics		
Thesis	**Antithesis**	**Synthesis**
Conscience (Determinism)		No choice and no autonomy, responsibility, or accountability
Will (Indeterminism)		Total freedom of choice; however, still no responsibility or accountability. Anarchy.
Conscience	Will	Reason and intuition. Confined but free choice, autonomy, responsibility, and accountability. Relative limited 'free will' and limited 'guiding conscience'.

(Van der Wal 2000:506)

As Table 3 indicates, if we were subjected to conscience only we would live a life of complete determinism. We would have no choice but to act according to the dictates of conscience. Under such conditions, we could not be held responsible for our acts and omissions. The same applies if we have no conscience but only a totally free will: indeterminism. If no limitations were set to our free will, there would be no standards of right and wrong against which the rightness and wrongness of our acts and omissions could be assessed. However, if we place conscience and will in dialogue, the situation changes completely. We have confined freedom of choice, a choice between what we will and what we ought to do. This choice gives the individual autonomy, responsibility and accountability, the pillars of professional and answerable conduct.

Meaning

The question remains: why do some caregivers maintain an altruistic humanistic will orientation and a social conscience while others apparently do not? According to Harrison (1990:125), the answer is that caring itself is a process of creating meaning. Indeed, for Heidegger (Steiner 1989:26 and 101), it is care (*Sorge*) that makes human existence meaningful. It is the fact that something matters, that intentionality is qualified by the caring ethic that makes human life meaningful. Caring makes sense and gives meaning only to those who value the caring ethic and who have the will to care.

Reason and intuition

The outcome of the interconnectedness of intentionality, will, conscience and meaning attribution takes on two forms, namely reason (as reasoned decisions) and intuition (as an educated guess). Reason and intuition should not be seen as opposites. Concurrent or immediate reflection is what differentiates intuition from reasoned decisions as the sources of reason and intuition are the same (Van der Wal 2001:7). Both these human capacities are of the utmost importance in practising ethics in nursing, in the context of either intuitively knowing what to say or do, or coming to a rational decision via the process of ethical decision-making.

Virtue

The final quality attributed to the individual as ethical (or caring) agent, is virtue. If the outcome of the actions, attitudes and conduct informed by reason and intuition continuously serve as a source of positive feedback to us, then such a positive incentive can only result in caring becoming a virtue (Dent 1986 and Meilaender 1984 cited in Klimek 1990:179). Virtue is the power of acting exclusively according to one's true nature. The degree of virtue is the degree to which one is striving to, and is indeed able to affirm one's own being - in this instance our authentic caring being. 'It is impossible to conceive of any virtue as prior to the striving to preserve one's own being' (Tillich cited in Van der Wal 2000). To act unconditionally out of virtue is the same as to act under the guidance of reason, to affirm one's essential being or true nature. Here we enter the realm of virtue ethics where the character of the individual is an important determinant of ethical and moral behaviour and decision-making. The virtuous character and virtue ethics combat the reduction of ethical behaviour to the application of rules and calculus of good and right as is the case with the application of a pure deontological and teleological approach to ethics (Mautner 2000:593). Character determines how we perceive of and frame situations. It allows for the flexibility that deontology and teleology lack.

There is, however, a concern in some circles of female-dominated professions such as nursing. Historically, for women to be virtuous meant to be submissive, obedient, and self-sacrificing (Chinn and Kramer 2004:165). As we have indicated earlier, this is a totally outdated viewpoint of caring and the caring professions and of the relationship between the women-dominated caring professions within the health care arena and the male-dominated curing professions. It is, nonetheless, important to ask who defines what is virtuous and who benefits from virtuous behaviour.

The role of knowledge, skill and experience

The contents of the four components above and the outcome of the debate among these components (intentionality, will, consciences and meaning attribution) are all founded on experience and presuppose being informed about others and things and being in touch with oneself. One's experience, meaning attribution, knowledge and skills, are interwoven and constantly changing. All three domains of learning, namely the *cognitive* (intellectual), *affective* (emotional) and *psychomotor* (skill) are involved in creating and sustaining the caring ethic. This leads to the concept of competence as a defining attribute of caring. Though competence is often thought of as mere dexterity (the psychomotor), the concept also includes knowledge and thinking skills (the cognitive) and interpersonal, social and emotional skills (affective).

With regard to ethical and caring behaviours, knowing what to do, how to do it and when to do it seem powerful building blocks in enhancing the conscience of the morally-inclined individual, as well as enhancing the willingness to involve self in situations. Competence leaves the nurse and other health professional prepared to involve herself in the affairs of fellow human beings when called for. However, competence does not automatically lead to anticipated moral and caring behaviours. Not acting according to one's level of competency constitutes immoral and unethical behaviour and is directly related to acts of omission, carelessness and negligence. It is ultimately the individual nurse's or other health professional's decision (informed decision) whether to abide by their better judgement, and ethical and caring concern, or whether they are going to succumb to immoral behaviour encouraged by bribery, blindly abide by political correctness, adulation, conceit or mere indifference (apathy). On the other hand, abiding by the caring ethic and a model of the individual as an ethical and caring agent, the individual nurse and health care professional will experience what Watson (1999:129) perceives as the outcome of a post modernist view on the transpersonal *caring-healing model*. By equating caring with healing, Watson professes that:

■ Caring releases the potential for healing and wholeness.
■ Caring consciousness is primary for the caring-healing practitioner.
■ An expanded view of the person and what it means to be human is created.
■ Caring processes are revered.
■ Caring is a moral imperative for the survival of both humans and the planet earth.
■ Caring is a converging global agenda for nursing (and other health sciences and professions) and society alike (Watson 1999:129).

Concluding remarks

Although caring is, by its very nature, considered good, and the caring experience fulfilling to the caring person, the negative effects of caring - the demand it places on the individual, and the threat of co-dependency that can develop - have also been noted (Van der Wal 2000:119). Keeping personal boundaries, protecting personal integrity and personhood, combating loss of personhood and the development of co-dependency; all these demand pertinent structures to accompany courses in ethics and caring and to sustain the individual nurse and health professional. The involvement of the cognitive, affective, psychomotor and conative (will) domains in the caring ethic demands that equal attention be given to each domain. It is the truly educated rather than the merely trained professional who should be the product of a course in nursing and health-care ethics. Consequently ethics courses and supportive programmes need to:

■ invest in different intelligences. Nursing and other health sciences curricula should no longer be teeming with contents that develop only the rational/academic intelligence of students. Emotional intelligence, social intelligence and spiritual intelligence should be developed equally. Life-skills development, the self-curriculum, reflective practice, stress maintenance and the like should form part and parcel of an ethics and caring programme.
■ foster connectedness by allowing caregivers to care. This is especially true for students in nursing and other health professions.
■ foster directedness by designing, and living by, institutional philosophies, visions, missions and policy statements founded in the caring ethic.
■ create an educational milieu and work environment that is conducive to ethics and caring and which reflect ethical conduct and caring in action.

Critical thinking activities

1. Within the broader definition of the term 'bioethics' (see Chapter 1) identify an issue of vulnerability in each of the following relationships and indicate how you would alleviate vulnerability in each: intra-personal (relating to one's self), inter-personal (relating to others) and extra-personal (relating to things, animals, nature).

2. With reference to caring as a relational activity, consider the implications that each of the attributes of caring in Table 2 has for the individuals involved in the relationship, that is the caregivers and the receivers of caring.

3. Give an outline of the supportive subjects you would include in a continuing education program in the area in which you are working.

4. Reflect on how the educational programmes you have been involved in, or are presently involved in, formed your conscience, fostered your will orientation within the ethical dictates of the programme, attributed meaning to your life and led to connectedness to the 'objects' towards which the programmes are directed. If the outcome of your reflections is in any way negative, question yourself regarding this negativity before questioning aspects relating to the programme, others or circumstances.

part 2

Perspectives on ethical theory, principles and decision-making in health care

If a nurse can develop the ability to objectively justify ethical decisions, she has, by that very fact, developed the ability to make appropriate decisions. But it seems impossible that she could develop an ability to consistently make appropriate decisions if she does not possess the ability to justify decisions

(Husted & Husted 1995:25).

Ethical theory and decision-making in nursing and health care

Silvia Pera

Outcomes

Studying this chapter will enable you to:

- differentiate between moral and non-moral guides in ethical decision-making
- distinguish between subjectivism, objectivism and relativism in making moral judgements
- identify two major ethical theories
- critically discuss consequentialism or teleology
- describe non-consequentialism or deontology
- name four major ethical principles which guide moral action in health care
- identify several moral rules derived from major ethical principles
- describe Kohlberg's hierarchy of moral development
- name four decision-making models/processes in nursing and health care
- discuss one decision-making model which you can apply in your work environment.

Introduction

Decision-making in health care is guided and influenced by theories of ethics and ethical principles. A brief overview of two major theories of ethics is presented in section one of this chapter that can assist in clarifying the ethical dimensions of dilemmas encountered in nursing practice. Each approach looks at dilemmas from an ethical point of view and suggests reasoned ways of analysing or conceptualising decisions and choices in the ethical dimensions of nursing practice. Perspectives on ethical principles are also provided for consideration by nurses who find themselves in situations where they are unsure of the right decision to make in conflicts between rights and duties. Ketefian (in Oermann 1991:221) believes that ethical theories and principles provide the decision-maker with cognitive methods or viewpoints that will assist in determining whether actions are morally appropriate.

Moral development theory is concerned with the reasons for actions and decisions. Knowledge of basic ethical theory and principles will not make decision-making easier but it will be of value in analysing various responses to moral dilemmas. A number of decision-making processes and models developed by various nurses are presented to assist ethical decision-making in day-to-day professional health-care practice.

Basic ethical theories and principles

Ethical theories and principles should not be regarded as clear-cut formulas for resolving ethical dilemmas in health-care practice, but rather as aids to the analysis and understanding of such dilemmas. What follows is a simplified account of ethical theory which, together with the degree of acquaintance with the moral foundation of nursing provided in the previous chapter, will be helpful in understanding and working with practical problems in daily health-care practice.

Theoretical considerations

Before discussing the traditional theories, it is necessary to give a brief account of what makes some dilemmas and judgements moral, and whether moral judgements are subjective or objective. The question about what makes any given normative standard moral rather than religious, legal or political should not be seen as merely theoretical, since according to Beauchamp and Childress (2001:3), this has practical implications.

Moral and non-moral action guides in decisionmaking

Several contemporary philosophers have tried to identify criteria for distinguishing between moral and non-moral considerations. They maintain that there are three main conditions for moral action guides, two of which are considered formal conditions while the third is concerned with moral judgements, rules and principles. According to the first condition, a moral action guide is whatever a person or society regards as supreme, final or overriding. The second condition is universality, which is a widely accepted condition for moral action guides. The third condition is that a moral action guide must have moral content. Some philosophers also believe that it should contain some direct reference to the welfare of others.

Beauchamp and Childress question these conditions and argue that it cannot be said that every overriding action guide is necessarily moral, since to hold that supremacy is a necessary condition of morality is to prejudice the weight that moral action guides should carry when they are in conflict with political, legal and religious action guides. Beauchamp and Childress also contend that, while universality may be a necessary condition of moral thinking, it is not sufficient for distinguishing moral judgements from other action guiding judgements that also meet this requirement. Universality does not imply that only one moral system of principles and rules is correct and universally applicable, regardless of social context. To a certain extent, universality makes a formal point about the logic of moral judgement. It should be possible for any person who accepts any moral judgement to apply that judgement universally in similar circumstances. Beauchamp and Childress also maintain that the contention that moral action guides should have reference to the welfare of others does not necessarily indicate that the welfare of all parties should carry the same weight. Most principles and rules of interest in biomedicine, whether moral or not, also involve some direct reference to human welfare (Beauchamp & Childress 2001:3-4).

It is clear, therefore, that while many people *believe* they can recognise moral action guides when they encounter them, it may be very difficult to distinguish between moral and non-moral considerations in arguments about moral issues.

The nature of moral judgements

The fundamental question raised in the area of analytical or meta-ethics (see Chapter 1) concerns the subjectivity of moral judgements. Judgements are said to be subjective when they are considered to be merely expressions of opinion and, therefore, neither right nor wrong. In the field of moral discourse subjectivists believe that an act is right because the individual or group judges it to be right. Subjectivists maintain that human judgements create morality and that there is no set of objective moral truths.

Relativism holds that all values are relative and differ according to the individual culture or society that holds them. Individuals or cultures have immunity against the judgements of others no matter how distasteful or repugnant their values and practices. The female genital mutilation practice in some African cultures is a good example of this (Bandman & Bandman 2002:43). Objectivists, on the other hand, insist that human judgement discovers rather than creates morality. They perceive right and wrong to be independent of what people think and believe. It is the function of human judgement to discover the right and wrong inherent in a particular course of action (Deloughery 1991:180).

McConnell (1982:9-13) asserts that there are good reasons for holding that moral judgements are objective. He advances four arguments to show that most people believe moral judgements to be objective. Firstly, moral arguments are regarded as a serious matter. Subjectivists, he maintains, would regard moral arguments as inconsistent or irrational. Secondly, when a moral dispute occurs, advice is often sought. If subjectivism were true, then seeking moral advice would be regarded as inappropriate or irrational. Thirdly, people sometimes experience moral doubt after they have acted on a decision which they had deemed appropriate and rational. But if subjectivism were true, moral doubt would be perceived as inappropriate or irrational. Fourthly, if subjectivism were true, one could not criticise the moral view of a racist like Hitler, for example, assuming his views were consistent. If Hitler's moral views were considered to be wrong, the consequences of subjectivism could not be accepted.

Traditional ethical theories

If one accepts that moral judgements are objective, then there are criteria of rightness and wrongness. Several ethical theories exist in which these criteria are discussed. Two notable theories are consequentialism and non-consequentialism. It is important to understand the differences between these two theories.

Consequentialism or teleology

Teleological (derived from the Greek *telos*, meaning 'end') theories, also known as utilitarian or consequentialist moral theories, hold that the rightness or wrongness of an action is solely dependent on the results the action produces.

There are three kinds of consequentialism: egoism, utilitarianism and limited consequentialism.

■ Egoism

For the egoist the morally right thing to do is whatever promotes self-interest. According to Deloughery (1991:181) egoists believe that one should always act to produce the greatest happiness (good) over unhappiness (evil) for oneself.

As a theory of morality egoism has no place in health care. Bandman and Bandman (2002:42) are of the opinion that health-care professionals who accept egoism look only for the good they can get for themselves. They believe that such professionals will select work environments where, for example, they do not have to attend to patients who have AIDS, TB or other infectious diseases.

It is evident that, even if feelings of altruism are taken into account, egoism has no place in nursing because it implies that while one may do things for others, one's own pleasures or comfort are the chief end of moral action.

■ Utilitarianism

According to Beauchamp and Childress (2001:340-341), utilitarianism is one of several ethical theories that measure the value of actions by their ultimate ends and consequences. Utilitarianism assumes that one can weigh and measure harms and benefits, and produce the greatest possible balance of good over evil for most people. Utilitarians argue that one should always act to produce the greatest amount of long-term happiness for everyone.

Utilitarianism can be either act-utilitarianism or rule-utilitarianism; in other words, the rightness of an act or the rightness of a rule is judged by the consequences which the act or rule brings about. Loewy (1989:18) argues that the trouble with either form of utilitarianism is that it makes an action good only because of its consequences and ignores the role that motives or intentions might play. Two additional problems with utilitarianism are, firstly, that it is difficult to assess the amounts of happiness likely to be yielded by either individual action or general rules and, secondly, the happiness of the greatest number may in fact involve the unhappiness of the minority.

■ Limited consequentialism

Not all consequentialists judge the morality of an act by the consequences it holds for oneself (egoism) or for the greatest number (utilitarianism). For many people, the consequences for a specific individual or limited number of individuals are the deciding factor in determining the morality of an act. McConnell (1982:15) calls this version patient-consequentialism where the good of a selected group of people is maximised.

Beauchamp and Childress maintain that the utilitarian tradition is often quoted when decisions have to be made about health-care delivery. They cite the example of a hospital where a decision was taken to permit heart transplants because it was felt that 'in an age where technology so pervades the medical community there is a clear responsibility to evaluate new procedures in terms of the greatest good for the greatest number' (1983:21).

Davis & Aroskar (1997:57) argue that utilitarianism is in direct conflict with medical ethics, where everything possible is done for the individual patient. If, for example, every hospital decided to have a renal dialysis unit for kidney transplants, for example, the consequences for primary health-care services would be devastating. The principle of justice should be added to the principle of utility when making ethical decisions about how widely the 'good' ought to be distributed throughout society.

Non-consequentialism or deontology

The views of non-consequentialists are usually called deontological moral theories. According to the deontological position it is the good intention to do one's moral duty which determines whether an action is morally praiseworthy.

Deontological theories, sometimes called formalist theories, hold that some features of acts other than or in addition to their consequences make them right or wrong. Frankena (in Beauchamp & Walters 1978:23) maintains that deontological theories deny what teleological theories affirm. Deontologists believe that it is possible for an action or rule of action to be morally right or obligatory, even if it does not bring about the greatest balance of good over evil for oneself or society. An action may be right or obligatory simply because of some other fact about it or because of its own nature. For example, keeping a promise is right not because of any consequences of such a rule but because it is right in itself. Loewy (1989:19) asserts that deontological theories are often denounced for being inflexible and worthless as guidelines to daily decisions. An action such as lying is, according to the deontological position, considered wrong under all circumstances. Davis & Aroskar (1997:55) point out that, in health-care practice, the deontological position does not resolve dilemmas for the professional who must decide between telling or withholding the truth. The professional knows that the truth will undoubtedly hurt a particular patient in a given situation where the principle of telling the truth conflicts with the principle of doing no harm.

There are different versions of deontological theories, which not only contend with each other but also with teleological theories. Some deontologists appeal to divine revelation such as the Ten Commandments, while others appeal to principles of Natural Law Ethics, according to which an action is good if it is in accord with human nature and bad if it is contrary to that nature.

Act-deontologism is a kind of deontological ethics that has developed in reaction to appeals to divine revelation or Natural law. In a given situation in the home environment, for example, the moral values of a community health nurse would influence decisions about the kind of information provided to the family. A moral judgement made in one situation would thus apply to any other similar situation regardless of the time, place or persons involved. In any home environment, for example, given a similar situation, the nurse would give the same kind of information about birth control methods (Davis & Aroskar 1997:50). Act-deontologists are committed to the principle of universality, and according to this theory, one has only rules of thumb to go by. There are no criteria, standards or guiding principles: one simply gathers all the facts and then makes a decision. An act is right simply by virtue of its being chosen and by the commitment to universality.

Rule-deontology holds that there is a non-teleological standard consisting of one or more rules. Rule-deontologists hold that standards of right and wrong consist of specific rules, such as keeping promises and never telling a lie.

Many tenets of the health-care profession are deontology-oriented; for example, the emphasis that is placed on confidentiality or having respect for all people. Commitments made between health professionals and individual patients are important – they should be honoured and cannot be broken to maximise the good for others. Ketefian (in Oermann 1991:222) maintains that those commitments often result in ethical conflicts, especially concerning staffing and resource allocation. She cites an example where a nurse in an understaffed unit wishes to meet the needs of a seriously ill patient but must also meet the needs of the other patients who demand her care and attention.

Ethical theories are difficult because moral problems often overlap. Deloughery (1991:185) asserts that the majority of ethical questions that nurses face will raise the same problems repeatedly because of the unlikelihood that a completely satisfactory solution to a problem will be reached. Although no solid evidence exists that nurses should choose one ethical theory over another, she warns against slipping into pragmatism/relativism in an irresponsible manner, since situations vary and are often extremely complex.

As far as health and nursing care are concerned, conflicts easily occur when consequentialists and non-consequentialists together try to reach an ethical decision for treatment. Differences in moral beliefs and the steps that are taken do not necessarily mean that one perspective is right and others are wrong. Of primary importance is that each health professional should understand where her individual beliefs, values and ethics are centred and then try to understand those of others (Smith 1989:184).

Ethical principles in nursing and health care

Ethics is the foundation of committed service to humankind and should not be considered a deterrent by professional health-care practitioners who take pride in their profession. Enlightened practitioners who are able to take a stand an ethical stand in the day-to-day routine care, and particularly during a crisis, help to carry the profession into the future with dignity.

From the brief description of the two most general ethical theories, it should be clear that the application of either theory to the same problem would have different results. Ethical principles are important elements in the formation of moral judgements in professional practice. Ethical principles provide guidance for thinking and acting in order to determine what should or should not be done in particular situations. Ethical principles may also be viewed as rules or codes of conduct, or as generalisations that provide a basis for reasoning. These principles may be based on religious traditions, on worldviews or on normative ethical theories such as utility and duties or obligations (Davis & Aroskar 1997:49). While theoretically the number of principles is unlimited, many can be grouped together under a few headings. Deontologists, for example, hold that certain major principles such as autonomy, non-maleficence, beneficence and justice serve as guidelines to moral conduct.

Smith (1989:184) contends that these major principles are intrinsic to nursing care. Fry (in Creasia & Parker 1991:151) believes that the most important ethical principles in nursing practice are autonomy, beneficence, justice, veracity, fidelity and the avoidance of killing. Some of these principles are dealt with in this chapter while others are addressed in greater detail in relevant chapters throughout the text.

The principle of autonomy

Autonomy is a term derived from the Greek *autos* meaning 'self' and *nomos* denoting rule, governance or law. This term was first used to refer to self-governance in Greek city states but as applied to individuals its meaning is quite broad (Beauchamp & Childress 2001:57-58).

In modern thought, autonomy expresses respect for the unconditional worth of an individual and respect for individual thought and action. Because people are rational beings, they should be treated as ends in themselves and never as a means to an end or as a means to the ends of others. To respect autonomy is to respect this capacity in other people. This allows them to make choices according to the principles that they will or legislate for themselves. To respect people in this manner is to treat them as ends in themselves and not as a means to one's own ends or the ends of others. Respect for individual thought and action means allowing people to make choices according to their convictions, as long as the choices made do not limit the freedom of choice of others and do not harm others (Fry in Fowler & Levine-Ariff 1987:41).

While autonomy is considered the highest of all principles, some people include informed consent, refusal of treatment and suicide. Others include truth telling, privacy and confidentiality (Thompson & Thompson 1992:32).

As a guiding principle, respect for autonomy is binding on all health professionals and should be adhered to unless it is overridden by another moral principle of greater weight or standing. It may not always be possible to allow patients, such as small children or the severely mentally handicapped, to make their own choices, or to allow patients to follow the course of action that they have chosen - for example, people in homes for the aged (Veatch & Fry 1987:102). In such instances the capacity of individuals to make autonomous choices may be questionable.

For health professionals in these situations, the obligation to prevent harm to others or to benefit the patient is perceived as having greater weight than the obligation to respect autonomy. Fry (in Fowler & Levine-Ariff 1987:41) believes that when a health professional respects the autonomous choices of a patient it implies that he/she should follow procedures for gaining informed consent before initiating procedures. A health professional respects a patient's autonomy by making sure that the patient receives all the information required to make an informed decision.

Autonomy is often compromised by the use of technology in the critical care environment; for example, where the autonomous action on the part of the patient is reduced. For example, when life-saving medications are administered, the patient's judgement and the severity of the patient's illness may be affected. While autonomy is a moral value that is highly prized by the professional, in certain situations the value of respect for people helps assure the basis of autonomy, particularly when patients are substantially non-autonomous.

The principles of non-maleficence and beneficence

Many types of ethical theory, both utilitarian and non-utilitarian, recognise the principle of non-maleficence. Some philosophers divide the principles of beneficence into four general obligations, namely:

- one ought not to inflict evil or harm
- one ought to prevent evil or harm
- one ought to remove evil or harm
- one ought to do or promote good.

Beauchamp and Childress contend that the first can be identified as the obligation of non-maleficence, that is, one ought not to inflict evil or harm. The other three they refer to as the obligations of beneficence, that is, the prevention of evil or harm and the promotion of good! They maintain that the three forms of beneficence require taking action by helping to prevent harm, by removing harm and promoting good. Non-maleficence, they maintain, requires *intentionally* refraining from actions which can cause harm (Beauchamp & Childress 2001:114-115).

The duties to avoid harm and to do good are rooted in the earliest traditions of health care. Ketefian (in Oermann 1991:223) maintains that while some authors treat these two major principles as distinct ethical principles, they may be viewed as opposites. According to these principles, treatment decisions in health care are based, firstly, on how to avoid harm to the patient and, secondly, on assessing how a patient can be helped. In clinical practice it is often impossible to separate these two principles.

From a health-care perspective, the infliction of harm takes on a much broader scope than from a medical perspective, where non-infliction of harm is focused on the use of medical therapeutics. The nurse or health professional, on the other hand, must avoid inflicting not only physical harm but also emotional, psychological, spiritual, moral or any other harm to the dignity of patients. Non-maleficence in health care ethics is a stringent principle that often overrides other principles. Non-infliction of harm is often discussed in terms of two such principles, namely the sanctity of life principle and the quality of life principle. According to the sanctity of life principle, life has value and everyone, particularly nurses and other health professionals, has an obligation to preserve it. This does not mean, however, that life is an ultimate value that must be preserved at any or all costs. The quality of life principle asserts that there are some lives that are not worth living. What a life not worth living actually is varies from individual to individual.

Davis (in Fowler & Levine-Ariff 1987:54) argues that while some critics attack the distinction made between killing and allowing to die, others favour it for moral and practical reasons. They believe that the distinction enables decision-makers to express and maintain ethical principles such as non-maleficence and to avoid certain harmful consequences. While some acts of euthanasia may not violate the duty of non-maleficence and are compassionate and humane, Fowler (1989:916) believes that a policy authorising killing would violate the duty of non-maleficence by causing a grave risk of harm in most, if not all, cases. While the principles of beneficence and non-maleficence, of doing good and avoiding evil, provide ready arguments to support those who wish to defend mercy killing, as well as to withhold or withdraw treatment, killing a patient under any circumstances is not an option for health professionals. A principle of avoiding killing – that is, the obligation not to infringe on the sacredness of human life or the obligation not to take human life – is needed for the nurse. Nurses are often uncertain whether or not their actions will contribute to a patient's death and whether or not such actions are morally wrong (Creasia & Parker 1991:156).

The principle of beneficence includes the principles of cost benefit analysis and paternalism. In situations of conflict the principle of beneficence does not always give guidance as to how good and evil or costs, including risks and benefits, will benefit from certain decisions that are required. In health care, such decisions range from determining the number and kind of hospital beds in a given geographic area to the justification of research involving human subjects. The problem of paternalism arises when health-care professionals must decide whether or not to intervene in the decisions and affairs of patients when they (the patients) choose harmful courses of action.

Smith (1989:186) argues that in health care the principles of non-maleficence and beneficence are often impossible to separate. The risk of harm and the actual occurrence of harm are often unavoidable if benefits such as cure, correction or relief are to be attempted and ultimately achieved. She cites an example of the treatment of an infant with hypoplastic left-heart syndrome. While some believe that the cost in pain and discomfort of treating the infant is too great in view of the unpredictability of the final outcome, others emphasise the potential for life that technology affords these infants and accepts the harmful effects of treatment. She maintains that the issues of avoiding harm and doing good become even more difficult when caregivers consider to whom they are responsible. Some assert that only the infant's interests are to be considered while others consider the interests of the parents as well. They acknowledge that the best interest of the parents may well be in conflict with those of their infant.

The principle of justice

The principle of justice is the unifying principle in health and nursing ethics. It includes principles of resource allocation and fairness. Three more or less standard positions have emerged for deciding how resources should be allocated. According to Veatch and Fry (1987:82-83) the most easily understood position simply answers the question of allocation of resources by reverting to the principles of beneficence and non-maleficence, that is, of trying to produce the most good on balance. For example, a nurse promises to help one of her patients but then realises that she might do more good, on balance, by helping another patient. A second group of philosophers, sometimes called libertarians, believe that the principle of autonomy or liberty, as they call it, provides an important counterweight to consequences. They believe resources should be allocated to the free choices of those who rightfully own or control them – if health care is provided for those in need, for example, not because they have a right to it but because the provider is willing to give the care out of a sense of charity. A third group rejects both these positions – they believe resources should be allocated according to the principle of justice.

In health care, the principle of justice mandates allocation of resources. But Smith questions (1989:186) the fairness of the allocation of resources for all members of society when the costs of heart transplants are calculated. Inequities in the distribution of basic health care affects the lives of thousands while relatively few benefit from organ transplantation or cardiac reconstructive surgery. Fairness is a provocative topic when health-care decisions are made, because while some individuals enjoy an overabundance of services, others lack even the most basic health care.

Levine-Ariff (in Fowler & Levine-Ariff 1987:111-112) states that the allocation of health-care resources is in line with suggestions that advocate the cautious evaluation of technology in the light of its effectiveness, safety, patient benefit and cost, but believes that the concern for health-care resources should be regarded as part of the cost. Policy decisions that promote physical facilities (i.e. buildings and equipment for health care), increase the level of available medical technology, improve research and provide medical education, often fail to focus on inadequate bedside equipment, staffing levels and staff skills. This creates dilemmas for nurses as they are expected to assume responsibilities greater than their professional conscience can allow. Ultimately, it is the nurse who sees the patient and family as the centre of concern and who must cope with the consequences. Nursing offers an essential health service but when nursing resources are scarce, the need of the patients for nursing care and their ability to benefit from that care are the criteria most often used by nurses. In today's economic environment, values deemed important for cost effectiveness must be balanced with the values necessary for the delivery of adequate nursing services for patients and families.

Moral rules derived from major principles

Several moral rules that have evolved from the principles of autonomy, beneficence, non-maleficence and justice, particularly in relationships between health-care professionals and patients, are fidelity, veracity, confidentiality and privacy. These moral rules are pertinent to problems that arise in the health-care environment (Beauchamp & Childress 2001:39). While some are dealt with throughout the text, brief reference to each of these moral rules or principles is relevant here because each is important to consider in the unique relationship between nurses and their patients.

■ Veracity and fidelity

The principle of autonomy, with its requirement for informed consent, is linked to the principle of veracity. This principle obliges both the health professional and the patient to tell the truth. Some ethicists question the absoluteness of this principle and argue that in the health-care environment there is such a thing as 'benevolent deception'. Francoeur (1983:24) believes that it may often be more beneficial not to give the whole story or even deliberately to deceive the terminally ill patient or the person at risk of developing an untreatable disease. An example of this would be Huntington's disease, which results in premature brain deterioration and death.

In the nurse-patient relationship, veracity is clearly linked with fidelity through the implicit social contract and covenant that binds nurses and patients in the moral community of the nursing-practice environment. The patient's trust in nurses – individually and collectively – to consider patient welfare first, is at stake. Fidelity to patients includes the moral requirement that patients should never be treated solely as a means to an end but always as an end in themselves (Aroskar in Fowler & Levine-Ariff 1987:86).

Fidelity in the form of making a promise is another aspect of respecting people. One kind of implied promise is to keep information that is disclosed in the course of providing health care confidential. Veatch and Fry (1987:138) maintain that if an explicit or implied promise exists as a result of well-established practices in the health-care profession and in codes of ethics to which health professionals are bound, then these professionals have a duty of fidelity to keep such information confidential.

■ Confidentiality and privacy

Another important aspect of fidelity is the confidentiality of information about patients. This principle may sound simple and uncomplicated but this is often an illusion. Health professionals almost always deal with more than one patient. As an example, Francoeur (1987:35) mentions the conflict between the rights and responsibilities of parents and their sexually active teenager's right to confidentiality when seeking a prescription for contraceptives from a doctor. Another example of this conflict may occur when a genetic counsellor discovers that a patient is a carrier of a fatal genetic disease and wishes to inform the patient's relatives of their risk, but is bound to confidentiality by the patient. It is evident that, in society, a patient's right to confidentiality often has to be balanced against the rights of others.

A dilemma that sometimes confronts the health professional is that she may find herself in the position where she has made two contradictory promises, namely to protect confidential information and to obey the law that requires reporting. For example, there is a specific law requiring that child abuse be reported. The health professional could, however, be convinced that reporting the abuse would hamper the parents' willingness to accept treatment and believe that she has a duty to the client rather than to society. This professional could be convinced that it would be immoral to report the case (Veatch & Fry 1987:153).

One viewpoint according to Beauchamp and Childress (2001:307) is that health-care professionals have a 'right' to break confidences in some circumstances but that they do not have a 'duty' to do so. According to this view they are permitted, but not obliged, to divulge confidential information. There are, however, clear legal duties to divulge confidential information when necessary, such as reporting contagious diseases, gunshot wounds and child abuse.

Privacy is the health-care professional's obligation to protect the patient from undesirable interactions. A very important part of this standard is, as outlined, the health professional's obligation to maintain confidentiality regarding a patient's affairs. A patient voluntarily gives up a part of his privacy to a health-care professional but this does not imply that the patient gives up all right to privacy nor does the whole world have the right of access to a patient's private affairs.

Widespread agreement is reached in various ethical codes that rules of confidentiality and privacy should prevail in relationships with patients. However, most codes and general theories hold that rules of confidentiality are not absolute (Beauchamp & Childress 2001:305).

Moral decision-making in nursing

Health professionals have to cope with numerous ethical issues and dilemmas that arise from scientific and technological progress. Such progress affects the interrelationships between nurses, patients and doctors, not only as individuals but also as members of an increasingly complex society. To make justifiable decisions, nurses and health professionals must have a strong ethical orientation towards work.

Moral reasoning and moral development

Moral reasoning is important for analysing situations of moral conflict. Moral development begins with the transition from what one might call the inborn or natural tendency to know what is right and wrong to a higher level of thinking based on logic. Social scientists have examined and studied moral reasoning and development from various perspectives, and moral reasoning is at present being used extensively in health-care practice (Ketefian in Oermann 1991:218).

Lawrence Kohlberg's prominent theoretical approach to moral development offers an understanding of why people do what they do, and serves as a useful tool in understanding and assessing moral decision-making processes. Kohlberg's theory evolved over a period of 20 years and extends other philosophical studies on moral reasoning. Kohlberg focuses on the moral development and cognitive processes involved in reasoning about moral choice which he believes structure a person's moral judgement. Kohlberg presents a hierarchical structure for understanding moral development, which is similar to Maslow's hierarchy of needs and Jean Piaget's stages of cognitive development (Lindberg *et al* 1990:297). An understanding of the theoretical stages of moral development is essential since people make decisions based on their level of moral development.

Kohlberg's hierarchy of moral development

Within the framework of his cognitive development theory, Kohlberg presents six stages of moral development which he groups into three major hierarchical levels: pre-conventional, conventional and post-conventional. Within each hierarchical level there are two progressive stages of moral development which reflect a distinct way in which moral problems can be evaluated. Progression through each of these stages varies greatly within society (Wright 1987:183).

■ Level one of moral development

The pre-conventional level of moral development occurs in early childhood. Most children under nine years of age and, according to Davis and Aroskar (1997:38), some adolescents and criminal offenders, are at this level.

In early childhood, the child is completely dependent on adults for nearly all aspects of existence – from physical needs, such as food, to emotional needs, such as safety and love. At this level an individual's moral choices are primarily hedonistic in that they are dictated by self-interest. Both stages of moral development at this level are equated with conformity to avoid punishment.

- Stage one individuals obey authority out of fear of punishment rather than from respect for authority. Right action is dictated by the avoidance of breaking rules for fear of punishment, or for the sake of obedience, or both. In nursing, an example of a stage one response is the nurse who, when faced with a choice either to stay and give nursing care in a grossly understaffed unit or to refuse to work under such conditions, decides to remain because she reasons that if she left she would be discharged and receive a bad reference. Moral behaviour is thus determined by the avoidance of punishment.

- Stage two individuals act in terms of what is called instrumental relativism. The individual reciprocates or retaliates within a relationship in order to achieve personal gain rather than to honour abstract concepts such as justice, duty or honour. Whatever provides personal satisfaction is viewed as right and what is right is to obey the rules when this is in the individual's immediate interest or when it involves an equal exchange, a deal or an agreement.

Fowler and Mahon (in Thompson & Thompson 1990:110) maintain that stage two persons are pragmatically opportunistic as they establish a tit-for-tat type of relationship that may involve bargaining but that is mostly directed at personal ascendancy or gain. The fear of physical consequences and of power exerted by those in authority determines the nature of right and wrong in both of these stages.

■ Level two of moral development

According to Kohlberg the conventional level of moral development occurs at a time when children move from concrete execution of formal operations to adult thinking (Lindberg *et al* 1990:297). At this level individuals conform to societal norms and try to maintain the *status quo*.

- Stage three in the conventional level involves mutual interpersonal expectations, relationships and conformity. Individuals establish interpersonal agreement or 'good boy – nice girl orientation'. They view conformity to social and peer pressure as a determinant of 'good' and 'right' behaviour. Fowler and Mahon (in Thompson & Thompson

1990:111) point out that for the first time the issue of motivation enters into the reasoning process. Attempts are made to meet stereotypical expectations of 'good' behaviour in individual and group situations. 'Good' and 'bad' become based partly upon the individual's ability or failure to meet stereotypical standards. In this stage the consequences of punishment or pain may be endured to meet the expectations of the stereotype.

■ Stage four individuals are oriented towards law and order. This stage is characterised by conformity to societal or institutional rules. Wright (1987:183) maintains that non-conformity to hospital policy, for example, may be construed as 'wrong', irrespective of moral duty to patients. Fowler and Mahon (in Thompson & Thompson 1990:112) cite an example of a nurse who refuses to discuss with family members the side effects of medication a patient is receiving because 'the doctor ordered us not to'.

■ Level three of moral development

The post-conventional level of moral reasoning involves more autonomous thinking in which reasoning becomes more complex. This last level, also labelled the autonomous or principled level, is where principles apply not only for their law and order values but because they express society's consensus about what is right.

■ Stage five of this level, according to Lindberg _et al_ (1990:298), 'is sometimes called the stage of national morality and has been identified as the governmental morality that affects national health policy'. Individuals have an awareness of the social contract and an appreciation of the law, which is directed towards rights and obligations, expressed in contracts between professionals and the parties they serve. Moral development in stage five recognises the interaction between, on the one hand, duty, the well-being of the majority, basic human rights, democracy and constitutionality with, on the other hand, what the conscience dictates as being 'right' (Wright 1987:183). Fowler and Mahon (in Thompson & Thompson 1990:112) maintain that stage five of moral development is apparent in the reasoning of a nurse who is caught up in the dilemma of dual loyalty – loyalty to the doctor and loyalty to the patient concerning a patient's prognosis. Hospital guidelines indicate that the nurse should support the doctor's judgement in this situation. The nurse supports the doctor's decision by giving evasive answers to family members but then decides to work towards changing the doctor's mind because she believes the family's right to the truth is a legitimate counterclaim.

■ Stage six of moral development applies to humankind in general. This is the highest stage of moral development where individuals have disassociated themselves from the rules and expectations of others, and define and choose their own values and universal ethical principles. These principles relate to universal principles of justice, such as the equality of human rights and respect for the dignity of human beings as individuals (Davis & Aroskar 1997:38). For example, a nurse may respond to conflict situations out of a sense of duty towards abstract ethical principles of justice, although these principles may not conform to established regulations or laws. An example is the nurse who has been given permission to use a comatose patient as a research subject. Although the patient's wife and the doctor have granted their permission, the nurse decides not to include the patient in the study because she feels that the patient's dignity would be violated by 'using him as an instrument rather than an end in and of himself' (Fowler & Mahon in Thompson & Thompson 1990:113).

According to Kohlberg certain circumstances may stimulate or account for a person's level of moral development, such as an individual's stage of intellectual/cognitive development and the social and educational climate to which the individual has been exposed. Ketefian (in Oermann 1991:219) states that environments which provide opportunities for group participation, the sharing of decision-making and the assumption of responsibility for the consequences of action will stimulate the development of higher levels of moral reasoning.

Various factors will also determine whether a particular person will live up to his or her stage of moral reasoning. Davis & Aroskar (1997:38) maintain that an individual's sense of justice is what is most distinctively and fundamentally moral. One can act morally while questioning all rules or the content of the greater good, but one cannot act morally and question the need for justice. Cultural variations in moral judgement also pose difficult problems because rules of ethical conduct are embedded in specific cultural patterns.

Gilligan challenges Kohlberg's conceptualisation of moral reasoning on the grounds that it is a male-oriented perspective on morality. Inherent in Gilligan's approach to moral development are integration and responsibility for others, whereas competition and fairness are integral to Kohlberg's conception of development (Hoyer *et al* 1991:171).

Gilligan's theory of moral development

In Gilligan's approach to moral development the focus is on the development of an understanding of responsibilities and relationships in terms of care and caring. According to Gilligan (in Kozier *et al* 1992:188), there are three stages in the process of developing an ethic of care. Each stage ends in a transitional period, which, according to her, is a period when the individual recognises a conflict or discomfort with some present behaviour and considers new approaches.

■ Stage one: caring for oneself

In this first stage of development the person is interested in caring for the self only and feels no concern or conflict with the needs of others. This stage is focused on survival and ends when the person begins to realise that there is a need for relationships and connections with other people.

■ Stage two: caring for others

During the second stage of development the person begins to understand the need for caring relationships with others. The selfishness of earlier behaviour is recognised and the person now approaches relationships with the aim of not hurting others. The person becomes more responsive to the needs of others. A transition period occurs when the person realises that this approach may cause difficulties when there is a lack of balance between caring for oneself and caring for others.

■ Stage three: caring for self and others

In this stage the person begins to realise that there is a need for balance between responsibility for the self and other people. In other words, the interconnections between the self and others is recognised during this final stage of moral development.

Both Piaget and Kohlberg assume that males and females see moral problems in the same light, namely justice and individual rights. During Gilligan's studies of how females perceive moral problems challenge this assumption, she found that women frame moral problems in terms of conflicting personal responsibilities rather than as conflicting rights. She found that, whereas boys like highly structured games with elaborate rules to resolve conflicts, girls preferred games that were less structured and less competitive. If conflicts arose, girls were more likely to stop the game to protect relationships. Adolescent boys first focus on developing their own identity by separating themselves from others and then develop their skill in intimacy and relationships at a later stage. Girls, however, generally learn the meaning of their own identity and intimacy simultaneously through their relationships. Francoeur (1983:21) maintains that 'Gilligan reminds us that the way people define moral problems, the situations they construe as moral conflicts in their lives and the values they use to resolve them, are all a function of their social conditioning'.

In Gilligan's study of women, gender differences became apparent. Men, for example, see morality in terms of individual authority, fairness and rights, and tend to devalue caring which they assume women will provide. Women, on the other hand, see morality in the context of human relationships and in their ability to care. Gilligan presents an alternative approach to moral reasoning that addresses an ethic of care where moral development is centred on the understanding of responsibility. In her study on women's experience of abortion, she concludes that 'a different voice guides their moral action and judgements' (Gibson 1993:2005).

According to Gilligan, the existence of these two distinct contexts for moral decision-making means that moral decisions depend on gender, which leads to a new understanding of responsibility and moral choice. However, the linking of these two paths with gender – caring in the case of women and justice in the case of men – is far from absolute. Instead, it appears that there is an interaction between these two moral voices, and that one or the other predominates in the beginning and gradually converges until a balance is achieved as a person's moral sensitivity matures (Francoeur 1983:25).

Ketefian (in Oermann 1991:221) states that no measurement tool exists at present to address this alternative perspective and that further research is necessary to validate these claims. Although Kohlberg's theory provides a useful tool for health professionals in practice, it will not make moral decisions easier. Professional health-care education and involvement in real-life dilemmas in health-care practice will promote critical thinking and the development of moral judgement.

Decision-making models and processes in nursing

Several decision-making models and processes in nursing and health care have been published since the early 1970s. Many are based on Kohlberg's moral development theory and decision-making theories. A selection is presented here in summary; for a more in-depth study it is advisable to consult the original text as indicated in the list of references. The general approaches to decision-making in most of these models closely resemble the approach to nursing known as the nursing process. The philosophy underlining this process acknowledges that people are individuals and that each person has needs and problems peculiar to himself or herself, but recognises that certain basic human needs are common to all people. Therefore patients have rights over their own bodies and should have a say in what is done to and for them (Rumbold 1993:49).

Thompson and Thompson's bioethical decision-making model

Joyce and Henry Thompson's decision-making model can be used to identify and analyse ethical dilemmas in health-care practice. For the successful application of the model, all participants in group decision-making are encouraged to be truthful in their responses to each step. An environment of trust, confidentiality and mutual respect is needed where each member of the group listens carefully to the others, tries to understand what is being said. Moral reasoning encourages discussion, which includes disagreement as well as the mutual searching for the reasons behind each individual's beliefs or values.

The first seven steps are part of the process of analysis. Step 8 includes the process of weighing and justifying, step 9 involves making a choice while step 10 involves reviewing or evaluating that choice.

1. Review the situation to determine health problems, the decisions required, ethical components, and key individuals.
2. Gather additional information to clarify the situation.
3. Identify the ethical issues in the situation.
4. Define personal and professional moral positions.
5. Identify the moral positions of key individuals involved.
6. Identify value conflicts, if any.
7. Determine who should make the decision.
8. Identify the range of actions with anticipated outcomes.
9. Decide on a course of action and carry it out.
10. Evaluate/review results of decision/action.

Thompson, Melia and Boyd's practical model for moral decision-making

When a nurse assesses a situation, she applies her knowledge of the principles and practice of nursing. This process is similar to the process involved in making moral decisions. Thompson, Melia and Boyd argue that moral considerations are inseparable from the nursing process. They suggest the following applications of their model to moral decision-making in nursing practice (Thompson *et al* 1988:211-214):

1. Assessment is the first step in moral decision-making and it involves getting clarity about different nursing environments, such as community or institutional environments. The needs of patients have to be identified as well as available resources. Then the relevant knowledge and skills need to be clarified.
2. Planning a course of action follows once the problem has been clearly assessed. This includes specific knowledge and practical procedures relevant to the problem, examining the ways in which similar problems were dealt with in the past, choosing appropriate means to achieve desired goals and, lastly, formulating a plan of action that includes contingency plans should things go wrong.
3. Implementing decisions depends on how effectively plans are worked out in practice. While implementation is the key part of 'action' it cannot be considered in isolation, but will involve moral deliberation at each stage of the process.
4. Evaluating a decision involves considering whether the actual consequences of an implemented plan of action are the same as the intended consequences, for example whether these consequences are better or worse than hoped for and whether the long-term effects of a course of action justify its becoming standard practice. Evaluation is

also concerned both with the success of individual steps in the process as well as with how successfully the whole process has been in practical and moral terms.

Husted's formal ethical decision-making model

For Husted and Husted (1995:30-31) the professional nurse's initial preparations for ethical decision-making are very important and, in this regard, they suggest the following:

- Care should be taken that ethical aspects of situations are not obscured by logistic and administrative concerns and the demands of 'hands on' nursing care.
- Insight should be gained into the actual aspects of a situation and the details of the health-care environment should be kept in mind. This will not interfere with ethical analysis but will help the nurse to remain within the context of the profession.
- The essential qualities of the ethical situation should be isolated with a view to drawing general conclusions which can then be applied to similar situations.
- Decisions should be based on stable permanent values and not on variable temporary ones.
- Finally, decisions should be made that will be of future benefit.

Husted's formal ethical decision-making model is based on a contextual application of bioethical standards (autonomy, freedom, veracity, privacy and beneficence) and is structured to help nurses make contextually appropriate (justifiable) ethical decisions.

Fig. 3.1   Husted's formal ethical decision-making model

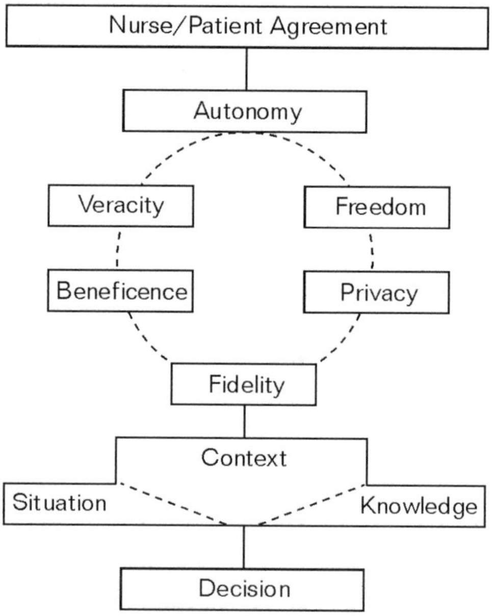

(Husted, G.L. & Husted, J.H. 1995. Ethical decision-making in nursing. St Louis: Mosby, 19.)

1. To understand the terms of the *nurse-patient agreement*, the nurse must be aware of the patient's unique nature (or autonomy) because every patient is a unique personality.
2. Every action that a patient takes arises from his *freedom*. A nurse who fails to respect a patient's freedom is not interacting with the patient. To understand the terms of their agreement the nurse must respect the patient's freedom.

3. The terms of the nurse-patient agreement are based on rational trust, which cannot exist unless the relationship is based on *veracity*.
4. Interaction based on agreement presumes self-ownership or *privacy* of the parties to the agreement. An agreement is invalid if it denies the self-ownership of one of the parties.
5. The final purpose of an agreement is for *beneficent* action. A nurse who fails to act beneficently towards a patient fails to fulfil their agreement.
6. An agreement calls for *fidelity*. An agreement that is not honoured is a contradiction in terms. No nurse can ever justify an ethical decision or action that breaches the implicit agreement with a patient.

Husted and Husted maintain that all these considerations form the context of the ethical interaction between nurse and patient. The ethical effectiveness of this interaction depends on the nurse's optimal awareness.

Ethics committee

The need to provide procedures for effective decision-making is recognised by all health-care professionals. Ethics committees are being formed by a number of health-care institutions in response to the difficult ethical decisions faced by patients, families and health-care providers. Ethics committees should be composed of ethicists, nurses, doctors, social workers, a minister and/or rabbi or priest, and possibly the institution's legal adviser. A multidisciplinary committee provides the broadest expertise and range of perspectives for dealing with ethical issues involving quality of life, terminal illness and use of scarce resources. Apart from the important role ethics committees play in making ethical decisions, they also function as consultants. They assist patients and their families in facing and resolving ethical dilemmas. They educate professionals on ethical issues and assist them in developing a systematically reasoned approach to ethical problem-solving.

While nursing has in the past been under-represented on most ethics committees, the trend currently is to include diversified nursing categories. Ethical concerns have thus become more readily recognised and addressed. In general the function of an ethics committee is to write or review policies, to consider complex cases carefully and to make recommendations to the appropriate person when required.

Husted and Husted give valuable guidelines regarding the type of person who should serve on an ethics committee and the type of questions members should consider during bioethical discussions. They maintain that persons who have an immediate answer to every ethical dilemma or those who cannot come to an ethical decision will hinder the work of the committee and produce harm to the patient. The person who best serves the interest of the committee is the nurse who works with the patient and has first hand knowledge of the situation. (Husted & Husted in Deloughery 1998:238-239)

Guidelines on the functioning of an ethics committee and the type of questions that should be considered will be dealt with more fully in a subsequent chapter.

Concluding remarks

While many people believe that they can recognise moral action guides in ethical dilemmas and judgements, in disputes it is generally very difficult to distinguish moral from non-moral considerations. Ethical decision-making presumes an objectivist approach, because a discussion on ethical principles can be meaningful only if morality is objective in some way or another. The two major theories of objective morality are consequentialism and non-consequentialism.

Moral reasoning and decision-making are vital and are like the practice of nursing with its emphasis on identifying and critically analysing its ethical dimensions. Ethical nursing practice requires nurses to respect people, obtain informed consent, preserve quality of life, prevent harm, remove harmful conditions, do good for patients and not inflict harm. These values, as Fowler (1989:964) maintains, are among the norms of obligation that will guide ethical analysis and judgement. They are the substance of models for ethical decision-making. While ethical theory and reasoning will not solve ethical dilemmas, they provide the framework for structuring and clarifying them. Regardless of the model applied by the nurse or ethics committee, ethical decision-making remains a rational and analytical process consisting of six generic steps:

1. Recognising and defining the dilemma.
2. Identifying alternatives.
3. Evaluating the alternatives.
4. Choosing the appropriate decision.
5. Converting the decision into action.
6. Evaluating the action to determine whether it was effective and whether it conformed to relevant moral principles.

A nurse should be able to engage in moral reasoning based on moral principles that are separate from institutional norms and authority because each moral situation requires an independent moral judgement. When choosing between alternatives, values hold a key position in the decision-making process and include not only personal values but also professional, societal and cultural values (Gibson 1993:2006).

Critical thinking activities

1. Which three conditions have been identified and serve as action guides in moral decision-making?
2. Why are moral judgements regarded as objective?
3. How do rule-deontologists differ from act-deontologists in moral decision-making?
4. What is the difference between the principles of non-maleficence and beneficence?
5. Give examples of the application of the principle of justice in health care.
6. Which moral rules are derived from major ethical principles? Give one example of each rule as applied in nursing practice.
7. Why is a knowledge of moral development theory necessary for nurses?
8. What are the differences between Kohlberg's pre-conventional, conventional and post-conventional moral development stages?
9. How does Gilligan's theory of moral development differ from both Piaget and Kohlberg's assumptions about the moral development of males and females?
10. How many steps are there in Bandman and Bandman's nurse-patient decision-making process? Give a brief description of each step.
11. What is the main function of an ethics committee?

Ethical principles and rules in moral decision-making and professional-patient relationships

Silvia Pera

Outcomes

Studying this chapter will enable you to:

- describe the importance of respect for autonomous choice in health care
- appraise the mechanism of informed consent in nursing practice
- explain the necessity for confidentiality in health care
- describe the advocacy role of the nurse as caregiver
- debate the importance of truth telling in nursing practice
- differentiate the forms of accountability in nursing practice.

Introduction

The ethical principles of autonomy, beneficence and non-maleficence were outlined in the previous chapter with reference to their role in ethical decision-making. In this chapter we consider the important ethical norms or rules, which are based on these principles and which guide and influence both decision-making and professional-patient relationships in health care. Fundamental to the principle of autonomy, for example, is respect for autonomous choice, the right to informed consent, the right to confidentiality and professional advocacy in nurse-patient relationships. Veracity, or truthfulness in professional-patient relationships, is grounded in the principle of beneficence, which provides specific guides to action. Professional accountability in health care and nurse patient relationships, on the other hand, is based on the principle of non-maleficence.

Respect for autonomy

The term autonomy means having the freedom to make choices about issues that affect one's life and it is closely linked to respect for persons (Burkhardt & Nathaniel 2002:41). Autonomy is further defined as the individual's freedom to determine his/her own objectives and to act accordingly. This implies that a person should be free to decide for him/herself, on condition that his autonomy does not encroach upon the autonomy of others. The concept is further simplified by saying that it is the freedom to decide whether or not action can or will be taken (Oermann 1991:222).

In health care the principle of autonomy embraces patient self-determination according to which patients are considered to be in charge of their own destiny in matters of health and illness (Deloughery 1995:230).

To acknowledge a person's right to hold views, to make choices and to take actions based on personal beliefs and values is to respect a particular person's autonomous choices. This is the fundamental right in health care and in professional-patient relationships.

Beauchamp and Childress state that 'respect for autonomy is not a mere **ideal** in health care; it is a professional obligation'. They hold that autonomous choice is a right and not a duty of patients (Beauchamp & Childress 2001:63).

Autonomy and the patient

A patient who seeks medical or nursing assistance entrusts his/her body to health practitioners. This does not mean, however, that in doing so, the patient forfeits his/her right to autonomy (Martin 1993:29). Indeed, society attaches great value to the patient's autonomy. It must be borne in mind, however, that the ethical principle underlying respect for the patient's autonomy does not guarantee that the patient will make the right decision if he is left to his own devices (Quinn & Smith 1987:33).

In health care autonomy also means that the patient has the right to information, the right to agree or to refuse to undergo treatment or to participate in research. In practice, however, there are limits to autonomy. Some patients, because of their physical or mental conditions, have diminished autonomy (Davis *et al* 1997:105).

Autonomy and the nurse

An experienced professional and conscientious nurse is knowledgeable and usually better able than the patient to make objective judgements. The nurse should discuss a patient's choices with him/her and so help the patient to arrive at a more informed judgement than he/she might do alone. However, an effective nurse always recognizes the patient's autonomy and freedom (Deloughery 1995:118).

Informed consent

All procedures in health care require that a patient has given his/her permission. To be able to grant consent, the patient must be fully informed about the procedure, its possible advantages or disadvantages, as well as any alternatives to the proposed treatment. Rowson (in Tschudin 1993:33) regards consent as one of the cornerstones of health care from a legal and moral point of view. It is necessary from a legal point of view because it enables the practitioner to defend him/herself, after consent has been given, against a possible charge of assault; and from a moral point of view because it displays respect for the patient's autonomy and right to self-determination.

According to Beauchamp & Childress (2001:78), there are two meanings of informed consent. The first meaning is where the person does not merely express agreement or comply with a proposal but must actually authorise something through an act of informed or voluntary consent. The second meaning of informed consent is tied up with formal procedures that institutions have to follow before proceeding with diagnostic, therapeutic or research procedures.

Legal validity of consent

Volenti non fit iniuria (a willing person is not wronged; he who consents cannot be injured) is the legal maxim that expresses the defence of consent (Neethling *et al* 1999:97). In order to be legally valid, consent must be based on information that has been provided to explain the relevant treatment.

Strauss (1992:10-11), an authority on medical law in South Africa, points out the following interesting legal aspects of informed consent:

■   Consent to a dangerous experiment or illegal abortion will not indemnify the doctor and his helpers against prosecution.

■   Consent may occur in writing, verbally or tacitly (i.e. through conduct). In this regard, however, the person must be in his/her right mind, 18 years of age or older, and fully informed of the nature, consequences and possible complications of the intervention or treatment. If the person meets these requirements, co-operates fully, and does not offer any objections or resistance, it may be assumed that he has consented. An important aspect in this regard is that mere acquiescence is not accepted as consent.

■   A minor of 18 years and older may grant or refuse consent independently (Child Care Act, 1983 (Act 74 of 1983), section 39(4)). This Act also provides for consent by the superintendent of the hospital in cases of emergency where the parents or legal guardians are not present (Strauss & Mare 2001:74).

■   Spouses may grant informed consent independently of one another, even if they are married in community of property. This principle also applies where a woman consents to a sterilisation in the absence of any medical indication.

■   A man does not have the right to oblige his wife to undergo an operation or a medical examination against her will.

Therapeutic privilege

More room has recently been allowed, legally speaking, for the discretion of the professional person who must provide the patient with information. In the past, the principle of disclosure of all relevant information, whether detrimental to the patient or not, was rigidly adhered to.

Legal exceptions to the rule of informed consent allow health professionals to proceed without consent in cases of emergency, incompetence and waiver. While these three conditions are not controversial, an exception occurs in the therapeutic privilege accorded to doctors. A doctor may legitimately withhold information based on sound medical judgement when divulging information would be potentially harmful to a depressed, emotionally drained or unstable patient. The precise formulation of this therapeutic privilege varies according to legal jurisdictions (Beauchamp & Childress 2001:84).

The right to refuse consent

When a patient refuses treatment, it is the duty of the professional to recognise the autonomy of the patient and to display the necessary responsibility by finding out the reason for the refusal. If the refusal is based on an informed and rational decision, the decision should be respected. But if the patient is in an emotional state or has not properly understood the information, it is the responsibility of the professional to convey the information more clearly. The situation becomes more complex if the professional believes that the patient is mentally unbalanced and is not competent to make the decision. A very clear distinction should be drawn between competence in the case of informed consent and competence in the case of informed refusal (Rumbold 1993:124-125).

In the case of informed consent, the patient must understand the information before consenting to the proposed treatment. Rumbold (1993:121-122) distinguishes between informed consent and educated consent, where the former does not necessarily mean that the patient has understood. A patient may have a language problem, be prejudiced or panic-stricken and, consequently, not absorb the information; or he may simply not have the necessary intellectual capacity. In this regard the professional conveying the information plays a decisive role. Ingelfinger (in Wright 1987:200-202) says that in the case of research, for example, the ideal is that a patient who is about to participate in the research is fully informed about what the research involves. However, it is virtually impossible for a layman to understand everything about highly technical procedures. For that reason, even if the researcher has obtained informed consent from the patient, it still falls short of educated consent. Consequently, the patient is wholly dependent on the conscience and goodwill of the researcher for his protection.

Cases in which consent cannot be obtained

Some patients are genuinely not in a position to form an informed opinion. Examples of such cases are:

- The *unconscious patient*. If the patient is unconscious, the family may give their consent or, in an emergency where the family is absent and there is no time to contact them, the law authorises the superintendent of the hospital to grant consent (Strauss 1992:155).
- *Children under the age of* 18. Informed consent cannot be obtained from minors of 17 years and younger. In these cases the parents or legal guardian must give consent. In cases of emergency, where the parents or guardians are not present and there is no time to contact them, the superintendent is once again authorised to grant consent.
- *Mentally handicapped and brain-damaged patients*. Moral guidelines for obtaining consent can be laid down only if the assumption is that all human rights also apply to this group of people. These patients are entitled to respect, just like any other person, and they should be protected against harm or injury (Rumbold 1993:122-123). If the patient is not in a position to grant consent, the court will appoint persons to decide on his/her behalf (Strauss 1992:10-11).

The role and responsibilities of the nurse

The process of obtaining informed consent is complex and nurses must be sensitive to the fact that the mere act of asking a patient to sign a form giving permission to particular treatment may constitute a form of coercion. The nurse must make the patient aware of all options, the possible outcomes of each option, the likely outcome with no treatment and the implications that each option will have on future life-style. If the nurse thinks that the patient does not understand the implications of treatment, of alternative options or non-treatment, or is unable to consider various options, it is the nurse's responsibility to intervene. Legally the nurse must notify the doctor and ask for further information for the patient. The primary concern of the nurse is to ensure that all criteria for autonomous decision-making are met before obtaining the patient's signature on a consent form. Witnessing a patient's signature on a consent form implies accountability on the part of the nurse. Burkhardt & Nathaniel (2002:211-212) add that although the nurse is legally required to ensure that there is proper informed consent, there is no clear course of action when a nurse believes that the patient has not been informed and the doctor is unco-operative in remedying the situation.

Confidentiality

A confidential relationship arises whenever one person entrusts confidential information with another person. In popular usage this confidential information is known as secrets. Where the person to whom the information has been entrusted is a nurse, the patient has the right to believe that this confidential information will not be conveyed to others without the patient's consent and that it will be used only for the purpose for which it has been given (Rumbold 1993:130). Melia (1988:37) claims, however, that despite the moral correctness in the keeping of secrets, the basic philosophical question remains: why is it good to keep secrets? Does keeping secrets mean that the patient receives more effective care?

McHale (1993:74) identifies two important aspects of confidentiality, namely limiting access to information and making provision for communication about intimate and other sensitive, personal matters. Vulnerable patients, especially dying patients, are particularly susceptible to revealing personal information. The relationship between the person telling the secret and the one listening to the secret is very intimate and should never be betrayed by repeating the secret (High 1989:8). This is precisely where the dilemma arises for the nurse, since she has to decide what should and what may not be repeated. In the execution of her professional accountability she will not disclose any information, except with the consent of the patient or a person who may make decisions on behalf of the patient, or if the court requires such a disclosure (Lee 1987:24).

Confidentiality and the law

The point of departure of any dispute about confidentiality must be the fact that confidentiality is a patient's right (Tschudin 1993:2). Nurses and other healthcare personnel are obliged both legally and ethically to maintain strict confidentiality in respect of the patient. If this obligation is not met, a serious ethical offence is committed and disciplinary steps may ensue (Strauss 1992:15). Deloughery (1995:208) agrees and maintains that most institutions lay down strict policy measures for the confidentiality of patient information and that it is the nurse's duty to acquaint herself with these measures. Beauchamp & Childress (in Rumbold 1993:133) warn that the disclosure of confidential information bears a burden of proof, which cannot be denied.

Strauss (1992:15), however, mentions some circumstances under which confidential information may be disclosed, namely:
- with the patient's consent
- without the patient's consent with a judicial order
- without the patient's consent when the disclosure is in the public interest.

Confidentiality and privacy of patient information

Computerisation

Information technology makes patient information alarmingly easy to obtain. A counter-measure is, according to Curran & Curran (1991:47), necessary to protect the patients' confidentiality and privacy. The trend in hospitals and clinics to computerise data has brought about a new awareness of the confidentiality of patient information and a great deal of attention is now being paid to the question of who may or may not examine the data.

Patient access

A patient's access to his/her own report remains a controversial issue. Ownership of patients' reports vests in the health institution, and the patient, or an authorised representative, may not remove these reports. However, the patient's right to information on his/her diagnosis and treatment is currently more widely recognised, and so the patient may no longer be refused access to his/her own documents. In some states of the USA an authorised third party is allowed to study the patient's documents. In South Africa the chief executive officer of the relevant institution decides whether or not a patient may have access to information about him/herself (Bruce 1988:161-172).

It is obvious that thoughtless and careless conduct in respect of sensitive information (for example, a patient who tests HIV positive) can have serious economic and social consequences for the patient, his family and the community. Nurses must ensure that patient information is not accessible without supervision and control. Any person who has access to this information, be it a nurse or doctor, should be bound by a code of ethics. The main consideration should be to protect the patient against unauthorised and unnecessary invasion of his/her privacy (Milholland 1994:19-24).

Advocacy

A nurse's role in advocacy is often erroneously viewed as a role in which he/she is in a position of power. He/she supposedly speaks and decides on behalf of the patient in the face of the doctor's (or anyone else's) alleged prejudice.

The relationship that exists between a nurse and a patient is a special one. Some of the duties and obligations of such a relationship often run deeper than the normal scope of social interaction (Rumbold 1993:128).

Unlike other health professionals the nurse is in an ideal position to experience the patient as a human being with unique strengths. Furthermore, the nurse, more than any other professional, is in a position to act as link between the medical team, other health professionals and the administration. As patient advocate the nurse never loses touch with the patient's autonomy. In the role of caretaker, protector and advocate the nurse is always available to help the patient win the final battle of life over death (Bandman & Bandman 2002:22).

Advocacy as an ethical component of nursing practice

A nurse's value system is reflected in the way she approaches her role as the patient's advocate. According to Curtin (in Tschudin 1992:97), one of the most important characteristics of advocacy is that it embodies the ideals of the ethics of caring. It is within this ethics of caring that the relationship between people develops.

According to Brown (in Tschudin 1992:98), there are four reasons for a nurse acting as a patient's advocate:

- The first is the quality of the care that the patient receives.
- The second is the patient's access to care.
- The third is the patient's awareness of the care, which he/she receives, its effects and side effects.
- The fourth is the patient's understanding of the alternatives to the proposed treatment.

The role of the nurse as patient advocate

The most important argument in favour of advocacy is that the patient should have sufficient information to enable him/her to act as his/her own advocate (Tschudin 1992:98).

The nurse's role as advocate includes the following:

- to inform the patient of his/her rights and to ensure that he/she has all the necessary knowledge to make an informed decision
- to support the patient in the decisions he/she makes
- to safeguard the patient against abuse and violation of his/her rights (Bandman & Bandman 2001:23).

To do these things, the nurse needs a thorough knowledge of the relevant Acts and codes of ethics of the nursing profession. Kohnke believes, moreover, that the most important characteristics a nurse should have are open-mindedness, impartiality and a sound knowledge of people.

The nurse's most important role in advocacy is to inform the patient so that he/she can make his/her own decisions. If a patient is not able to do so, the nurse should act only after a thorough assessment of the situation.

Veracity (truthfulness)

The principle of veracity involves the practice of telling the truth. Health-care professionals have the responsibility to tell the truth and truthfulness is a cornerstone of the respect that exists in the professional-patient relationship.

According to Beauchamp & Childress (2001:284) there are three arguments in favour of veracity or truth telling.

- Firstly, veracity is based on respect owed to others.
- Secondly, veracity is closely connected to obligations of fidelity, or loyalty and promise-keeping. Communication with others implies speaking the truth and not lying. Patients have the right to the truth regarding diagnoses, prognoses and health care interventions.
- Thirdly, adherence to rules of truthfulness is essential in fostering trust. Relationships between health-care professionals and patients ultimately depend upon trust.

Truthfulness in nursing care

In nursing, veracity or truthfulness engenders respect and open communication between nurse and patient. The violation of the principle of veracity shows lack of respect. Professionals are ethical which means that they have a responsibility to tell the truth. Veracity refers to the objective transmission of information as well as the way the professional fosters the patient's understanding. Caring professionals should, therefore, not forget that there are gentle and harsh ways of telling the truth. Other principles such as mercy and compassion form an integral part of the truth-telling process when dealing with vulnerable patients (Burkhardt & Nathaniel 2002:52).

A clear distinction should be drawn between withholding the truth and distorting the truth. In the case of informed consent it has already been established that there are exceptional cases in which the truth may be suppressed. However, no justification can be found in the literature for the distortion of the truth.

Deception, in whatever form, implies broken confidence, since the person who listens trusts that the person speaking is telling the truth. Lying not only robs the patient of reality, but also destroys the confidential relationship between the patient and the practitioner.

Whenever a patient is robbed of reality, he is robbed of his freedom, leaving him even more helpless and vulnerable than before (Curtin & Flaherty 1982:326-327).

Another form of deception is the avoidance of questions by way of vague answers. For example, a patient asks about his blood pressure reading and the nurse tells him that it is normal when in fact she knows that actually it is normal for a hypertensive patient. She may believe that this half-truth is not a distortion of the truth. However, she would not only be deceiving herself, but the patient as well and would be tantamount to lying.

Accountability

Accountability forms an integral part of professional practice since the nurse has to continually evaluate a wide variety of circumstances and then accept accountability for her judgement. Accountability not only implies responsibility when something goes wrong; it is built into the nurse's everyday professional conduct. She is primarily accountable to the patient and the public, but also to colleagues - particularly if she has delegated tasks to them - and to her employer, her profession and herself (Tschudin 1992:110-111).

Different forms of accountability in nursing practice

The exercise of accountability involves investigating a situation, setting out the different options available, demonstrating an expert understanding of the possible consequences and making an informed decision (Tschudin 1993:131).

Professional accountability

A professional practitioner is constantly faced with ethical decisions. The code of ethics of his/her profession serves as a guideline for deciding on the correct professional conduct, but the final decision will still have to be made by the practitioner him/herself. Marks-Maran (in Tschudin 1993:129-130) points out that an action that is professionally correct is not necessarily administratively or legally correct.

Moral accountability

Marks-Maran (in Tschudin 1993:130-132) states unequivocally that there is no regulation, law, code or job description for moral accountability. An action, which is morally defensible, is not necessarily lawful. A morally responsible decision is based on one's own personal value system, which in turn is based on knowledge. Moral accountability is therefore not transferable. The nurse who decides to give a patient an injection of an additional dose of analgesic could justify her decision morally, but not legally or administratively.

Legal accountability

Conflict may arise in nursing practice between the nurse's legal accountability and her moral accountability. A nurse caring for a patient for whom an analgesic has been prescribed every four hours but who complains of severe pain after two hours, could experience conflict in that she would wish to administer an additional dose or to increase the dosage. If she were in fact to do so after one of the other nurses had signed the necessary records with her, she would be breaking the law and would be held accountable for her actions. Morally speaking, she could argue that she had the patient's interests at heart and that caring is supposed to relieve suffering (Tschudin 1993:124-126).

Administrative accountability

Here the nurse is accountable to her employer or the institution for which he/she works. As an employee, the nurse has a responsibility to her/his employer to meet her/his obligations in terms of her contract, job description and the policy procedures of her employer or institution. Marks-Maran (in Tschudin 1993:127-128) once again underscores the possibility of conflict, which may, for example, occur in decision-making, which, in a given situation, according to the nurse is not to the benefit of her patient. Here, too, the practitioner must make an ethical decision for which he/she will be held accountable.

Accountability and responsibility

Although these two concepts are closely related, it is also important to understand the difference between the two. Manthey (1989:17) makes the following distinction: '*Responsibility* is the allocation and acceptance of an instruction where everyone involved knows who does what, while *accountability* is a retroactive review of decisions that have been made, actions that have been carried out and then establishing how effective they were.'

Accountability has to do with the justification of actions by understanding their reasons and possible consequences, whilst responsibility may be an indication of actions, which should be carried out in a certain situation without the need for the actions to be understood or explained. A person may be responsible for certain actions without being expected to account for these actions. Whenever an action is carried out simply because the chief professional nurse or the doctor has ordered the action, it is a responsibility, but whenever the practitioner who must carry out this action wishes to know the reason for the action and its possible consequences, it is a matter of accountability. Accountability therefore never involves actions, which are carried out automatically.

Accountability and responsibility are very closely related since responsibility involves the person's obligation to be able to account for his/her actions by providing satisfactory reasons. Searle & Pera (1992:183), however, point out that an important difference between accountability and responsibility is that responsibility is the duty to perform some function or another satisfactorily, while accountability refers to the person's responsibility for his acts and omissions.

Responsible conduct, according to Holden (1991:398), is associated with freedom. This freedom does not imply unrestrained behaviour, but is in fact associated with self-control. Feinberg (in Holden 1991:398) regards people who act impulsively or compulsively as powerless and irresponsible because such people are unable to choose freely.

Concluding remarks

Consideration of ethical principles in patient care suggests the development of a more reflective morality in nursing and health care practice. Respect for an individual's autonomy recognises that the patient is a member of a community which implies that decisions made affect others. Informed consent grounded in the principle of autonomy acts to safeguard patients by preventing them from harm. Protecting the patient's right to confidentiality and privacy is recognising the patient's worth and dignity as a human being. In the role of patient advocate the nurse asserts the patient's choices and desires on his/her behalf. Ultimately, the goal of the advocacy role is to promote the autonomy, self actualisation and individual uniqueness of the patient. In the nurse-patient relationship veracity, linked with fidelity, binds care-givers and patients in the practice setting. Accountability in nursing is the foundational value on which the values of autonomy and advocacy find sustenance in nursing. Accountability helps to define the relationships of patients, nurses, other health-care professionals and the community at large

Critical thinking activities

1. Describe the role of the nurse with regard to respect for autonomy.
2. Critically discuss informed consent in nursing practice, highlighting the doctor's and professional nurse's roles.
3. Discuss the importance of confidentiality in patient care.
4. Appraise advocacy in nursing practice.
5. Debate the virtue of veracity in health care.
6. Define the different forms of accountability in nursing practice.

part 3

Perspectives on rights and relationships in health-care practice

To talk about nurses' and patients' rights without working to make them a reality is to surrender to passivity and continuing dependence on others. This is not the vision of what professional nursing can and should be for nurses as moral agents and for patient care

(*Davis, Aroscar, Liaschenco & Drought* 1997:99).

Human rights and legal liability in nursing practice

Rita-marie Jansen & Teuns Verschoor

Outcomes

Studying this chapter will enable you to:

- define the Bill of Rights and explain the most important human rights
- indicate how the Bill affects the nursing profession
- distinguish between the horizontal and vertical operation of the Bill
- suggest remedies for the violation of human rights
- explain the requirements of legal liability and the distinction between private-law and public-law liability
- distinguish between professional liability and legal liability
- give a detailed explanation of liability on the grounds of negligence.

Introduction

Few professions are more affected by the law than the nursing profession. The reason for this is that nursing (albeit with honorable intent) encroaches upon precisely those aspects of human life that are protected by the law. The protection of physical integrity, human dignity and privacy are among the primary objectives of the law. In the case of nursing interventions, such as thorough physical examinations, interviews and something as common as the administering of an injection, it is for the most part only the fact that the patient has given permission or that the action is being taken in his interest without his knowledge (where, for example, he is unconscious) that prevents claims against nurses.

In this chapter we consider the Bill of Rights and its influence on nursing practice, and then turn to the legal liability of nurses and related matters.

The bill of rights

What is a bill of rights?

A bill of rights is a legal document in which the fundamental values and needs of the population or nation are entrenched against violation by the government. It may also specify certain actions that are desired of the government (the so-called **vertical** relationship). The South African 1996 Bill of Rights performs this traditional task, but goes further. It recognises that the private abuse of human rights may be as injurious as violations perpetrated by the state. For this reason the 1996 Bill of Rights also protects individuals against abuses by other individuals (the so-called **horizontal** relationship). In this respect the 1996 Bill goes further than the Bill contained in the Interim Constitution of 1993.

Different types of human rights (also referred to as fundamental rights)

A distinction is made between three types of human rights:

■ **First-generation human rights (so-called civil and political rights)**

This group consists of all those fundamental rights which the government may not violate. Rights such as the right to life, the right to human dignity, the right to privacy, the right to language and culture, the right to freedom of religion, the right to freedom of speech and association, the right to equality and the right to property are some of the rights that fall under this category. These rights are sometimes known as 'blue rights'.

■ **Second-generation human rights (so-called socio-economic rights)**

In this category, an obligation is placed on the government to render assistance. These rights consist, *inter alia*, of the right to work, to education, to housing, to medical care and to state-aided care of the aged.

In contrast to the 'hands off' approach in the case of first-generation rights, the government is obliged to intervene in the case of second-generation rights. These interventions, which originated in socialist thinking, may be defined as obligations or ideals and are sometimes referred to as 'red rights'.

The potential for conflict between the two types of human rights is very real. The problem revolves around the right to property (a first-generation right) in particular. In order to comply with second-generation rights, the government requires funds which, in turn, may lead to higher taxes and, in extreme cases, to the nationalisation of private property. Different countries' bills of human rights give precedence to one group or the other, depending on the underlying ideology of the specific country.

The South African Bill consists mainly of first-generation human rights, but certain second-generation rights are also entrenched, such as the right to housing (s 26) and of access to health-care services (s 27). People have the right to social assistance only if they are unable to support themselves. Children are afforded special protection. Only the right to basic education and social services for children under eighteen and for detainees are stated in unqualified terms and can be enforced directly. Section 35(2)(e) contains a right of detained persons to adequate medical treatment. Every child has the right to basic nutrition, health and social services (s 28). Otherwise there is no direct right to health-care services, but only a right of access to such services. The state has a duty to take reasonable legislative and other measures to achieve the progressive realization of these rights. This must be done within the available resources of the state. Government departments must provide the Human Rights Commission with information about measures they have taken towards the progressive realisation of these rights every year.

The effect of the Constitutional Court's judgement in *Government of the Republic of South Africa and Others v Grootboom and Others* 2000 11 BCLR 1169 (CC) is that the allocation of health-care service resources must include effective access to health-care services by the most vulnerable members of the community. It opens up to the courts the actual resourcing and organisation of health-care services so that the courts are able to ensure that those services fulfil their constitutional obligations.

■ Third-generation human rights

These rights generally pertain to groups. These include the right to an environment that is not harmful to one's health or well-being (s 24). A duty is placed on the state to prevent pollution (amongst other things) for the benefit of present and future generations. These are the so-called 'green rights'.

The division into three categories does not imply a hierarchy of rights. The division is also not watertight and does not apply rigidly.

The South African Bill of Rights

The Bill of Rights (contained in Chapter 2 of the Constitution of the Republic of South Africa, 1996 (Act 108 of 1996)) embodies the basic principles that have always been fundamental to the ethics of nursing.

Basic human rights, such as the right to life, the right to privacy, the right to human dignity and to equality are emphasised in the Bill. These concepts are not new or foreign to nursing practice but because they are mentioned in the Bill they have greater legal force. The ethics of nursing is now supported by the constitutional order. The so-called *Grundnorm* of the South African Bill is apparently that of equality. This right is confirmed at least three times in the Bill.

As far as the basic principles are concerned, there is no problem, but their formulation in the Bill lacks some clarity. The right to life, for example, receives unqualified protection. Section 11 reads: 'Everyone has the right to life.' Unlike the bills of rights of other countries, our Bill makes no provision for exceptions. Subjects such as capital punishment, abortion and euthanasia are directly affected. The Constitutional and other High Court decisions have already provided clarity in some of these problematic cases.

In S *v Makwanyane* 1995 3 SA 391 (CC) the death penalty was declared unconstitutional as it conflicts with the right to life and can no longer be imposed or carried out.

The constitutionality of the main features of the Choice of Termination of Pregnancy Act (92 of 1996) was confirmed in *Christian Lawyers Association of South Africa v Minister of Health* 1998 4 SA 1113 (T). The High Court found that a foetus cannot be a bearer of the right to life, because a foetus does not form part of 'everyone' (as used in s 11 of the Constitution).

Draft legislation on euthanasia has been tabled, but not passed. Both future and present legislation will be measured against the Bill of Rights. Legislation by Parliament is therefore no longer unassailable.

The Bill operates primarily between the individual and the state. This is known as the **vertical** application of the Bill: the individual in relation to the government. Fundamental rights have full vertical application (section 8(1)). The citizens of the country are protected by them against legislative, executive and administrative acts by the state (at all levels of government) that violate their basic human rights. The policy, rules and conduct of the staff of a state or provincial hospital therefore fall directly under the Bill.

Horizontal application means that an individual may enforce these rights directly against another person. Section 8(2) states that natural persons and juristic persons (that is non-state entities) are bound by the Bill of Rights to the extent that is applicable for them to be bound by it. In deciding whether this is the case, a court must take into account the nature of the right, the nature of the duty imposed by the right, the nature of the private conduct in question and the circumstances of the particular case. The right to citizenship (s 20) is, for example, not of such a nature that it can be applied between individuals. But the right to equality (s 9) is: If the owner of a private hospital decides that a person of a certain race is not allowed in the hospital, such a person may enforce his constitutional right to equality against the hospital owner. A court will find that the right has full horizontal application and that the hospital owner's conduct was unconstitutional in that he violated the person's right not to be discriminated against unfairly. The formulation of section 9(4) indicates that the right not to be unfairly discriminated against will always apply to private conduct.

The right of access to health-care services (section 27(1) and (2)) probably does not apply horizontally. Since the conduct of private persons/entities has to be funded from their own pockets, the same duties may not be imposed on them as can be imposed on an organ of state which relies on public funds. Unlike a state hospital, a private hospital cannot be saddled with the duty to provide every child with basic health-care services (section 28(1)(c)) and provide everybody with access to health care.

However, the right not to be refused emergency medical treatment (section 27(3)) probably does apply horizontally. This section reads: 'No one may be refused emergency medical treatment.' What this section requires is that remedial treatment that is necessary and available be given immediately to avert the harm. The right does not extend to routine medical treatment and it does not guarantee free services. Emergency treatment may not be refused because of lack of funds, but payment for treatment may be sought after treatment has been provided.

The state's duty under section 27(3) is 'not to refuse ambulance or other emergency services which are available and not to turn a person away from a hospital which is able to provide the necessary treatment'. This available-and-able qualification makes it clear that section 27(3) does not create a positive constitutional obligation on the state to ensure that emergency medical facilities are made available so that no one in an emergency situation can be turned away.

In *Soobramoney v Minister of Health, KwaZulu-Natal* 1998 1 SA 765 (CC) the court held that the situation of a person suffering from chronic renal failure and requiring dialysis two to three times a week to remain alive was not an emergency demanding immediate remedial treatment. Instead it was an ongoing state of affairs resulting from an incurable deterioration of the applicant's renal function. Accordingly, section 27(3) did not give such a person a right to be admitted to the dialysis program at a state hospital. The court was concerned that a decision to the contrary would have the consequence of prioritising the treatment of terminal illnesses above other forms of treatment, including primary health care. The court did not rule out interfering with 'rational decisions taken in good faith by political organs and medical authorities' but would 'be slow' to interfere.

Section 28 of the Bill affords every child (under the age of 18) the right to, *inter alia*, basic health and social services. Basic health care is defined as follows by the World Health Organization (WHO): 'Primary health care is essential health care based on practical, scientifically sound and socially acceptable methods and technology made universally accessible to individuals and families in the community through their full participation and at a cost that the community and the country can afford to maintain at every stage of their development in the spirit of self-reliance and self determination. It forms an integral part both of the country's health system of which it is the central function and main focus, and of the overall social and economic development of the community. It is the first level of contact of individuals, the family and community with the national health system bringing health care as close as possible to where people live and work and constitutes the first element of a continuing health-care process' (1978 Declaration of Alma-Ata.)

In the Bill, no further reference is made to health services or the right to them. The policy document of the African National Congress (drafted with technical assistance from the World Health Organization and the United Nations Children's Fund (UNICEF)) was published in May 1994 and provides more details about a national health plan for South Africa. Free health care would be provided in the public sector to, *inter alia*, children under the age of six, pregnant women, the aged, the handicapped and certain categories of the chronically ill. The health plan as a whole integrated with the Government's then Reconstruction and Development Plan (RDP).

The National Health Act, 61 of 2003, presently also serves as a policy document. This Act came partially into operation on 2 May 2005.

Remedy in the case of violation of human rights

If for example an individual feels that an organ of state is violating his human rights, his legal representative will institute legal proceedings against the state in the High Court. The High Court is competent to adjudicate on all alleged violations of human rights, with the exception of those instances in which the violation is contained in an Act of Parliament. The High Court can therefore also rule on provincial legislation. If the litigant does not obtain satisfaction in the High Court, he may lodge an appeal with the Constitutional Court. Moreover, only the Constitutional Court is competent to rule on parliamentary legislation. Draft legislation is at present being prepared which will extend the jurisdiction of the courts, and the possibility exists that even magistrates' courts will in future also be able to adjudicate on certain unconstitutional conduct (thereby establishing a far less expensive process).

Litigation costs money. Various institutions currently provide legal assistance to underprivileged persons in deserving cases. The institutions that may be approached for assistance are Lawyers for Human Rights, the Legal Resources Centre, the Legal Aid Board and the Human Rights Commission.

Legal liability of the nurse

If one were to ask a group of nurses who the most important person in their profession was, they would probably reply in unison: 'the patient'. From a legal perspective, nurses should place themselves directly alongside the patient. The scope of nursing care and knowledge is expanding, specialist disciplines are emerging and more skills are required. Amid the hotchpotch of claims, obligations and increasing responsibility, the possibility of legal liability is rapidly increasing. If each nurse does not look after her own position, no one else will do so for her. A basic knowledge of those legal principles affecting the nursing profession is therefore indispensable to every nurse.

Legal liability

Briefly, the term legal liability means that the perpetrator must bear the punishment for his act or compensate the aggrieved party. To incur private law or criminal liability, certain requirements must be met:

- A nurse must have **acted** illegally and, therefore, not have been in a state of automatism as, for example, a sleep-walker is. In practice this requirement usually does not pose a problem. An act may consist of an act (commission) or an omission. (Compare, for example, section 35 of the Nursing Act, 1978 (Act 50 of 1978).)
- It must be proved that it was a nurse's conduct that **caused** the harmful consequence, which is sometimes problematic. It may, for example, be very difficult – but not impossible – in a case of alleged cross-infection to prove that it was in fact the negligent conduct of the nurse, and not other factors, that caused the infection.
- The conduct must be **wrongful/unlawful**, and therefore unreasonable in the eyes of society.
- **Culpability, intention** or **negligence** must also be present. Virtually all the court cases in which nurses are involved, deal with the question of culpability and, more specifically, with whether the nurse was negligent. This aspect will be discussed in greater detail later.
- For private-law liability and for consequential crimes, there must also be **damage** or **prejudice**. If for example a nurse gave a patient the wrong medication but he did not take it, no damage and therefore no liability would arise. The South African Nursing Council could, however, find a nurse guilty of unprofessional conduct in such a case.
- Lastly, a nurse must also be **culpable**. There must be no doubt that the perpetrator possesses the necessary mental capacity to distinguish between right and wrong and to act in accordance with this insight.

Classification of the law

South African law is only partially codified. This means that certain legal rules are contained in laws but certain unwritten rules apply also.

The portion of our law that is codified is referred to as **statutory law**. This law has been included in Acts (statutes) and established by the legislature.

The unwritten legal rules come from **common law**, which for the most part arose from custom and has been conveyed from generation to generation since the earliest times. For example, no written legal rule exists which provides that one may not kill another, and yet such an act is unlawful and punishable.

Both common law and statutory law may be divided into three groups, namely **private law**, **public law** and **formal law**. **Formal law** largely has to do with the procedure in terms of which lawsuits are instituted and disposed of and therefore does not require further discussion at present. The distinction between private law and public law relates to the type of liability that the nurse may incur.

Public law is that part of the law in which the authorities act towards the subject in a relationship of authority. Public law is chiefly directed at the protection of the public interest. The state takes the initiative in instituting a criminal case. Should a nurse therefore have **negligently** caused the death of a person, a charge of **culpable homicide** could ensue. Although it seldom happens, crimes based on **intentional** conduct have arisen from nursing practice. Examples of these are **murder** (the unlawful and intentional causing of the death of another person – usually as a result of the application of euthanasia), **assault** (the unlawful and intentional infliction of harm upon another – where, for example, awkward and ill-mannered patients sustain injuries as a result of deliberately rough treatment) and *crimen* *iniuria* (where the nurse offends the dignity of the patient by, for example, revealing intimate details to outsiders or through unnecessary sexual handling).

In the case of intentional crimes it must be proved that the nurse performed the act **knowing** that it was wrong and nevertheless **willing** it (hence the term 'wilfully and knowingly').

Nurses can also be charged as accomplices where, for example, they assist a doctor whilst being aware of the fact that he is committing a crime. Where a nurse cannot withdraw without harming the patient's health, the criminal conduct should be reported to her senior as soon afterwards as possible.

If a nurse is found guilty of the commission of a crime, an appropriate punishment is meted out, either in the form of a fine or a prison sentence, or both. Community service under supervision is also considered as a sentencing option.

Criminal liability does not normally involve financial advantage to the individual (as complainant) for his violated interests. **Private law, or civil liability**, is at issue when the aggrieved party must be compensated. This type of liability is most prevalent. One and the same act may lead to both criminal and civil liability. The court record in the criminal case may be introduced as evidence in a civil case in which damages or satisfaction are claimed from the nurse or her employer.

Private law therefore regulates the relationships between individuals and protects private interests. When a nurse has, for example, negligently (or intentionally) caused the death of a breadwinner, his/her dependants may institute a claim against the nurse (or her employer) in terms of private law for loss of maintenance.

In other instances the patient may even claim for, *inter alia*, his/her increased medical expenses, pain and suffering, disfigurement and reduced life expectancy.

A nurse's employer (for example, the province or owner of a private hospital) may be held vicariously liable for her conduct if the act is performed in the course of her duty. Civil claims could total enormous amounts and it would therefore be better for the aggrieved party to act against the employer. The employer may, in turn, recover his damages from the nurse, but this is not customary at provincial or state hospitals.

Professional and ethical liability of nurses

In addition to legal liability, the South African Nursing Council can also take action against unethical or unprofessional conduct on the part of a nurse.

The South African Nursing Council has set out a number of types of conduct which would be regarded as unprofessional or unethical conduct and against which the Council may take action. A nurse's name could be struck from the register, which would mean that she would no longer be allowed to practise the nursing profession. In the case of less serious offences a nurse is merely given a warning or reprimanded or suspended from nursing practice for a period of time. Note that the conduct of a nurse need not necessarily meet the requirements of civil liability (in a court). The Council could, for example, find a nurse guilty of unprofessional conduct if she gave a patient the wrong medication but he did not take it (and therefore no harm resulted).

Legal liability on the grounds of negligence

In South African law an objective test, namely the test of the **reasonable person**, is used to establish negligence. In *Kruger* v *Coetzee* the Appellate Division gave this authoritative formulation:

(a) would the reasonable person in the position of the perpetrator –
  (i) have foreseen the possibility of damage; and
  (ii) have taken steps to prevent such damage;
(b) did the perpetrator's conduct deviate from the above-mentioned standard? If so, the offender was negligent. If not, the offender is not culpable.

The reasonable person is not a physical person, but a fictitious being which the law has fabricated to establish a workable norm. The reasonable person comprises all those characteristics which society requires of its members in their conduct towards one another. The reasonable person is an average person, not exceptionally gifted or over-cautious, but neither would he/she take reckless chances or fail to display discretion.

Where the conduct of an expert has to be evaluated, the test of the reasonable person is adapted and one works with the standard of a **reasonable expert** in that specific field. The test would therefore be that of the **reasonable nurse**, the reasonable doctor or the reasonable electrician, for example. It is only reasonable, where an expert performs an activity, to expect a higher degree of skill, caution and care than would otherwise be the case, in order not to be negligent. Who would undergo a brain operation if they knew that the skill and care of the surgeon were measured against those of the average person in the street?

■ The measure of expertise is described as 'reasonable'. A nurse is not expected to possess the highest possible measure of expertise existing in the profession. As early as 1924 the Appellate Division expressed it as follows in *Van Wyk v Lewis*: 'In deciding what is reasonable the Court will have regard to the general level of skill and diligence possessed and exercised at the time by the members of the branch of the profession to which the practitioner belongs.'

■ Furthermore, greater care and expertise are required of a specialist than of an ordinary expert. A theatre sister would be measured against the standard of the 'reasonable theatre sister'.

■ The reasonable nurse is expected to keep abreast, to a reasonable extent, of developments and new knowledge in nursing.

■ A nurse would also be found negligent if she were to undertake a specialist activity knowing that she did not possess the necessary knowledge and skill. In accordance with the maxim *imperitia culpae adnumeratur,* ignorance is regarded as negligence. An example is when a sister from the ophthalmic ward works an extra night in the intensive care unit to earn overtime (knowing full well or at least foreseeing that she does not possess adequate knowledge and skill).

Nurses should guard against becoming involved in risky situations. In nursing practice staff shortages are frequently experienced and it may happen that a nurse is sent to another section to assist. If she does not possess the necessary knowledge or skill, she should inform her senior accordingly, otherwise it would appear as if she regarded herself as competent to perform the task. Should she nevertheless have to work there, and something goes wrong, it would be clear that she did so under protest and at the insistence of her senior. If the relevant skill and knowledge could in fact be expected of her in terms of her service contract, she must bring herself up to date in that respect without delay. A further example is that of a nurse working night duty in the theatre being persuaded by a doctor to assist with an operation at short notice. Should something go wrong, it would be a case of each one for himself and her ignorance would be regarded as negligence unless the circumstances could be regarded as an emergency situation.

■ Conduct in an emergency situation is evaluated differently. The test for negligence requires that the reasonable person (or reasonable expert) be placed **in the same circumstances as the perpetrator** to determine the norm of conduct. The reasonable person is not superhuman and the law therefore makes provision for errors of judgement in an emergency situation. There must, however, be no doubt that it is a reasonable error before the offender will emerge free of the reproach of negligence. In addition, a nurse may also undertake certain tasks in an emergency situation which would normally fall outside the scope of nursing practice, such as assisting with an operation. Should such a situation arise, the Nursing Council must be provided with a report on it as soon as possible.

It could not, however, be regarded as an emergency situation if a staff shortage regularly arose and circumstances demanded using a nurse without the necessary knowledge or skill. If a nurse without the necessary training were obliged to work in an intensive care unit on a regular basis and to perform tasks for which she did not have the necessary knowledge or skill, she should lodge an objection in writing. If there were no response to her objection, the correct procedure would be for the nurse to report the problem to the Nursing Council via her professional association (e.g. Denosa) and to send a copy of her letter to the chief executive officer of the institution. Were she simply to remain silent, it would be assumed that she approved of the situation and that she regarded herself as competent to perform the tasks.

■ There are circumstances that require greater care from nurses, such as when they work with things that are dangerous in themselves (for example certain medications or apparatus) or where they have to care for someone who suffers from some incapacity or disability (for example children, the aged, the blind, unconscious persons or persons having a clouded consciousness).

■ A nurse would not necessarily be able to rely on the fact that she merely carried out a doctor's request or instruction. If a reasonable nurse would have known that it was an erroneous request which could be detrimental to the patient, such a defence would not succeed. The reasonable nurse is, for example, considered to be familiar with the effect and recommended dosage of the medication she administers.

■ The importance of record-keeping cannot be overemphasised. Accurate and written records of patients' treatment are the first line of defence in any claim that may be instituted against nurses or their employers. Claims are often instituted only months and even years after the treatment complained of, when no one is able to attest with certainty to its precise details. However, when it can be proved that notes of the treatment were made on the patient card shortly after the application of such treatment, and that notes on patient cards are in general accurate and complete, this would facilitate the case of nurses and their employers considerably. The only exception is when it is clear from the notes that the wrong treatment was applied!

■ It is apparent from court cases that nurses often come off second-best in comparison with doctors when they find themselves in the same situation and negligence is at issue. The nurse should always act as the reasonable nurse and never rely on the assumption that she could depend on the doctor. Should something go wrong, it would be a case of each one for himself. *Administrator of the Orange Free State v Soumbasis*, a 1992 Appellate Division judgment, provides a good illustration of this matter.

In this case a seventeen-year-old boy broke his leg in a soccer match. An orthopaedic surgeon performed a reduction and put the leg in a plaster cast. A necrotic condition of the muscles and tissue in the lower leg led to the leg having to be amputated below the knee some three and a half months later. The necrosis was caused by the development of a so-called compartment syndrome. The restriction of blood supply was not relieved quickly enough and irreversible tissue damage resulted.

The surgeon and the provincial administration (as employer of the nurse concerned) were sued for damages. It was contended that the surgeon had been negligent in that he had allegedly failed to examine the patient after the operation before granting permission for his discharge, and had also negligently failed to inform the patient of the possible dangers and danger signals. On evidence it was found that the surgeon had acted as the reasonable surgeon in relation to the post-operative care, and he got off scot-free. The court found, however, that the nursing staff had been negligent. The nurse had failed to warn the patient when it had become clear to her that the doctor had not warned the patient or that the patient had not been aware of his warning. The court furthermore found that she had been particularly negligent in not letting the surgeon know about the change in the patient's condition or about his complaints. The nurse had been dealing with him from the time she came on duty in the morning until he was discharged at 12h00. She could not even recall that he had been in her ward and upon giving evidence in the trial court (six years later) she simply had to rely on the scant notes that had been made in the file. She admitted that the patient could possibly have complained of pain but that this had not been of such a nature as to cause warning lights to flash for the reasonable nurse. The Appellate Division found that the reasonable nurse would have ensured that the patient was not discharged from the hospital before his complaints had been conveyed to the surgeon and he had responded to them.

Concluding remarks

If a nurse does not wish to incur legal liability, it is as well to remember the following basic principle:

It is better to ask many questions beforehand than to have to reply to many questions (in court) afterwards.

Critical thinking activities
1. What is a bill of rights?
2. Identify the most important types of human rights.
3. How does the South African Bill affect the nursing profession?
4. What is the distinction between the vertical and horizontal application of the Bill?
5. Explain the content of a person's right not to be refused emergency medical treatment.
6. What remedy does a person have if his human rights are violated?
7. What are the requirements for legal liability?
8. Distinguish between legal liability and professional liability.
9. Distinguish between private law and public law liability.

9. What is the test for negligence?
10. How does the normal test for negligence differ from the test in the case of negligent conduct by nurses?
11. Explain the operation of the maxim *imperitia culpae adnumeratur* in nursing practice.
12. What influence does an emergency situation have on the test for negligence?
13. What is the importance of accurate record-keeping?
14. What explanation would you give to a junior colleague in answer to the question of whether it is always safe to simply respond to a doctor's instructions?

Ethical concerns in relationships between nurses, patients, family members and members of the health-care team

Anne-Mart Oosthuizen

Outcomes

Studying this chapter will enable you to:

- highlight a number of factors that contribute towards the development of the nurse-patient relationship
- discuss the importance of mutual trust in the nurse-patient relationship
- identify factors that have a negative influence on the nurse-patient relationship
- give at least two reasons why it is important for nurses to have a good relationship with the family of patients
- describe the factors that could affect relationships between nurses, doctors and other health-care professionals.

Introduction

The nurse-patient relationship and the nurse-doctor relationship have undergone tremendous changes during recent years. At first nurses were prescribed to in an authoritarian manner about how patients should be handled. Prior to 1950 the nurse's role was primarily to render physical care on the instructions of the doctor. The focus of the profession was not social intervention. Nevertheless, the interpersonal component of nursing was recognised by some nurses. As early as 1938 the nurse was described as the link between the doctor and the patient (Ramos 1992:496). Blue and Fitzgerald (2002:314) maintain that although there are still authoritarian elements in the nurse-doctor relationship, nurses have developed their own disciplinary knowledge, based on notions of care rather than medical cure.

The relationship between nurses and patients: the basis of nursing

Technological development, specialisation in nursing and medicine, and the disproportional distribution of health personnel are factors which contribute to a reduction in personal nursing and health care. Castledine (2004:231) argues that the nurse-patient relationship is threatened by the ever-demanding technical skills that nurses are expected to master. The nurse-patient relationship forms the basis of nursing. It is an intimate and trusting relationship that often extends to the family of the patient. In this relationship nurses are committed to caring for patients and their families. This care may involve long hours with the patient and their families during periods of intense vulnerability (Haynes, Boese & Butcher 2004:111). It is a dynamic relationship in which the humanity of both the patient and the nurse plays a role. The nature of a nurse-patient relationship is determined by the needs of the patient and the nurse's response to these needs. Because it is dynamic, it changes continually (Curtin & Flaherty 1982:87).

Throughout the history of nursing, the image of the nurse-patient relationship has formed the basis of attempts to understand the nature of nursing. Without the central characters of the patient and the nurse, nursing cannot exist. Nurses perform the roles of patient advocate, nurturer, adviser, educator and co-ordinator of services.

Not all patients respond in the same way to illness or injury and the degree of dependence on the nurse varies. The nurse's task of co-ordinating and managing care gives her the opportunity to be in continual close contact with her patients. Nurses are the people who spend the greatest amount of time with individual patients and who therefore establish deeper relationships with patients than other members of the health-care team. Tschudin (1999:16) maintains that 'nurses could be the key to positive patient outcomes'. The author cites Vaughan (1996) who found that these outcomes are not the result of good management, enough resources or a stable environment, but of human contact – a caring relationship between nurse and patient.

Rights and duties in nurse-patient relationships

In nurse-patient relationships, legal and ethical rights and obligations are at issue. A legal obligation arises when a contract is entered into between a nurse and a patient or between a nurse and a health service. An ethical obligation, on the other hand, arises in the nurse's relationship with the patient, the hospital, other health-care workers and even the patient's family (Thompson & Thompson 1990:10-11).

A nurse can play a key role in creating a climate in which the rights and needs of patients are recognised and respected. As advocate for the patient, a nurse can make decisions to protect the rights of patients. Patients are often defenceless and nurses can, on the basis of their knowledge and experience, support and assist patients in making decisions.

It is an unfortunate fact that often patients feel obliged to subject themselves to what the health team prescribes because they are not aware of their rights, or because they are not in a position to express their needs. Patient advocacy is an essential nursing function and nurses are in an excellent position to act as advocates for patients to ensure that their rights are recognised and protected.

The importance of the nurse-patient relationship

Castledine (2004:231) maintains that the nurse-patient relationship is important for ten reasons, namely to:
- help patients make decisions
- avoid isolating and dehumanising patients
- act as an advocate for vulnerable patients

- nurture co-operation and understanding
- help in patient assessment and problem-solving
- help patients cope with their problems
- help patients undertake, or carry out for them, activities of living and human needs
- nurse dying patients and those with terminal illnesses
- teach and promote health education
- learn about new ways of nursing and caring for people in a changing world.

Development of the nurse-patient relationship

Questions often arise about the development of relationships with patients. These patients are people in relation to whom a nurse will have the normal range of human feelings. However, in the socialisation process, the emphasis is always on professional conduct.

A nurse's feelings towards specific people can cause problems and conflicts. It is accepted that, in the daily course of events, a nurse will meet people whom she likes or dislikes, or for whom she does not have any particular feeling. After all, there are many types of people on earth and the same variety of people appears in the nursing situation. It goes without saying that nurses cannot be forced to like everyone and may experience natural feelings of preference or dislike for particular patients. Because this can have both good and bad consequences, nurses are warned not to become too involved with patients.

Because patients should feel that they can trust nurses with private and personal information, it is clear that the relationship between the patient and the nurse is of the utmost importance. A relationship of trust is non-judgemental, warm, sincere and empathetic. If one person in the relationship is sincere and warm, there is potential for the other to be the same. The human dignity of each is recognised and confirmed, and this forms the basis of care and physical and emotional health. It is in the interests of both parties to have good relations (Tschudin 1993:7).

Nurses enter into relationships with patients in order to fulfil their professional responsibilities. Both patient and nurse bring a variety of personal values, beliefs and moral points of view to their relationship (Thompson & Thompson 1992:75-76). However, a nurse has a commitment to the patient which extends beyond her own personal feelings and moral points of view. She must know what values and beliefs the patient and his family subscribe to in order to respect them.

Factors that contribute towards the development of a nurse-patient relationship

Therapeutic reciprocity

Therapeutic reciprocity is a mutual exchange of feelings and ideas between nurse and patient with the aim of strengthening the outcome of the relationship. There are, however, certain environmental factors which can have a negative influence on therapeutic reciprocity, factors such as noise, lack of privacy or time, and language and cultural differences. An attempt should be made to eliminate these interfering factors as far as possible to encourage meaningful interaction between nurse and patient. It is part of a nurse's skill in the establishment of therapeutic reciprocity to rise above environmental factors which may hamper a relationship.

According to Marck (1990:49-57), the results of therapeutic reciprocity are positive. Nurse and patient share responsibility for and control over the outcome of their relationship.

Mutual respect for values and beliefs in nurse-patient relationships

Nurses enter into relationships with patients in order to provide nursing care whenever it is desired. Depending on the nature of the nurse-patient relationship, a nurse's values and the integration of these values into daily nursing practice influence the quality of the care. Where nurse and patient do not share the same values and beliefs, the relationship can be seriously threatened. The code of ethics for nurses defines, *inter alia*, the principle of respect for a patient's human dignity and uniqueness. This implies that nurses should be familiar with the beliefs and values of their patients. What is important is that nurses and patients do not try to impose their values upon one another. Respect for the values of patients, whether or not nurses share them, is essential (Tadd 1998:6-9). Respect for others transcends cultural differences, gender issues, religious differences and racial concerns (Guido 2001:56).

Mutual trust in nurse-patient relationships

In a relationship where one person depends on another person for competent, quality nursing care, trust is essential. Nursing is a caring profession (Haynes *et al* 2004:363) and caring implies maintaining communication and ensuring that trust is established. This means allowing patients to make decisions for themselves and trusting those decisions. Mutual trust, as opposed to unilateral or one-sided trust, should not be underestimated.

It is clear that trust forms the basis of successful and effective health-care relationships. If a patient wishes to derive maximum benefit from nursing care, it is not only essential that the patient trust the nurse, but also that this trust be cultivated and nurtured through the nurse's trust in the patient. Haynes *et al* (2004:111) maintain that the intimate, trusting relationship that exists between a nurse and a patient serves as the core for ethical decision-making.

Negotiation in the nurse-patient relationship

The importance of a nurse-patient relationship in which the patient is involved in decision-making relating to his care is endorsed in nursing literature. In the past, most health care followed the 'medical model' which advocated domination by the professional providers of care. Patients were regarded as passive recipients of care and decisions relating to health and illness were the domain of the doctor. It would be naïve to believe that this idea has disappeared entirely. It holds serious ethical implications for nurse-patient relationships if the consumers of health care cannot exercise choice and express opinions on the care which they are receiving. Nurses should never lose sight of the fact that patients are 'consumers' and should be actively involved in their health care. Thus the idea of a partnership between nurses and patients plays a key role in nursing today. Within this partnership nurse and patient share responsibility for decision-making (Trnobranski 1994:733-737).

Accountability within nurse-patient relationships

A nurse has elected to nurse, and therefore accepts the responsibilities associated with nursing practice and, accordingly, develops a set of professional obligations and values. A nurse must be accountable for her conduct. Health-care consumers nowadays are more informed and expect expert care in all facets of the health-care system. To a greater extent than ever before, patients and their families are holding nurses accountable for rendering effective, safe and ethical health care (Searle 2000:175; Snowdon & Rajacich 1993:7).

Relationships with difficult and unpopular patients

People see nurses as caring, compassionate and nurturing professionals. The public expects nurses to be there for the vulnerable and sick 24 hours a day, and to care for them unconditionally. There are, however, some patients who are less likeable than others and are, therefore, difficult to care for.

Issues such as race, religion and economic status can affect the caring relationship. Problematic factors include situations in which there is too great a like-mindedness between nurse and patient, where the patient's conduct is unacceptable to the nurse, or where the patient himself is guilty or can be held responsible for the condition in which he finds himself. Potentially vulnerable patients are smokers with lung cancer, drug addicts, alcoholics, patients who have contracted AIDS through high-risk behaviour, patients who do not co-operate, patients who have attempted suicide or patients who use violence (Olsen 1993:1696-1699). Difficult patients (Duxbury 2000:5) are those who make nurses feel uncomfortable, frustrated or ineffective.

Unpopularity impacts seriously on nurse-patient relationships. Both patient and nurse are likely to suffer harm in such a relationship. A nurse who often has to care for difficult and unpopular patients may experience job dissatisfaction and frustration, which could ultimately lead to her leaving the profession. Another possibility is that a nurse may have problems dealing with her personal feelings and consequently feel antagonistic towards an unpopular patient. She may even feel that her time can be put to better use by caring for other patients instead. According to Kus (in McCloskey & Grace (1990:554)) this hostility may find expression in many ways, such as ignoring call signals or being cool and detached instead of warm and sensitive towards the patient. Unpopular patients are at risk of not having their psychological or physical needs met. Patients are vulnerable. Duxbury (2000:20) maintains that the best way of ensuring that the needs of the difficult patient are met is to focus on the positive challenge facing the nurse and the difference he or she can make. To view patients solely in a negative light can only do harm and perpetuate the 'difficult patient syndrome'. Instead, the nurse must try to put subjectivity aside and recognise that the patient may be experiencing a degree of distress such as fear, anxiety, uncertainty, frustration, anger or ignorance, and objectively try to intervene by addressing the underlying distress.

Relationships with patients from culture groups that differ from that of the nurse

Every nurse must sometimes nurse a patient who belongs to an ethnic or religious group that differs from her own. A nurse who is not aware of the influence cultural differences can have on the nurse-patient relationship can deprive a patient of the therapeutic value of a caring nurse-patient relationship. According to Bonaparte (in Murphy 1993:449) the potential therapeutic relationship between nurse and patient can be adversely affected if the nurse is ethnocentric. Ethnocentrism of the cultural mainstream affords support, status and security to members of the group but sometimes results in the stereotyping and stigmatisation of non-members (Germain 1992:2). Mistrust and prejudice make a caring nurse-patient relationship impossible (Oosthuizen 2002:12).

A nurse who renders nursing care across cultural boundaries should be mindful of communication differences (verbal and non-verbal), differences in values and beliefs, and differences in dealing with sickness and death. Hospital rules do not always provide for the cultural customs and conventions of specific groups and therefore a greater measure of sensitivity and flexibility is demanded of nurses. An ethical obligation therefore rests on nurses to provide patients with culturally acceptable care (Oosthuizen 2002:12).

Relationships between nurses and families of patients

The principles of nurse-patient relationships reside in various other interpersonal relationships which affect the dignity of patients. A holistic approach to nursing must include the patient's family. Anyone who is a significant part of the patient's normal lifestyle is considered a family member (Hudak, Gallo & Morton 1998:21). Very often a patient experiences primarily a biological crisis whereas the rest of the family experiences an emotional crisis. By expanding the concept of patient to include the family, the patient's total well-being will be enhanced.

There are at least two reasons for devoting attention to patients' families. Firstly, families make a valuable contribution towards the life experience of each member of the family. Secondly, some health problems can have an adverse affect on the family's ability to function (Curtin & Flaherty 1982:108).

Families are valuable resources. They can provide information that has a bearing on a patient's situation. The family also often has access to many resources which can directly influence the patient's recovery or adjustment to a particular health crisis. It is a fact, however, that the family often requires assistance to recognise the resources it has and to utilise them to the maximum degree. Although the nurse can assist the family to mobilise its resources, this does not imply that she accepts responsibility for obligations which are really those of the patient or family.

The stages in the relationship between nurses and family members

Oermann (1997:105) describes family relationships with health-care professionals, based on a study by Thorne and Robinson (1988), as an evolving three-stage process. The first stage is naïve trusting, which refers to family members' trusting that the nurse and all other health care professionals will act in the sick member's best interests. If discrepancies arise between family members' views and the nurse's view about the best interests of the patient, family members realise that their trust was founded on naïve assumptions. The second phase, the disenchantment phase, is characterised by dissatisfaction with care, leading to frustration and fear. Families view the sick member as vulnerable and in need of protection and wish that they could be involved in his/her care. The third phase is guarded alliance, where families renegotiate trust with health-care professionals. In this phase families actively seek the information they need, demonstrate understanding of the differences in perspective, state their own perspective and expectations more clearly, and negotiate towards mutually satisfying care. It is said that even though families have reached the third stage in the relationship they often do still experience the frustration of waiting, the fear of not knowing and the anger when they realise that their own expertise is devalued.

The nature of the nurse-family relationship

A nurse-family relationship arises when a nurse recognises the family's need for support. Often it is the needs of only one family member that give rise to the development of a relationship between the nurse and the family. Nurse-family relationships are more complex than nurse-patient relationships because they include person-to-person relationships with at least two members of a family, and often many more.

The nature of a nurse-family relationship is determined by the relevant health problem. Where patients are hospitalised for an acute illness, the nurse-family relationship is often linked to the nurse-patient relationship. The relationship between the nurse and the family becomes far more important, however, if the health problem is of a long-term nature, or of an irreversible nature, both of which require difficult decisions that affect the patient's quality of life.

Factors that affect nurse-family relationships

Although nurse-family relationships are affected by the relevant health problem, this is not the only factor that affects the relationship. The relationship is affected by the place in which it develops. In other words, a nurse-patient relationship in the case of a hospitalised patient would differ from a relationship where the nurse visits the patient at home and other members of the family are included in the relationship. Another factor that may affect a nurse-family relationship is the quality of interdisciplinary work relations. A spirit of co-operation between doctors and nurses ensures the flow of information to the patient and the family, whereas a lack of co-operation may result in confusion and obstruct the primary objectives of care. Family problems may also affect a nurse-family relationship and it goes without saying that a family with many problems poses a greater challenge to the nurse than a family with few problems. The type of assistance rendered by the nurse also affects a relationship, be it direct physical care, instruction in health matters and self-care, or guidance in the use of available community services (Curtin & Flaherty 1982:103-121).

Regardless of the form of the nurse-family relationship, a nurse may not forget her role in establishing a supportive environment for the patient and his/her family. A nurse will have to use her discretion and decide what the family requires – sometimes merely emotional support and sometimes far more. The demands made by such relationships are very great, but the potential rewards are even greater. As relationships grow, the patient, the family and the nurse grow and develop.

Relationships between nurses

The ethical principles involved in keeping promises, telling the truth and respecting people as individuals apply as much to the members of the health- care team as they do to patients. The attitudes people have towards their work are influenced by the quality of their relationships with their colleagues (Tadd 1998:127). Nurses have professional relationships with one another which include certain responsibilities such as co-operation, self-development and support. They belong to the same profession and identify with their peer group. Nurses are part of the health-care team and they contribute towards the nursing profession and, therefore, they work with their colleagues towards the realisation of defined goals, namely to promote the welfare of the public (Curtin & Flaherty 1982:125-128, 131-132).

In their relationship with one another, nurses respect one another's knowledge, experience and rights. Rights include friendliness, compassion and sympathy as well as a nurse's right to use her abilities, to express her feelings and to be recompensed in a fair manner. By applying this rule nurses will have respect for one another because they are compassionate, sympathetic, competent, accountable and responsible. They respect one another's rights and have an obligation to promote the welfare of the public (Thompson & Thompson 1990: 125; Searle 2000:144). Nurses live in a multicultural society and should be aware of cultural differences. Today's health-care team is culturally diverse and some factors that influence relationships are cultural. Respect for one another's culture and acceptance of differences that might exist between nurses with different cultural backgrounds will promote positive relationships.

Factors that affect relationships between nurses

Problems are sometimes experienced in relationships between nurses. Spengler (in Pence & Cantrall 1990:116) has identified certain problem areas in relationships between nurses:

- lack of group co-operation
- forming of groups
- pressure applied by peers to adhere to traditional behaviour
- fear of success
- lack of support for other colleagues in their efforts to achieve.

Typical problems in relationships between nurses are rooted in poor professional ties, for example by keeping quiet about errors made by other nurses. Other problem areas that have been identified are favouritism and an absence of support and co-operation. Whenever positive professional relationships are poor or absent, both the nurse and the profession will suffer (Pence & Cantrall 1990:261, 265).

As a solution to potential problems in relationships between nurses, Trandel-Korenchuk and Trandel-Korenchuk (in Pence & Cantrall 1990:116) propose that nurses should develop a sense of self-love and respect. By doing so, nurses will learn to admire, appreciate, trust and respect their colleagues.

Nurses should develop a professional identity, with a sense of duty and responsibility towards their work and towards one another. Nurses should achieve higher academic qualifications and foster the value of achievement among student nurses. Professional relationships between nurses should be based, first and foremost, on respect for one another's rights. Nurses should avoid situations which endanger these rights. The best way in which the quality of nursing can be improved is for nurses to offer one another the necessary co-operation, guidance and criticism. Withholding support leads to loss of trust, not only on the part of colleagues, but also on the part of patients, because it reduces the quality of nursing care (Curtin & Flaherty in Pence & Cantrall 1990:258, 264). In order to prevent poor professional relationships, nurse educators and leaders should ensure that professional relationships are encouraged and maintained.

Nurses can enhance professional relationships by supporting one another's efforts to deliver quality nursing-care and working collaboratively with nursing administration. They should affirm the nursing strengths of others, and constructively address nursing deficiencies (Taylor, Lillis & LeMone 2001:291). Mutual respect is essential in the relationship between nurses.

Relationships between nurses and other members of the health-care team

Health care is complex and demands the skills of a variety of professional health workers. It is important that all members of the health-care team work together to enhance the well-being of the patients in their care. Nurses (Taylor, Lillis & LeMone 2001:291) have to co-ordinate the inputs of members of the multidisciplinary team and serve as a liaison between the patient and family and the health-care team. Northouse (in Oermann (1997:152) maintains there are three interdependent factors that promote effective relationships among members of the health-care team. In order to understand the roles of other members of the health-care team it is necessary to clarify the roles of each member of the team. Misunderstandings and under-utilisation of every member's unique expertise can then be prevented. Equally important is the process of sharing control in which health-care professionals attempt to have a mutual influence without one group dominating the other. By frequently communicating with doctors and other members of the health-care team, effective inter-professional relationships are promoted.

Relationships between nurses and doctors

It is generally accepted that nurses and doctors have a common goal, namely the health and well-being of the patients in their care. They co-ordinate their contributions to health care, provide information and give recognition to one another and exchange knowledge where necessary. Each has an ethical responsibility towards the other to protect their professional reputation (Searle 2000:207).

Blue and Fitzgerald (2002:320) maintain that according to international research, nurse-doctor relationships have not yet reached their full potential in the sense that there continues to be mutual mistrust and a perceived dominance of medicine over nurses and nursing work. However, research conducted in the last decade of the 20th century reveals that nurses are less dependent on and subordinate to doctors. It was found that collaboration with doctors increased when nurses were both assertive and co-operative in their relationships.

The role-socialisation of nurses – that is, the socialisation of nursing students into the role of professional nurses – came about two decades ago through various nursing educational bodies (Jones 1994:38). Student nurses used to be taught how to act in relation to doctors; that doctors, for example, had more knowledge than they did and that they should therefore respect them. Nurses were told that they were important assistants to doctors in the treatment of patients and that they should help the doctors in every way possible (Stein in Pence & Cantrall 1990:162-163). The socialisation of doctors and nurses has occurred as a result of technology, consumer awareness and limited expenditure and has contributed to changes in the relationships between nurses and doctors. Nowadays nurses assert themselves and may be described as self-reliant, independent and accountable (Jones 1994:38-39).

Nursing training in the form of apprenticeship used to require minimum educational qualifications. In contrast, medical training could be obtained only through intensive and expensive university education (Trandel-Korenchuk & Trandel-Korenchuk in Pence & Cantrall 1990:113, 115). Today nursing students study at universities and autonomous colleges and enjoy proper student status. Early nursing schools attempted to recruit sophisticated women as student nurses but from their early days they attracted only working-class women. Today people who have successfully completed twelve years of school training are taken into consideration.

Over the years a well-known game of role-socialisation has developed in hospitals. This is known as the 'doctor-nurse game'. A hierarchy has developed with the doctor as the more dominant person. Doctors are taught to approach nurses from a position of superior knowledge. In this way the hierarchical class relationship between nursing and medicine is maintained (Baker & Diekelmann 1994:65). Both Stein and Trandel-Korenchuk and Trandel-Korenchuk (in Pence & Cantrall 1990:115) hold the view that the objective of the 'doctor-nurse game' is that the nurse appears self-assured and responsible while the authority of the doctor is supported and protected. The doctor possesses knowledge and is responsible for the treatment and prescription and controls all information about the diagnosis and treatment of the patient. At times nurses are given only limited information about their patients—the information the doctor wants nurses to know.

Recent studies (Snelgrove & Hughes 2000:661) indicate that the straightforward hierarchical relationship which underpinned the 'doctor-nurse game' no longer exists as the predominant form of interaction between doctors and nurses. These studies suggest that old stereotypes are being broken down, and that role boundaries are shifting to reflect such influences as work pressure, differences between clinical areas and the changing knowledge context of nursing. It is argued that doctor-nurse interactions are more diverse and situation-specific than those described in traditional models of doctor-nurse relations, which emphasised dominance and subordination.

Types of nurse-doctor relationships

There are various types of nurse-doctor relationships.

Collaborative relationships

According to Northouse (in Oermann 1997:154-155), collaborative relationships imply continuous interaction between health workers in which everyone participates in problem-solving. Collaboration distributes control and prevents one health worker from dominating another. Investigations have shown that there is better co-operation between nurses and doctors in primary care and critical-care units.

Collaboration is built on respect for the contributions of others. Professionals realise that expertise and input from a variety of health-care professionals are needed to solve the complex health-care problems confronting patients today (Northouse in Oermann 1997:155). Pike voices a similar view and says that collaboration displays trust and respect for others. She also says that collaboration forces nurses and doctors to share responsibility for patient care and that collaborative relationships precede reasonable, comprehensive, creative and humanistic care whenever a moral dilemma arises. Such relationships are difficult and there are various points of view on them. The objectives remain to increase patient satisfaction, to reduce resources and to shorten the period of hospitalisation (Pike 1991:352-353, 361).

Collegial relationships

Searle (2000:172) maintains that the relationship between a nurse and a doctor is a collegial one between two practitioners who share responsibility for the patient. Partnership between nurses and other health workers is, according to Northouse (in Oermann 1997:153), essential for good health care.

Trusting relationships

Caring and confidentiality are essential for trusting relationships. All parties to a relationship must trust one another. Genuine care encourages spontaneous trust and creates relationships which are based on open-handedness and mutual respect (Tschudin 1992:7). The mutual trust and respect which are present in collaborative relationships also help to develop cooperation.

Factors that affect relationships between nurses and doctors

Problems arise in interprofessional relationships when friction and misunderstandings occur among members at work. The 'difficult' doctor can negatively influence relationships and cause team members, frequently nurses, to feel hurt and alienated rather than respected members of the team. This can influence the outcomes of patient care. Maintaining positive relationships with a 'difficult' doctor presents a challenge to the nurse. Traditionally nurses have less difficulty with other health team members while many difficulties with doctors have been reported (Davidhizar & Dowd 2003:9). Although health workers co-operate closely with one another, they sometimes do not understand one another's roles. This creates problems as a result of demands made on one another (which may not be in accordance with a particular professional role) and consequent misuse of unique expertise (Northouse in Oermann 1997:1152). The relationship between doctors and nurses is often complicated by stressful situations and long years of prevailing stereotypes (Ashworth 2000:127). Better communication and the ability to handle conflict more effectively will result in better cooperation between doctors and nurses. Davidhizar and Dowd (2001:12) state that negative communication is one of the most destructive forces that can be present in the health-care team. By using positive communication techniques the nurse can enhance interpersonal interactions with the doctor.

Rapid changes in health care have brought new challenges to the nurse-doctor relationship. Ashworth (2000:128) maintains that many nurses now have relationships where there is mutual respect and recognition of one another's expertise even when disagreements based on different perspectives occur.

Concluding remarks

It is clear that nurse-patient-family relationships can be beneficial to all parties concerned. Where mutual trust and respect for values are present within a caring relationship, the nurse is no longer merely the benefactor but also a beneficiary, because both nurse and patient benefit from what the one learns or receives from the other. The nurse, doctor and other members of the health-care team are mutually dependent on one another. If they fulfil their responsibilities towards one another and work together as a team, this can only lead to healthy relationships and an excellent service can be rendered to humanity.

Critical thinking activities

1. Discuss ethical relationships among nurses.
2. Write notes on the following:
   - collaborative relationships
   - collegial relationships
   - trusting relationships.
3. Make a list of your personal feelings whenever you have to nurse a potentially vulnerable patient such as a smoker with lung cancer or a patient who has attempted suicide. Do you respect the dignity of the patient at all times?
4. Discuss the importance of mutual respect and trust in a nurse-patient relationship.
5. Explain the importance of collaborative relationships between nurses and other health-care professionals.

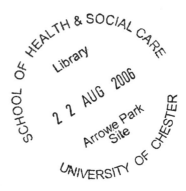

Ethical concerns in relationships between nurses, their employing authorities and trade unions

Nelouise Geyer & Thembi Mngomezulu

Outcomes

Studying this chapter will enable you to:

- describe the nature of contracts between nurses and their employers
- critically discuss the underlying ethic fairness and justice embodied in legislation
- describe working conditions for nurses in South Africa
- discuss the ethical conflict that can arise in a bureaucratic environment
- debate the role of unions in ensuring that justice prevails in labour practices in nursing
- debate the concept of essential services and how it impacts on nurses and health services.

Introduction

In South Africa the rights of health-care users have been widely discussed and well established – and formally included in the National Health Act (61 of 2003). **All South African citizens, including health-care professionals, have rights. Nurses, however, have to take into account their responsibilities and duties and the vulnerability of the people in their care. The challenge is clearly how the rights of the parties involved in the health-care situation should be balanced.**

Nurses in South Africa offer their services to employers in either private or public facilities. These facilities vary in scope and complexity, from corporate bureaucracies, such as large multi-purpose hospitals, to small clinics and doctors' surgeries.

The employment relationship is reciprocal. Employers, in this case health-care facilities, hire employees, including nurses, to provide a service on behalf of the employer. In the private sector the objectives include profit-making. Nurses, in turn, provide their labour in return for remuneration and the opportunity to exercise and improve their marketable skills. When parties conclude an employment contract they incur certain rights and obligations. The employer becomes entitled to the nurse's skilled labour who, in turn, is obliged to provide it. The nurse on the other hand, is entitled to remuneration and the employer is obliged to pay it. This employment relationship of course entails more than simply an exchange. It is a continuing relationship in which the parties interact as human beings. The nurse's entitlement to remuneration cannot be adequately provided for unless the employer provides an environment that is conducive to work and tools that allow the nurse to perform to the best of her/his ability.

Justice and legislation

The value that is enforced in legislation is fairness or justice. The underlying ethic is to treat other people the way they would want to be treated (Hall 2002:229). This principle applies to all persons, whether employee or employer. The further lawmakers stray from enforcing a minimum ethic, and the more the law is delegated to rule-makers to write the details, the harder it is for the employer or employee to anticipate the content of the statute. For example, from the knowledge that one should be fair to one's employees, one would not automatically predict that accident records must be kept, which is an Occupational Health and Safety Act (OHSA) requirement. But if one is fair to one's employees, one would make the workplace as safe as possible, which is a more important OHSA requirement. Technical violations of the law, such as violations of record-keeping, are far less serious than substantive violations, such as having dangerous conditions for workers. Violations of the right contained in sections 23 and 24 of the Constitution of the RSA, 1996 to just and favourable work conditions can lead to death and disability. Although there is detailed legislation in this regard, it is not properly enforced and, as a result, nurses and other health workers are not properly protected.

A variety of new laws to enshrine and protect the rights of all parties have been passed in the new South Africa. Some of the legislation makes provision for infrastructure to support the implementation of legal solutions, but many of these mechanisms still have to be put into place. The challenge for the young democracy in South Africa is to translate progressive pieces of legislation into practice for the benefit of its citizens.

Enforcing justice through legislation

The laws that enforce the ethical value of fairness include the law of due process and antidiscrimination and labour laws.

- Due process means appropriate procedure. Appropriate procedure must be followed before the state can take your life, freedom or property. This determination is written into section 33 of the Constitution of the Republic of SA and the execution of the section is provided for by the Promotion of Administrative Justice Act (Act 3 of 2000). Due process is important when the licensing capacity of the SA Nursing Council (SANC) is threatened. Licensing impacts on the professional's freedom to practice and has economic value, which is regarded as a property right. The professional's freedom and property are protected by the Constitution (sections 21, 22 and 25). Because of these determinations the SA Nursing Council cannot interfere with the professional's license, except by using due process or appropriate procedure, which is spelt out in the Nursing Act (Act 50 of 1978) and its regulations. Due process means, amongst other things, that the professional must be given notice of the charges levelled against him/her within a reasonable period to allow him/her to prepare and defend him/herself against the charges/allegations, and must be given a fair trial in terms of both procedure and substance.
- Antidiscrimination is enforced by section 9 of the Constitution as executed by the Promotion of Equality and Prevention of Unfair Discrimination Act (Act 4 of 2000) and the Employment Equity Act (Act 55 of 1998). These laws have specific determinations on the prevention of discrimination that is unfair, such as discrimination based on gender, age, disability, race and religion. It must be kept in mind that discrimination is not always bad or negative - we sometimes have to discriminate in favour of things that are good for

us or else we will indiscriminately choose things that are bad for us. Similarly it is not unethical to dismiss an employee who steals from or harms health-care users and other workers.

■ Labour laws enforce a minimum of the value of fairness to protect employees. Some examples are fair labour practices, collective bargaining and the right to organize into unions (Constitution 1996, and Labour Relations Act (LRA) (Act 66 of 1995)); the right to safety in the workplace (Occupational Health and Safety Act (Act 85 of 1993)); the right to be compensated for occupational injuries and diseases (Compensation for Occupational Injuries and Diseases Act (Act 130 of 1993)); fair employment conditions and conditions of service (Basic Conditions of Employment Act (BCEA) (Act 75 of 1997)); insurance against unemployment (Unemployment Insurance Act (Act 63 of 2001)).

Nurses must be familiar with these laws and ensure that their provisions are applied to ensure justice in the workplace – these laws protect and provide recourse or assistance to all parties involved in the health-care environment.

Autonomy and the nurse as employee

Autonomy applies not only to health-care users, but also to nurses and other clinicians. The autonomy of the nurse is, however, not without its legal boundaries as provided for by the Nursing Act (50 of 1978) and its regulations, which determine the ability of certain nurses to make decisions that are not subject to authoritative review by those outside the profession. The professional autonomy of the nurse therefore means the right and the responsibility of the nurse, as a member of the nursing profession, to act according to the shared standards of the profession (MacDonald 2002:196; Frith 1996:196; Fry 1994:30). Kant (in Hall 2002: 215) believed that people must be able to reason in order to act autonomously. Three conditions are required for an action to be characterised as autonomous (Hall 2002:211):

■ intention to perform an action
■ understanding of the intended action (the person knows what s/he is doing)
■ the person acted freely, without control by another person or thing.

Section 15(1) of the Constitution 1996, protects the right of nurses to choose not to participate in specific procedures - such as termination of pregnancy (TOP) - that violate their morality. As with any other rights, there is an obligation - the nurse has to inform her/his employer timeously that s/he is not prepared to perform or participate in procedures related to TOP. The nurse has to inform the employer in writing that s/he has a conscientious objection to participating in the termination of pregnancies and therefore will not be participating in any such procedure. These procedures include, but are not limited to, the administering of oral or intravenous medication to terminate the pregnancy, or taking the table into theatre to assist the surgeon with a termination of pregnancy or to do a vacuum extraction. Nurses may, however, not discriminate against women who exercise their choice to have the pregnancy terminated and may not refuse to provide general nursing care to these health-care users. This statement does not adequately provide direction to the nurse in clinical practice, as it does not adequately delineate where 'general care' tasks stop and tasks relating to the TOP procedure starts. One such example is setting up an infusion for a woman who is going to theatre for a TOP. The nursing profession needs to debate this matter further.

Autonomy also means that a nurse has the right to refuse to perform any procedure or action that seems wrong to her. The nurse must be able to justify such actions and inform the relevant parties of such a decision. For example, a registered nurse employed by a pathologist as a phlebotomist has an ethical responsibility to ensure that a client sent to the laboratory by a medical practitioner for HIV testing has been informed of this request and has received suitable counselling. If this is not the case, the nurse may not obtain a blood sample for HIV testing as it will constitute assault and the health-care user has the right to recourse and could institute legal proceedings against the nurse. Even if the pathologist as the employer of the nurse issues an instruction to the nurse to take the blood sample without having obtained the necessary informed consent and counselling, the nurse has a right not to perform this task, not only because of the health-care user's right to informed consent, but also because of the nurse's role as an advocate for health-care users. Occupational health nurses in industry often find themselves challenged by a situation where they are required to obtain a urine sample from an employee to test for substance abuse. The employee is then sometimes dismissed for other reasons, although everyone knows that it is actually related to the outcome of the urine test. Nurses should not be subjected to a situation where they cannot maintain confidentiality of the outcomes of investigations done for employees who visit the clinic. The role of the occupational nurse as an independent practitioner must be protected and respected by all parties.

Employment contracts

When nurses start working at an institution, they are obligated to that institution and an employment agreement/contract should be drawn up and signed by both the employer and the employee. The agreement must be freely entered into by both parties who must be fully aware of the nature of the duties, rights and obligations agreed to at the time of contracting. It is possible for a contract of employment to arise tacitly, such as when an employer allows a person to work for some time without entering into an express contract. There is a legal requirement that contracts of employment should be in writing in terms of the BCEA, for the sake of clarity and the prevention of ambiguities and disputes. The BCEA further requires employers to provide employees with certain information in writing which gives clarity to a written contract. However, the non-observance of this formality will not necessarily render the contract null and void. Nurses must ensure that they obtain a copy of the contract so that they can use it for reference purposes.

Common obligations should be embodied in an employment contract and the provisions of the agreement bind both parties. Both parties (employer and employee) may terminate the contract providing valid reasons and giving notice as provided for the contract of employment. No party may alter the conditions of employment unilaterally and if one of the parties does not abide by the conditions of the agreement, that party has committed a breach of contract and legal steps can be taken against such a party.

The main obligation of nurses as employees, under the contract of employment, is to place their personal services at the disposal of the employer. Failure to render such services may take many forms, ranging from desertion through to absenteeism and poor timekeeping. The nurse's duty to render service is the corollary of the employer's duty to remunerate, the maxim being 'no work, no pay'. The reverse, of course, also applies, namely 'no pay, no work'

– employees who have not been paid may legitimately refuse to work without breaching their contracts. If a number of employees engage in a concerted cessation of work for the purpose of obtaining some concession from their employers, they are deemed to be on strike. These employees may not be dismissed for breach of contract, but the employer need not pay them for the time not worked. Other obligations of nurses as employees include the obligation to maintain reasonable efficiency; to further the employer's business interests; to conduct oneself in a proper and acceptable manner; and to refrain from behaviour that may be detrimental to both the employer and the employee (Grogan 2003:45-50).

Psychological contract

The psychological contract is an unwritten, individual agreement between the employer and the nurse, which places an ethical obligation on both parties. The contract has two components to it. It covers the expectations of the employer of the nurse as an employee and the nurse's attempt to meet those expectations. It also incorporates the nurse's expectations and the employer's willingness to realise these (Bezuidenhout, Garbers & Potgieter 1998:7). The nurse accepts the job in good faith and the expectations of the employer are that s/he is competent and will apply him/herself diligently to the job to enhance the business of the employer while the expectations of the nurse are that s/he will be given the necessary support and guidance as well as be provided with developmental opportunities to further her career. Should these expectations and aspirations not be realised a feeling of disappointment sets in between the parties that affects the relationship.

Breach and termination of a service contract

It is unfair and unethical not to abide by a service contract that both parties agreed to. A contract is breached every time that a primary obligation is not met by any party to the contract. The right to terminate summarily is affirmed by the BCEA. Where the nurse has breached the contract of employment through serious misconduct or negligence, for example, the employer may not only terminate the contract summarily, but could also sue the employee for losses incurred as a result of the breach. In such cases, however, the onus rests on the employer to follow a proper procedure, which may include providing proof that he/she is not vicariously liable for the incident that led to the misconduct.

A contract can be terminated by the nurse resigning from the institution by giving notice as determined in the contract. The termination can be due to mutual agreement; the death of either party; insolvency of an employer; or when one party, in a case such as the nurse's continued absence as a result of disease, cannot fulfil her/his obligation. Obviously in any of these actions the principles of fairness and justice must apply. Where official action by the state renders either party incapable of performing his or her obligations, the contract of employment will lapse. This will be where the employee is, for example, sentenced to a long period of imprisonment. The employer may also terminate the contract for operational reasons (Grogan 2003:75-80).

A disturbing trend is developing in South Africa where nurses are being held accountable for a failing system over which they have no control. There has been a notable increase in the number of disciplinary hearings involving nurses. These include both workplace hearings and SANC professional conduct hearings. On closer scrutiny it is clear that nurses are being punished because of a failing health system; the staffing ratios are totally inadequate which predisposes nurses to making mistakes. In addition, some government employers are not dealing with misconduct in the workplace but refer all cases to the SA Nursing Council. This confuses the role and autonomy of the SA Nursing Council.

Working conditions

Job satisfaction is essential for good staff relations. Labour unrest will occur wherever personnel are not happy with working conditions. Good salaries and working conditions, security, and competitive employment benefits promote job satisfaction. To ensure that nurses as employees are happy in their jobs, good labour relations have to be established and maintained. Labour relations include the involvement of three stakeholders, namely the employees (who are usually represented by their unions), the employer and the government (who provides the legal framework within which labour relations take place) (Bezuidenhout *et al* 1998:6).

Over the past decade, the transformation of health-care institutions, under the pressure of managed care and mergers, has had a dramatically negative effect on the working conditions of nurses. In many hospitals, efforts to reduce costs are achieved by reducing the number of nurses, increasing workloads, and expanding the responsibilities of nurses. As a result nurses work overtime to provide proper nursing care. The employer very often turns a blind eye to the fact that nurses work far more than the legally allowed 45 hours plus only 10 hours' overtime per week. The nurses therefore find it easy to obtain a second job to supplement their income, often at the cost and quality of life of their families and themselves.

With a reduced workforce, nurses have been required not only to work increased amounts of overtime but also to function across multiple units and multiple specialties. The systematic understaffing within hospitals has led to a diminution of job satisfaction and morale among nurses and, more critically, has had an adverse impact on patient outcomes which is often difficult to measure in monetary terms. A profit or saving may be made at a cost to human lives.

Workplace violence

The high prevalence of violence in the workplace of South African health-care workers is of particular concern. Health-care users and their relatives are the main perpetrators of physical violence, while staff are the main perpetrators of psychological violence, which includes verbal violence, bullying, sexual and racial harassment. The tables below indicate the prevalence of the five different types of workplace violence that were found in the study. The low prevalence of sexual harassment is probably the result of poor reporting (Steinman-Marais 2002).

Table 1   Prevalence of physical violence

Description	Public health services	Private health services
Subjected to attacks	17%	9.1%
Witnessed attacks	25,5%	10,1%
Preventable	70,3%	29,7%

(*Steinman-Marais* 2002:4)

Table 2   Prevalence of psychological violence

Description	Public health	Private health	Average	
Verbal abuse	60,1%	38,7%	51,7%	1 in 2
Bullying/mobbing	24,4%	6,3%	20,5%	1 in 5
Sexual harassment	4.8%	4.4%	4.6%	1 in 20
Racial harassment	27.1%	17.4%	22.3%	1 in 5

(Steinman-Marias 2002:4)

In South Africa there is a high prevalence of verbal abuse of nurses (mainly female) by medical practitioners (mainly male), which is quite often ignored by management. This constitutes a gross violation of the rights of nurses to respect and dignity and should not be tolerated. The Democratic Nursing Organisation of South Africa's (DENOSA) research on nurse emigration indicated that workplace violence is one of the top five reasons why nurses are leaving the country (Xaba & Philips 2002). Management has an important and crucial role to play in dealing with and preventing workplace violence. Workplace policies that are enforced consistently have proven to be effective.

Ownership of records

Records created by the nurse in a health facility, belong to the health facility and should be retained as proof of the care that has been provided. Records of the nurse in an occupational health clinic of any industry belong to the nurse or doctor in charge of the clinic and may not be accessed by the employer for any reason and certainly not for disciplinary purposes. In both instances, if the health-care user agrees to make his record available to another party for whatever reason, the nurse can make the record available. The Promotion of Access to Information Act (Act 2 of 2000) does provide an opportunity to other parties to apply formally to have access to certain documents that may include health-care user records.

Moral distress

As professionals, nurses are engaged in a moral endeavour and, as a result, confront many challenges when making decisions. When they cannot do what they think is right, they experience moral distress that leaves moral residue. Moral distress is a major problem affecting nurses in health-care systems in South Africa and, indeed, the rest of the world.

Most health-care users are vulnerable and therefore require protection and competent and timely care. Nurses may not, for a variety of reasons, always be in a position to provide protection or all the care that is needed. When this happens, they suffer moral distress. In 1984 Jameton (in Corley 2002:636) defined moral distress in the nursing context as painful feelings and/or the psychological disequilibrium that occurs when nurses are conscious of the morally appropriate action a situation requires, but cannot carry out that action because of institutionalised obstacles such as a lack of time, lack of supervisory support, lack of adequately trained staff, insufficient staff, abuse of medical power and institutional policy. In 1993 Jameton distinguished between initial and reactive moral distress (Jameton 1993:544). In initial distress, the person feels frustration, anger and anxiety when faced with institutional obstacles and interpersonal conflict about values. Reactive distress is defined as the distress that people feel when they do not act upon their initial distress. This eventually leads to 'wounded' nurses who have lost their ability to care and be involved with health-care users and their relatives, burnout or, finally, resignation.

Webster and Bayliss (2000:217) recommend that the definition of moral distress be broadened to include the failure to pursue 'the right course of action' (or failing to do so to one's satisfaction) because of an error in judgement, some personal failing or circumstances beyond one's control. They propose that moral distress can lead to compromised integrity.

Moral distress is more serious than job dissatisfaction and it is imperative that nursing service managers are aware of this and deal with the situations leading to moral distress. Major sources of moral distress include harm to health-care users in the form of pain and suffering; the treatment of health-care users as objects when meeting institutional requirements; inadequate staffing; health-policy constraints; the medical prolongation of dying; the definition of brain death; and the effects of cost containment (Corley 2002:639).

One of the consequences of moral distress is that nurses may avoid health-care users or be over-solicitous to them because the nurses feel guilty about what is happening to them.

Increasing salaries and improving working hours are not sufficient to resolve the situation and other strategies should be developed, such as shared governance, increased autonomy for registered nurses, and the empowerment of nurses to serve on ethics committees and develop problem-solving skills and strategies to prevent moral distress. Nurse education often concentrates only on ethical principles, but this does not adequately prepare students for institutional realities. From an organisational perspective the literature provides the following guidance (Corley 2002:649-50):

■ Nurses who have high levels of work satisfaction and believe that they are in a more constructive work culture will have lower levels of moral distress.

■ Nurses who have good relationships with their peers, health-care users, managers, the hospital administration and physicians will have less moral distress.

■ Nurses who have more influence in their work environment and thus are more likely to take action to resolve ethical dilemmas will have less moral distress.

■ Nurses who work in health-care organisations that do not provide a supportive environment and mechanisms for addressing complex conflicts with physicians will experience more moral distress.

■ Nurses who work in health care organisations that encourage collaboration with physicians and the development of trust with them will experience less moral distress in ethically complex situations.

Nurses as ethical mediators

Woods (2001:404) argues that nurses are ideally placed to undertake the role of mediator between medical staff and health-care users and/or their representatives. The very fact that nurses occupy a central position between all parties may actually enable them to bring about a more collective process of moral decision-making. It has been maintained that nurses find ways around these contextual problems because they are more than capable of using their 'in-betweenness' as a very effective strategy to promote good care. Nurses are, therefore, ideally positioned to respond to the need for ethical mediation for the following reasons (Woods 2001:405):

■ Nurses continue to maintain a position of public and personal trust through their work in more intimate aspects of care.

- They represent a 'human face' in a world of advanced medical technologies and specialised procedures.
- They perceive their work as 'a moral endeavour' supported by a 'mission to care'.
- They are guided by a relational and strongly contextual ethic that predisposes them towards a high degree of ethical involvement and commitment in caring for the health-care users in their care.
- They have a stronger mandate towards advocacy for their health-care users than sometimes 'blind loyalty' to the medical profession.

For similar reasons, nurses have to act as ethical mediators to protect colleagues from verbal abuse from doctors, health-care users and their relatives, and even from politicians. Nurses must accept and cherish their role as ethical mediators since nursing provides continuity of care often not possible to other categories of health-care workers.

Moonlighting

Moonlighting is the general term used for the practice of accepting employment with another (secondary) employer outside 'normal' working hours. The income generated is for the nurse's own account. Although moonlighting may breach the limitation on the working hours determined in the BCEA, the practice of moonlighting as such is not unlawful. The employer does not own the employee, but the employer must keep it in mind that the essence of the employment relationship is the control of the employee's labour potential. If there is no interference with the nurse's performance in the primary job, and it does not interfere with the interests of the employer, there is no reason why she cannot undertake additional work in her own time. This additional work may be a job that is remunerated or it could be voluntary, such as working at one's church or school activities. However, if the extra work creates a situation that makes the employment situation intolerable, for example, when the nurse is so tired that s/he falls asleep on night duty, the employer will have a legitimate reason to complain and even challenge the practice.

Employment contracts often contain a blanket statement that employees may not take another job outside of working hours without permission from their employers. Labour consultants believe that such a blanket statement is problematic and would probably not be enforceable. Employers can, however, reasonably require that their employees inform them if they wish to work after hours to ensure that there is no conflict of interest with the business of the employers, or conflict with the hours for which the employers have contracted them. Some unacceptable activities would include:

- Moonlighting during the night at one hospital while having to be on duty at the primary employer at 07:00 the following morning. The nurse still has to travel from one hospital to the other and will certainly be late on duty for your primary employer. This will conflict with the hours for which the primary employer has contracted the nurse.
- The employer would usually not object to approving the request for nurses who want to start a private practice with the intention to deliver home-based care after hours. The employer will certainly have a serious objection if the nurses use equipment (e.g. baumanometer, thermometers) or stock (e.g. injections and swabs) that belong to the employer – the nurse can be charged with stealing from the institution if this happens. If the health-care user is a client of the hospital and the nurse goes to see the health-

care user after hours at his/her home and gets paid for services rendered, the moonlighting is in competition with the primary employer.

■ If health-care users are treated with a product manufactured by a company for which the nurse has worked and if the nurse now starts an independent practice where health-care users will be treated with products manufactured by the same company, a conflict of interest will arise. Companies often place a restriction of trade clause in their contracts with staff, which means that nurses who resign from the company are prohibited from divulging trade secrets of that company for a predetermined period.

Serious ethical issues are at stake here. The BCEA states clearly what the limit for overtime is, but it is not clear who is responsible for ensuring that employees adhere to these requirements. There is no doubt that the nurses have a responsibility towards themselves, their families, their employers and the health-care users they care for; that they should get sufficient rest to perform a good day's job and spend quality time with their loved ones. The OHSA further requires the employer and employee to ensure that a safe workplace is maintained – this would include ensuring that employees are not overworked. The nurse therefore has an ethical responsibility not to overwork intentionally.

Using the phone and time of the primary employer to arrange moonlighting is a plain conflict of interest and breach of the duty of good faith. Any employees who conduct their own business during their employer's time, or do not give their full effort and attention to their employer's interest, are in breach of their obligations.

Ethical conflict in a bureaucratic environment

There are four potential sources of conflict between obligations and loyalty:

■ In an environment like a large hospital nurses quickly form an idea of where they fit into the bureaucratic pecking order and, accordingly, they decide what their obligations are. One thing they realise quite quickly is that it is in the interests of the institution to discourage or ignore criticism. However, the efficiency of nurses can give rise to conflict with other health-care personnel because nurses are driven by the belief that care should be exclusively based on the principle of 'concern for the health-care user'. The increasing use of technical aids can also become a source of conflict in large hospitals in the sense that technology becomes more important than patient care (Thompson & Thompson 1990:61-62).

■ Conflict may arise in the context of conflicting loyalties. The most common ethical conflict occurs when a doctor and health-care user has differences of opinion on treatment and the nurse is requested to take sides. Sometimes nurses have to prevent conflict between health- care users and health-care authorities by deciding to support their employer because their post is so important to them (Thompson & Thompson 1990:62-63).

■ As a result of nurses' employee status in a hospital, they become part of the hierarchical network of power. They have different responsibilities towards health-care users, the employer and colleagues and requests from any one of them may be in conflict with the ethical and legal responsibilities to the others. Because they have so little power, nurses are regularly expected to carry out instructions from others (doctors and health-care users) without themselves participating in the decision-making process or without their knowing why the decisions have been made. Such difficult circumstances could lead to poor care for health-care users. Nurses learn from experience to identify situations of potential conflict and consequently prefer work in environments where such conflicts occur less frequently (Thompson & Thompson 1990:63-64).

■   The nurse herself may be a cause of potential conflict in that her personal ideas may differ from her obligation to render a professional nursing service in an ethical manner. Furthermore, nurses choose, consciously or unconsciously, not to be in control of the job. There are usually many people who are ready and willing to assume control should nurses wish to relinquish their autonomy (Thompson & Thompson 1990:65).

Trade unions

A trade union is defined as 'an association of employees whose principal purpose is to regulate relations between employers and employees, including any employers' organisations, (LRA section 213). The use of the term 'principal purpose' merely means that regulating the relationship between employees and employers is only one of the functions of a trade union - unions may engage in any activities to ensure that their members' interests are represented and protected.

The primary function of trade unions is therefore to ensure that the ethical principle of justice or fairness is practised in the regulation between employees and employers.

The Constitution also protects freedom of association (section 18) and nurses can belong to any of the unions that have been registered with the Department of Labour. Most of the unions operating in the health services industry are general unions, with only two organisations having only nurses as members, namely the Democratic Nursing Organisation of SA (DENOSA) and the SA Democratic Nurses Union (SADNU).

The challenge facing unions that organise nurses is acknowledging the complexity of the environment within which they operate and keeping themselves abreast of rapid developments in the sector. At one stage or other we are all users of health services and, as such, are concerned about the kind of reception we get when we enter a health facility and the contribution we can make to ensure that nurses feel adequately protected and motivated. Unions need to create an awareness amongst all stakeholders of the complexities of the health-care profession.

Solutions to grievance, differences and disputes

Trade unions have diverse functions, but their primary role is to engage in collective bargaining with their members' employers in order to improve conditions of employment and to represent their members in grievance and disciplinary matters. Keeping abreast of changes in labour laws ensures that unions and employers are in a position to utilise the legal framework to ensure good labour practices.

Strikes

Section 23(2)(c) of the Constitution of South Africa determines that everyone has the right to strike. The LRA (section 213) entrenches this right provided that correct procedures have been followed and the employees are not employed in essential services. Essential services personnel can take part in strike action only where a minimum service agreement is in place.

The gap in the legislation is that it assumes that parties will always co-operate and conclude such an agreement, and there are no prescribed penalties in law for offending parties who may frustrate the process and abuse the system. Nurses in the public sector are denied the right to strike and yet their employment issues appear to be ignored at the bargaining table and, therefore, there is a degree of frustration and low morale amongst nurses that has led to many of them leaving the country.

Essential service and the right to strike

Various forms of industrial action and strikes have become common among health workers. Traditionally nurses have never resorted to strikes to resolve disputes. The reason for this could be that withholding nursing services is in direct conflict with the very core and ethics of nursing. Nursing is about caring, relieving pain and suffering, and nurturing. When there is no prospect of healing the patient, nursing remains the only service for helping the patient to deal with his/her condition and allowing him/her to die with dignity. In the past strikes were criminal offences in South Africa in terms of the Nursing Act (50 of 1978) as amended. According to Thompson *et al* (1988: 185) it is the idealism and dedication of nurses that exposes them to blackmail in negotiations on salaries. The non-striking stance of nurses makes them vulnerable to exploitation by their employers. It is nevertheless impossible to separate the care of health-care users from the bargaining power of nurses in respect of fair and equitable conditions of service in the public sector. Then there also is the Constitutional determination in section 23 (2)(c) that all workers, including nurses, have the right to strike.

When Curtis (1981:145) refers to the right of the health-care user to health care, she distinguishes between special and general rights. The special right to health care arises when a nurse accepts a patient. The nurse accepts certain obligations towards the health-care user and the health-care user receives the right to nursing. Should the nurse, therefore. withhold or stop nursing, the rights of the health-care user will be infringed. Curtis points out, however, that if a proposed strike is announced in good time and provision is made for both those health-care users who are already in hospital and for emergency cases, the scope of the infringement of the user's rights could be limited to a certain extent. Yet if the health-care user's right to health care is a general right, which has the same status as the right to life or freedom, the withholding of nursing can never be justifiable. It is, however, debatable whether the health-care user's right to health care can be regarded as a special or a general right. If the nurse has made provision for emergency cases and for the health-care users currently in hospital, the right of the health-care user cannot, according to Curtis (1981:146), be a strong enough appeal against strikes. Curtis also believes that when employers disregard certain rights that nurses have as employees, nurses have the same right as others to protect their rights. Where negotiations and less drastic measures have failed, nurses may resort to strikes. The problem is that the nurses' right to strike is in conflict with the user's right to nursing. Of the two rights it would appear that the latter is more important than nurses' right to strike.

When the issue of strikes is regarded from a moral point of view, one cannot simply regard the role of the nurse as an unselfish, self-sacrificing service to humanity. However, when the treatment of health-care users is reduced to a risky life-threatening level, nurses must respond. According to Thompson *et al* (1988:185) the nurse's prescribed duties are set aside by this response. This is not to say that when nurses are exploited, they are not entitled to take steps. The steps that are taken must, however, correspond proportionately to the risks to which their health-care users are exposed to or the degree of exploitation or intimidation which the nurses are experiencing. According to Thomson *et al* (1988: 186), in such circumstances the principle of justice takes precedence over the principle of benevolence. It is fairly easy to plan for extreme situations. Yet, under less dramatic circumstances, it is difficult to determine whether the duty of nurses to provide care should enjoy priority over the decision to strike.

The International Council of Nurses (ICN), in its position statement that was adopted in Geneva, Switzerland on 19 November, 1999, noted the role of dialogue and negotiations while supporting the nurses' right to strike in extreme situations - nurses may strike when negotiations go nowhere. This position statement serves as a guide for the global nursing community in negotiating for improvements in the quality of care, the work environment and the recognition of the profession's contribution to society. In 1999 nurses took strike action in many countries around the world - including Denmark, Zambia, Canada, Israel, Australia, Colombia and for the first time, ever in Ireland.

Lucille Joel, ICN First Vice President and chair of the meeting that adopted the position statement on strike action, said: 'Nurses may choose to take industrial action when deficiencies in the quality of working life and economic rewards have become so serious as to affect the long-range prospects for maintaining high standards of nursing care.' The Vice President continued by saying: 'We recognise that social dialogue is the principal and most effective means of resolving workplace related problems. However, in extreme situations nursing employees may strike when negotiations with the employer have been unsatisfactory, unsuccessful or refused' (Press release ICN/PR/99 No. 21).

Special attention needs to be given to ways of improving negotiations for better salaries and working conditions. The formation of trade unions can empower nurses to a considerable extent, but Thompson (1988:190) warns that this power should be used with great circumspection within the bounds of professional morality. It is also useful to remember that the threat of a possible strike is often more powerful than a full-blown strike.

Nursing as essential service in South Africa

In South Africa nursing services in the private sector have been designated non-essential, which means that disputes of interest will be subjected to 'power play' by the parties. This means that nurses may embark on a full-blown strike for a dispute regarding a salary increase without any obligation to provide a skeleton staff for emergency nursing services. DENOSA believes that the private sector employer is happy to take this chance because of the perception that nurses are conservative, loyal and professional and therefore will not embark on strike action and abandon their patients. It has been DENOSA's experience, however, that instead of engaging in a full blown strike which can be devastating for health-care users and their relatives, picketing at the workplace is quite effective as the private sector employer does not like negative publicity. The public sector health system remains an option, or outlet, should services in a section of private sector collapse due to strike action.

The situation in the public sector is different because health and nursing services have been designated essential services since September 1997. Public health facilities are utilised mainly by poor people who have access to no other health care. Section 72 of the Labour Relations Act 66 of 1995 (as amended) states that in a service designated as essential the parties must negotiate and conclude a minimum service agreement (MSA).

The MSA gives clarity upfront and states how many staff members will be allowed to work when the rest of the staff embarks upon a protected strike. To date, such an agreement has not been concluded in the Public Health and Welfare Bargaining Council. In an interest dispute like a salary dispute, there has never been an award that has gone against the state. It is easy for the state to plead poverty and, therefore, the option of compulsory arbitration is ineffective for unions. The right to strike is entrenched in our Constitution as well as in the LRA. However, the employer so far has succeeded only in frustrating and stalling the process. It appears to DENOSA that the employer is once more abusing the loyalty and professionalism of health personnel. It should be noted that for the first time in history doctors mobilised themselves in June 2004 and marched to Parliament in Cape Town to demand better quality patient care. Thus, the stereotype of a conservative profession is being challenged.

DENOSA believes that problems of health-care personnel, particularly doctors and nurses, are not receiving the attention they deserve. Our health system is suffering as it is underfunded and understaffed, both of which make the work environment intolerable. In time employees will become desperate and will find strike action an option regardless of whether a MSA is in place or not. Exploitation and abuse need to be challenged one way or another. Vulnerable patients should be protected and this can be done only if health-care personnel themselves feel adequately protected. It must be remembered that the poor and unemployed as well as the most vulnerable of our society, the aged and the ill, vote the politicians into governance structures and expect to be protected. Justice must be seen to be done to all. The media is often guilty of selective reporting, and in this regard has managed to turn nurses into 'enemies' of the very community they seek to serve. This is not in the national interest; we all need balanced and responsible reporting.

The impact of strikes

Globally health-care workers, especially nurses, have found it difficult to go on strike. Strike action and potential strike action are regarded as important tools for workers, but it is important that adequate guidance and support are available for the workers involved. Nursing strikes that have been reported have all been caused by disillusionment with the structure and conditions of nursing, which include working conditions, nursing shortages, promotional opportunities, salaries and lack of educational opportunities (Clarke & O'Neil 2001: 351; Muula & Phiri 2003: 209). It is clear that nurses require a strong organisation to support them during strike action (Muula & Phiri 2003:211-12).

Media reporting on the 1999 Irish nurses' strike (Clarke & O'Neill 2001:350) appears to give higher value to masculine cultural codes and the performance of technical skills, whereas activities associated with feminine cultural codes of caring were considered of lower value. Nursing was described as a traditionally gendered activity and, because the gender was female, it was undervalued. Caring work was seen as a kind of philanthropy rather than a profession. It raised the familiar dinosaurs in health, namely 'power and patriarchy'. Nurses and nursing organisations need to articulate the complexity of caring in order to educate the public and the media about the value of humanistic caring.

In South Africa the role of trade unions in health-care services came to the fore in November 1985 during the strike of 900 student nurses at Baragwanath hospital (Bezuidenhout *et al* 1998:4). This trend has since been maintained.

Concluding remarks

When nurses feel deprofessionalised and dehumanized, and their pleas appear to fall on deaf ears, a vicious cycle of demoralisation is set into motion. Confidence in the system needs to be built up so that health-care workers believe that justice will prevail and that strike action is not the only means open to them to address legitimate demands.

Redman & Fry (2000:365) argue that the moral perspective of nurses must be respected, supported and incorporated into the fabric of institutions. Nurses, therefore, have to strengthen their voice by organising themselves into strong advocacy bodies. Nurses have to collaborate with co-workers to bring socio-economic concerns to the attention of their employers and members of the community and, if necessary, to participate in organised labour protest action to improve conditions for nursing practice (Redman & Fry 1994: 250).

Critical thinking activities

1. Debate the factors that impact on the rights of union members in the health-care environment and how the various stakeholders can address these.
2. Explain the importance of employment contracts for nurses in South Africa.
3. Discuss moonlighting as an ethical issue.

The rights of patients and nurses in health care

Sally van Tonder

Outcomes

Studying this chapter will enable you to:

- recognise and protect human rights as the rights of patients
- critically evaluate the rights, duties, responsibilities, privileges and special rights of nurses
- discuss human rights in the context of the rights of nurses
- explain the legal and moral rights of nurses.

Introduction

This chapter is concerned with the rights of patients and nurses in the health-care situation. For the patient what is important is the right to receive safe, high-quality nursing care. For the nurse the important question is the achievement of individual needs and the ability to function as an advocate for the patient.

In the past society emphasised the obligations of the community, but in recent years the emphasis has shifted to the rights of the community. Some of the important rights the community claims are the right to privacy, life, death, healthy environment and health care. It also claims some special rights for certain groups, such as children, the aged, the poor and the dying.

The rights of patients must surely be the most important moral issue nurses have to deal with, and for this reason the nurse's role is inextricably linked to the rights of patients. For this reason, too, the rights of patients are highly esteemed in the nursing profession. The patient is at the centre of all health services and health care. The patient is the reason for nursing and, therefore, the patient's interests are the nurse's first priority. Nevertheless, the fact remains that the patient sometimes becomes lost in the highly scientific world of contemporary health services. Medical progress and technological advancement have led to a situation where the quality of life and rights of patients are no longer given priority.

The importance of patient rights

As new developments take place in the medical field, the rights of patients are becoming a major issue. When one considers the issue of abortion, for example, it is clear that the rights of women and the rights of the foetus are in conflict with one another. In the case of euthanasia, the right of the patient to self-determination and the right to die are at issue.

Abortion has been legalised in South Africa and has become an everyday reality for some doctors and nurses. The free accessibility of legalised abortion can influence society's view of life. The value of life itself is questioned. According to Davis *et al* (1977:147) it is possible that the value society places on life is reduced and that the instinct to protect the vulnerable disappears. The possibility exists that the acceptance of abortion policy can also influence policies regarding the aged, mentally ill and retarded persons. Society may undervalue the right to life of those who are no longer productive and who are a burden, e.g. the aged, the chronically ill and the unemployed.

Rights and responsibilities

In talk about rights there are also other important concepts that must receive attention - concepts such as claims, duties, responsibilities and privileges. It is important to understand these concepts.

A **claim** is the right that controls the action of others.

A **claim** is the right of the patient not to be assaulted while receiving medical treatment. Thus the doctor has the **responsibility** not to assault the patient and a **duty** to prevent any injury to the patient.

The patient has a right, while he is in hospital, to safe nursing care and the nurse has a corresponding legal and moral **responsibility** to provide this.

Privileges and rights are not the same. A **privilege** can be seen as a **gain** allocated to someone, e.g. it is a privilege to be a member of a specific exclusive club (Davis *et al* 1997:85).

To ensure rights in a health-care situation, attention must also be given to the responsibilities of both the patient and the nurse.

Human rights as patient rights

Everyone lays claim to his or her own rights without considering how the exercising of these rights may affect others. It would appear that there is little understanding for the fact that all rights are not absolute. Rights are associated with duties and responsibilities. The nursing profession, like all other professions, always gives precedence to the rights of the community. Because nursing is the most important component of the health-care system, the nursing profession has a special responsibility to ensure and to protect the rights of patients at all times (Searle & Pera 1992:71).

The rights of patients are a subdivision of general human rights. Human rights arise from natural rights, which are rights that have a right of existence, irrespective of place or time. Natural rights are rights which people possess precisely because they are people. Husted and Husted (1991:217) point out that even if these natural rights are not recognised, honoured or protected, they are inalienable and cannot be denied. Human rights are therefore based on the principles of natural justice and for this reason patient rights also arise out of the general principles of natural law.

During illness the human rights of patients gain greater prominence, as does the importance of human rights in the nurse-patient relationship. The state of illness itself, and the proportions which it may assume, make the patient vulnerable to abuse. Furthermore, illness gives rise to new needs that must be met so that the patient's integrity as a unique individual is retained.

The right of the patient to know is included in the tacit contract between the doctor, the nurse and the patient. So too are the legal requirements and medical ethics questions about informed and voluntary consent to treatment a recognition of the right of the patient to know. The right to know is based on wider considerations than simply the legal right of the individual as a person. Because the patient is competent to make informed and voluntary choices him/herself, he/she is also held responsible for his/her actions.

According to Deloughery (1991:199), children, the aged, psychiatric and dying patients require special attention whenever their rights to information are considered. Because the patient is a child, it does not necessarily mean that he/she will not understand and, therefore, does not require information. Providing information only to the parents does not satisfy the child's right to know. The same aspects are applicable to the aged, mentally disturbed and dying patients. It follows that the nurse who is involved with these groups of patients should possess special communication skills.

Withholding of information and the truth

The principle of truth-telling, or of giving patients direct and honest answers, is a contentious issue. In the health professions truth-telling is an operational principle which is affected by the benefit the patient derives from being told the truth. When the truth can do more harm than good, there is no obligation to tell the truth. The problem is complex; it would appear that other moral values, such as concern and loyalty, are in conflict with the value of honesty.

Wright (1987:85) refers to the double standards the health services apply in truth-telling. Traditionally, health workers believe that they have the right, or even the duty, to decide what patients may or may not know. Even deception is justified when health workers assume the right to suppress or alter information, regardless of the patient's wishes.

Wright (1987:86) gives three fundamental reasons for withholding the truth:

- Patients do not really want to know about their illness.
- The truth will prejudice the patient.
- Only information that is beneficial to the patient is given.

Ways of withholding the truth from the patient are by providing false information, not correcting misunderstandings or incorrect ideas, and suppressing information. Deloughery (1991:202) points out that the reasons advanced for withholding information from patients cannot be supported by facts. Because doctors, nurses and family members cannot speak freely to the gravely ill or dying patient about death does not mean that they have been relieved of their obligations. If it is accepted that the patient has a right to information, this right places an ethical obligation on others to resolve the issue of who will tell the patient, when and how.

Rumbold (1989:87) asserts that a patient is done an injustice if he/she receives insufficient information. When this happens, the patient's dignity is disregarded and he/she is deprived of the little independence that the illness still allows. During treatment, the autonomy of the patient should be preserved and active participation in his/her own treatment should be promoted through open and sensitive communication.

The decision whether or not to inform the patient rests with the doctor; but the nurse, who is continually involved with the patient, naturally also becomes involved in this situation. On the one hand, she may respect the patient's autonomy and right to know, while on the other hand she may wish to protect him/her from bad news which may shock and harm. The decision to provide or withhold information should be taken with the greatest circumspection and responsibility because of the complexity of each unique situation.

The right to confidentiality and privacy

The ethical principle of confidentiality was discussed in Chapter 4. Here we consider the right to confidentiality and privacy. A person who has health problems is generally prepared to reveal his/her secrets, to make his/her body available and to display his/her vulnerability in order to receive assistance from someone whom he/she can trust. During nursing interventions a patient often shares personal information with the nurse. Nurses must learn to weigh the appropriateness of this information against the clinical state of the patient before providing the personal information to the doctor or co-workers. In order to keep communication channels open between the nurse and the patient, the nurse must, where the confidential information may prejudice the patient or others, inform the patient that confidentiality is impossible. Rumbold (1993:133) states that clinical information is confidential information, but it may be shared with the members of the health team involved with the patient. The patient has the right to complete secrecy and privacy of all personal information. This includes information in medical records, on the computer and in the nursing-care plan. He/she is also entitled to privacy relating to his/her treatment, case discussion, consultations and examinations.

The protection of confidentiality is one of the fundamental ethical requirements of professional health-care ethics. Unlike the principle of truth-telling, the protection of confidentiality is mentioned in virtually all codes of ethics, including those of nurses, as an absolute requirement.

The special relationship between the nurse and the patient comprises specific duties and obligations that entail more than is normally encountered in ordinary social interaction. These duties and obligations are recorded in the nursing codes. The most essential element in the nurse-patient relationship is that it must be based on complete trust. Rumbold (1993:129) also refers to the confidential relationship and asserts that the patient should trust the nurse's professional judgement, knowledge and skills. Similarly, the nurse should trust that the patient will provide her with all the necessary information to enable her to compile an adequate nursing-care plan. The nurse therefore possesses privileged information about the patient and it is her duty to keep this information confidential. The patient therefore has the right to expect confidentiality of the nurse.

Problems with confidentiality

Respect for the patient's secrets and his/her right to privacy are sometimes threatened by the predominant duty of the nurse to do what is best for the patient. Sometimes it is necessary to convey confidential information to fellow health workers to ensure that the patient will receive better treatment. It is important to obtain the patient's consent before confidential information is conveyed to others. It is when this consent cannot be obtained for some reason or another that the nurse is faced with a problem. The patient may also forbid the nurse to furnish information to fellow health workers and other people. If the patient's safety or wellbeing is threatened, however, the nurse may decide that her duty of caring takes precedence over the right of the patient to enforce his/her prohibition. Injudicious disclosure of confidential information is highly unethical and unprofessional (Thompson *et al* 1988:131).

Violation of confidentiality

The right to confidentiality and secrecy is not an unlimited right. Whenever, in the interests of justice, evidence must be submitted in a court to prove the guilt or innocence of someone, it is generally accepted that the principles of justice enjoy precedence over the patient's right to privacy. Doctors and nurses may not refuse to reveal information in a court. Nurses are also expected to disclose information on patients to the responsible authorities when the community's interests are endangered (for example during a serious epidemic), or when it is suspected that the patient's condition may endanger the lives of others. This also applies to patients with acquired immune deficiency syndrome (AIDS), when the patient's right to secrecy may be disregarded in order to protect others.

The right to privacy

The right to privacy encompasses both the right to respect for the dignity of the patient, namely his/her physical privacy, and the right to respect for the patient's secrets, namely confidentiality. The right to privacy does not, however, mean the right to a private room. Many people who are admitted to a hospital can expect to forfeit some of their privacy. Unfortunately it is also true that most hospital treatments and nursing interventions pay little consideration to people's sensitive need for privacy. Nurses should be familiar with policy relating to the patient's right to privacy. They should be continually encouraged to respect the privacy of the patient as a moral duty.

Legalising the rights of patients

Transformation elements in the new National Health Act 61 of 2003 refer to the rights of the population regarding health matters. These elements strengthen the rights of patients by legalising them. These rights include the right to:

- emergency medical treatment
- information regarding one's condition
- give informed consent for treatment
- participate in decision-making regarding one's health
- be informed when participating in research
- privacy
- access to health records
- submit complaints regarding health services
- be treated with respect (Appendix to *Finansies en Tegniek*, 8 September 2004:36).

Rights of nurses

The dilemma of the rights of patients does not lie with the identification of the rights, but with their protection. When examining the rights of nurses, the dilemma is that it is difficult to distinguish between the nurse's rights, duties and responsibilities.

Throughout the history and tradition of nursing, the focus has been primarily on the responsibilities of nurses and on nursing as a caring and helping profession. Autonomy and the rights of nurses have seldom been at issue. Whether nurses have rights or not is debated by many authors. It would appear that the rights and responsibilities of nurses cannot be separated and that there is still uncertainty about the terms *rights*, *duties* and *responsibilities*.

This lack of clarity about the terms indicates that nurses cannot exercise their rights without taking their duties and responsibilities into account.

Rights, duties and responsibilities

Wright (1987:34) grapples with the question of whether duties give rise to rights and whether rights result in duties. Is there a direct relationship between duties and rights? If a person has a duty, is this aimed at the right of another, or if a person has a right, does this automatically place a duty on another? Tschudin (1993:85) states very simply that one person's right places a responsibility and a duty on another person. Burnard and Chapman (1993:18) link the rights of nurses to what they possess, and their responsibilities to what they give. Rights are therefore related to aspects such as experience, recognition, status, gratitude and so on, while responsibilities include efficient nursing, individual care and the emotional support of patients. The nurse's responsibilities are found in the codes of nursing and the scope of practice. The responsibilities correspond with the work the nurse does and relate to the community, the profession, colleagues and patients/clients. These responsibilities are of a legal, personal and moral nature.

Tschudin (1993:116) finds it is difficult, however, to distinguish between the nurse's rights and her duties. According to Fagin (in Pence and Cantrall 1990:134), the nurse's rights and responsibilities cannot be separated and for this reason people confuse the two concepts and prefer talking about the nurse's rights and responsibilities. Elsie Bandman (in Pence and Cantrall 1990:140), on the other hand, asserts that as a result of the legal restrictions on professional activities, rights must support the nurse's responsibilities. She asserts that professional responsibilities must have corresponding special professional rights. Therefore, nurses have rights, and in order to function independently, they should claim their rights and make their voices heard.

Nurses' rights as privileges

Curtin and Flaherty (1982:129) also believe that the duties and rights of nurses cannot be separated and that the one is essential to the other. For this reason, whenever a person becomes a nurse, that person accepts a number of obligations and gains corresponding rights. These acquired rights differ from human rights in that they are privileges, which are necessary to perform professional obligations. These acquired rights are not rights that all people automatically possess; they are rights which a nurse acquires through training and experience and which enable her to nurse. If a nurse fails to fulfil her professional obligations, the legislative body, the institution or the profession may formally remove these rights. The nurse's colleagues, patients/clients and their families may disregard the rights at an informal level. These acquired rights of nurses can, according to Curtin and Flaherty (1982:130), be defined in professional and behavioural guidelines which are based on the ethical principles of the profession. Bertram Bandman (in Pence and Cantrall 1990:138) denies that nurses possess any rights whatsoever in their professional capacity. He asserts that a professional role assigns privileges and not rights. In respect of the patient the nurse, therefore, has privileges and not rights. These privileges emanate from the rights of the patient and with the consent of the patient. Rights belong exclusively to an individual and the nurse as an individual has rights, but as a professional practitioner the nurse has privileges.

Special rights of nurses

Some nurse leaders claim that nurses have no special rights but only obligations and responsibilities. In general, the rights of nurses are seen as privileges that arise from patient rights. According to Davis *et al* (1997:98) nurses have special rights that arise from their responsibilities to and relationship with the patient. Their social contract with the community also contributes to these special rights. Since nursing is seen as a right in relation to those in need of it and, indeed, as a social necessity, the nurse has a corresponding responsibility and special right to provide the service.

The Professional Standard of Nursing Practice, the American Nurses' Association code and nursing social contracts also support the idea that nurses have special rights. These special rights also help the patient to exercise his/her rights and responsibilities. The obligations and special rights of nurses require a new disposition regarding nursing ethics, decision-making and organising policies (Davis *et al* 1997:99).

Human rights as rights of nurses

Fagin (in Pence and Cantrall 1990:135) not only sees a connection between human rights and the rights of nurses, but also argues that because most nurses are women, there is a connection between women's rights and the rights of nurses. In the nursing situation the nurse's human rights should foster emotions such as compassion while her women's rights embrace freedom of speech, equality and respect. If human rights are assigned to the nurse in the nursing situation, these are indicative of the right to be heard, to question and to doubt, as well as to free participation and satisfaction. Rumbold (1986:140-141) indicates that nurses, like all people, have the right to freedom of speech, thought, conscience, opinion and religion. Nurses have already clearly exercised their right to conscientious objections by, for example, refusing to carry out procedures which are at variance with their religious convictions and freedom of speech.

Legal rights of nurses

The nurse's rights which are legally enforceable are, firstly, her rights as an employee and, secondly, her rights as a professional nurse.

Employees' rights

The same rights that are assigned to any employee are also assigned to the nurse. These are rights such as a safe, healthy working environment, regular payment of salary, and sick and vacation leave. DENOSA recommends that nurses be also entitled to a written employment contract and a job description, as well as information about the health service and equal treatment.

Professional rights

The International Council of Nurses (ICN) declares that nurses have the right to perform nursing according to the codes and ethics of a Nursing Act. The legal rights of nurses in South Africa are found in the Nursing Act (50 of 1978, as amended), and in other relevant health legislation. The professional rights of nurses are listed in Table 3:

Table 3: Professional rights of nurses

- Practising according to what is legally permissible for her/his specific practice.
- Refusing to carry out a task that is reasonably regarded as being outside the scope of her/his practice and for which she/he has insufficient training or for which she/he has insufficient knowledge and skill.
- A safe working environment, which is compatible with efficient care for the health-care user and which is equipped with at least the minimum physical, material and personnel requirements.
- A working environment which is free of threats, intimidation and/or interference.
- Proper orientation and goal-directed in-service education in respect of the modes and methods of treatment and procedures relevant to her/his situation.
- Negotiation with the employer for such continuing professional education as may be directly related to her/his responsibilities.
- Equal and full participation in such policy determination, planning and decision-making as may concern the treatment and care of the health-care user, in the case of a registered person.
- Advocacy for and protection of health-care users and personnel for whom she/he has accepted responsibility.
- Refusing to implement a prescription or to participate in activities, which, according to her/his professional knowledge and judgement, are not in the interest of the health care user.
- Conscious objection provided that:
  - the employer has been timeously informed in writing;
  - it does not interfere with the safety of the health care user and/or interrupt his/her treatment and nursing.
- Withholding participation in unethical or incompetent practice.
- Written policy guidelines and prescriptions concerning the management or her/his working environment.
- Disclosure to her or him of the diagnosis of the health users for whom she/he accepts responsibility.
- A medical support or referral system to handle emergency situations responsibly.

(SA *Nursing Council* 2004:15-16; ICN 2004 *b,c,d*)

Tschudin (1993:117) points out that regardless of where the nurse works, she has rights. She refers to individual nurses in certain areas of work who have additional rights such as, for example, the right to possess, to prescribe and to dispense specific medication. This right is, however, strictly defined and controlled by legislation, namely the Nursing Act and the Medicine and related Substances Act (101 of 1965, as amended) and its regulations.

Moral rights of nurses

For Tschudin (1993:117) the moral rights of nurses include the right to be heard by colleagues and supervisors. Nurses have the right to act according to their own personal convictions and value systems. They have the right to expect to be treated with respect and dignity. Nurses also have the right to expect that the personal reports and information which they have entrusted to supervisors will be kept confidential.

Concluding remarks

In the education of nurses all teaching in respect of ethics, professional practice, methodology and standards of nursing is centred on the rights of patients. Stated broadly, the population of South Africa has the right to access to unlimited nursing services. The right of the community to safe nursing vests in the right of each individual, group or community to health services. Rights of patients are not additional to nursing practice, they are the very heart of any decision-making in nursing.

To prevent the rights of nurses from being neglected in a context where doctors are held in high repute and nurses are viewed merely as the people who carry out the doctors' instructions, nurses must insist on their rights. In striving for the recognition of their rights, nurses should always be motivated by the improvement of nursing. It should also be borne in mind that the exercising of rights is inextricably bound to responsibilities and obligations. According to Curtin and Flaherty (1982:130), these rights and responsibilities not only ensure that nurses can do their work, but also that the work environment and conditions are conducive to nursing. Nurses also have privileges, such as the privilege of caring for sick, injured and vulnerable people. Davis and Aroskar (1983:86) point out that when the rights of nurses are recognised, patients are helped to exercise their rights.

Merely to talk about the rights of patients and nurses without practising and strengthening these rights is to surrender to passivity and remain dependent on others. Nurses can and must ensure the well-being of patients on all levels of service – at the bedside, in homes, schools, and the workplace and also at the policy-making level of organisations and government.

What nurses can do to ensure the rights of patients and nurses is to create an environment where patient and nursing values form an integral part of joint decision-making regarding patient care and the availability of health services.

Each nurse should view the rights of others as being just as valuable as her own rights. Within this context the nurse must critically evaluate responsibilities regarding herself/himself, the patient, the nursing profession and the employer.

Critical thinking activities

1. Explain the rights of patients according to the following:
   - the importance of patients' rights
   - rights and responsibilities.
2. Discuss human rights as the rights of patients.
3. Write notes on the following:
   - the right to treatment
   - the right to know
   - the right to confidentiality and privacy
   - legalising the rights of patients.
4. Explain the rights of nurses as:
   - duties and responsibilities
   - privileges
   - special rights.
5. Describe the difference between claims, duties, responsibilities and privileges.
6. Discuss the legal and moral rights of the nurse.

part 4

Perspectives on ethical issues in health-care practice

It has been asserted that knowledge and skills are fundamental to professionalism, but this is not the case. Although knowledge and skills do form an integral part of professional practice, the foundation of a profession consists of its declaration of its functions. These functions are acknowledged and faithfully adhered to by practitioners in the daily practice of their profession. The fidelity of practitioners lies at the heart of the relationship between individuals or the community and professionals. Without fidelity, trust cannot exist, and without trust, nurses cannot practise their profession
(*Curtin* 1982:101-102).

Nursing and health-care issues from the beginning of life to adolescence

Miemie Groenewald

Outcomes

Studying this chapter will enable you to:

■ discuss the issues relating to reproduction and antenatal care
■ explain the issues that arise in the different phases of life from birth to adolescence
■ identify and describe South African legislation relating to ethical issues.

Introduction

In this chapter we consider issues relating to reproduction and antenatal care, paediatric care and nursing care for adolescents. Since health-care practitioners come into contact with people at different stages of life, it is important that they have a working knowledge of everyday ethical problems to enable them to act within the ethical framework of the standards of their professions.

Reproductive and antenatal care

Throughout the world most people as the social norm accept the decision of two adults to enter into marriage and to start a family. All the major religions regard marriage as a sacred institution and reject adultery. Most legal systems in the world are intent on the protection of married couples and attach particular value to the nuclear family as the cornerstone of a healthy society.

Reproductive technology and infertility

Artificial insemination

Artificial insemination involves the placing of fresh or frozen semen obtained from the husband or a registered donor into the vagina or cervix of the woman. In South Africa, artificial insemination is controlled by the National Health Act, 2003 (Act 61 of 2003), and only a doctor or someone acting under his supervision may perform artificial insemination (Strauss & Maré 2001:155). Both the Act and the code of practice for medical practitioners (GN R1182 of 20 June 1986 as amended by GN R1354 of 17 October 1997, published by the Department of National Health) provide that artificial insemination may be performed on an unmarried as well as a married woman. Although consent of a married woman's husband is not a requirement, without it the legal status of the child may be affected by virtue of the Children's Status Act 82 of 1987. The donation of semen is subject to the strict measures of the Act, requiring permission from the donor to undergo a physical examination and to conduct an interview with the doctor, as well as for the taking of gamete samples for testing, analysis and processing. The doctor meticulously records information on the donor and recipient, and certain prescribed personal details of the donor must be made available to the recipient and her husband, to the doctor who will perform the procedure and to the Director-General of Health. Donor files are kept in safe custody and no other person may be furnished with any information on these files. If a doctor knows or suspects that two or more pregnancies exist or five living children have been born from one donor's gametes, further gametes donated by the same donor may not be used for artificial insemination. Written permission must be given by the donor, his wife (if he is married), the recipient and her husband. With the permission of both man and woman, the child born as a result of artificial insemination is regarded as the married couple's legal child and they are legally responsible for the maintenance of the child (Strauss & Maré 2001:156-160).

Legislation cannot enforce ethical principles, and single heterosexual women and lesbians are increasingly insisting on their rights to have a child of their own. The traditional negative attitude of society towards unmarried mothers has relaxed considerably in the 21st century. So-called virginal births, which involve pregnancy with the aid of artificial insemination and a supposedly intact hymen, have received a great deal of publicity since the 1990s. Concerns about lesbian motherhood extend beyond the absence of a father and deal with the stigma associated with homosexuality and how it may lead to stigmatisation of the child by peers and others in society. Some believe that the unconventional role models surrounding the child will be detrimental to gender development and will lead to homosexuality. All the independent research studies on children raised by lesbian parents has shown the opposite, namely that in terms of social, emotional or gender development, these children fared as well as those from traditional families (Dooley, McCarthy, Garanis-Papadatos & Dalla-Vorgia 2003:164). In several American urban centres hundreds of children grow up with multiple parents where gay and lesbian couples and their friends of the opposite sex, involved in the conception and birth, all take an active role in rearing these children. Charo (2002:234-235) notes that these families are more significant than their numbers because they challenge the laws based on the heterosexual, nuclear family model.

Ethical arguments against artificial insemination are based on various views on marriage, parenthood and the family system that forms the core of a society. The Roman Catholic Church in particular regards intervention by a third party to bring about reproduction as morally unacceptable in particular (Rae 1996:46).

Artificial insemination can be viewed as degrading in the sense that the person is viewed as an object and deprived of values and human dignity. Artificial insemination in this sense is an 'artificial' procedure which eliminates the true meaning of sexual intercourse as an expression of marital love between two people. Artificial insemination from a donor could even be viewed as a form of adultery (Rae 1996:28).

The restriction on the number of times semen from the same donor is used (by several recipients) to eliminate the possibility of later incest between biological half-brothers and half-sisters, is viewed in a serious light (Hafez & Semm 1982:209; Hull 1990:50). The freezing of semen creates the possibility of using the semen of so-called superior fathers/donors for eugenic (race-improvement) reasons, for example donors who are Nobel prize-winners, renowned artists or gifted scientists.

The proponents of artificial insemination view the procedure as an aid to people with fertility problems who desire to have *a* child of their own (biologically and genetically the same as one or both parents). Parenthood is not regarded as a biological matter, but rather as the human function of commitment to the care and education of a child (Bandman & Bandman 2002:129).

Midwives who attend confinements of unmarried women, lesbians and virgins, who reproduce with the aid of donor-artificial insemination may not even be aware of the woman's unusual circumstances. Disclosure that disagrees with the midwife's beliefs about sexuality may pose a problem. Frith and Draper (2004:268) express concern about the care provided for lesbian mothers that is compromised by homophobia among midwives.

Just as nurses and midwives accept that not every marriage is happy and not every baby is wanted, so it is necessary to treat every woman as an individual without passing a value judgement based on personal prejudices (Heywood 1991:63).

In vitro fertilisation and embryo transfer

The definition of artificial insemination in the Human Tissue Act, 1983 (Act 65 of 1983), is broad enough to cover *in vitro* fertilisation as well. *In vitro* fertilisation is the joining outside the human body of a male and female gamete and the placing of the zygote into the uterus of a woman. *In vitro* fertilisation was primarily developed to relieve female infertility and the procedure involves the removal of an ovum (or ova) from a woman, fertilisation by sperm in a laboratory nutrient medium (*in vitro* means 'in glass') and the transfer of the newly formed human embryo to the uterus for implantation and gestation (Strauss & Maré 2001:162-164). During the sixties and seventies clinicians were under increasing pressure to find methods for the treatment of tubular infertility. The low success rate of surgical restoration of blocked oviducts gave rise to increased interest in an alternative method. Society's acceptance of single parents reduced the availability of babies for adoption and many infertile married couples, hoping to have children, turned to science (Marmaduke & Bell 1989:25; Devine 2000:102-103).

Two schools of thought have arisen in favour of embryo protection. The first school appeals for protection of the embryo on the grounds that the embryo is biologically alive, that development from embryo to foetus to child is continuous, and that embryos for transfer are deliberately created in the clinical context. Society's attitude towards children awakens a natural protective impulse on the part of adults and many people are opposed to tampering with embryos for fear of causing defects in children. This group believes that *in vitro* fertilisation ought to be banned in the event of a large number of children being born with genetic deviations. The second school bases embryo protection on a moral obligation towards the life of the embryo (Marmaduke & Bell 1989:26).

The answer came from science with the biomedical breakthrough on 25 July 1978, when Louise Brown was born in England. Ethicists and legislative authorities had to struggle to catch up (Campbell 1992:vii). Since the Brown baby was the product of her own biological parents' gametes, a similar case in South Africa would be legally permissible and ethically justifiable as a therapeutic intervention. The only reservation is that such procedures must comply with the provisions of the Human Tissue Act of 1983 (sections 22 and 23), and the regulations in terms of the Act (Strauss & Maré 2001:163).

Women who have been scheduled for *in vitro* fertilisation and embryo transfer are first treated with superovulation techniques so that more ova will be available for fertilisation.

The surplus of embryos not used for transfer has led to the development of cryopreservation. Not only is the prospect of available frozen embryos advantageous where problems for embryo transfer first have to be eliminated, but it also reduces the possible repetition of the withdrawal process of female gametes. Some people regard the preservation of embryos as an attractive alternative to family planning, but personal convenience is by no means the aim of *in vitro* fertilisation (Marmaduke & Bell 1989:27).

The reproductive revolution continues, although many ethical issues remain unanswered. Governments, media, scientists, ethicists, social workers and philosophers are trying to find solutions. Research is being conducted into the possible effects of reproductive technology on the individual, family and society of the future. Further investigations are important because the knowledge and insight that are gained will improve the nursing care and treatment of married couples with fertility problems (Carr, Friedman, Lannon & Sharp 1990:906-909).

Surrogate motherhood

Surrogate motherhood involves an agreement between a childless married couple (prospective or desiring parents) and a fertile woman, the surrogate mother, to be fertilised with sperm from the contracting man with the aim of undertaking a full-time pregnancy and surrendering the child at birth to the prospective parents. The surrogate mother furthermore undertakes to renounce her parental rights in respect of the child, who can then be adopted by the childless mother in countries in which this is a statutory procedure. Surrogacy is also defined as contract pregnancy (Pretorius 1987:275; Dooley *et al* 2003:55).

A distinction is made between partial and complete surrogate motherhood. Partial surrogate motherhood is more generally prevalent and involves the artificial insemination of the surrogate mother with sperm of the prospective father of the child. The surrogate mother is at the same time the genetic (or biological) mother of the child. Complete surrogate motherhood, on the other hand, involves *in vitro* fertilisation with ova and sperm obtained from the prospective parents, therefore genetic parents, whereafter the embryo is transferred into the uterus of the surrogate or host mother to bear the baby for the full term of pregnancy (Pretorius 1987:270).

One of the most difficult issues revolves around the legal relationship between the genetic parent(s) and the surrogate mother in relation to the legal validity and enforceability of the contractual agreement which the parties have entered into. Furthermore, numerous legal and ethical problems arise when the surrogate mother receives financial compensation for her services and the most contentious problem lies in the determination of the legal parents of such a child (Strauss & Maré 2001:164).

In South Africa, the Human Tissue Act of 1983 does not regulate the legal relationship between the genetic parents and the surrogate mother. A contractual agreement between the parties will probably not be regarded as enforceable in the case of the surrogate mother wishing to keep the baby. In terms of the Children's Status Act, 1987 (Act 82 of 1987), a child born of a surrogate mother is legally regarded as her and her husband's child and not as the child of the genetic parents. The Child Care Act further hampers surrogate motherhood, 1983 (Act 74 of 1983), which prohibits formal adoption if a child has been born to one of the prospective adoptive parents. Alternatively the couple can apply to the High Court for guardianship of the child. In its judgement the High Court, which is the guardian of children, may issue an order in the best interests of the child (Strauss & Maré 2001:164-165).

On 1 October 1987 history was made in South Africa with regard to surrogate motherhood when a married grandmother from Tzaneen gave birth to triplets in Johannesburg. The genetic parents were her own daughter and son-in-law. This example of a 48-old grandmother's compassion for her childless daughter had a happy ending in spite of the dramatic twist in timing. Just thirteen days before the promulgation of the Children's Status Act 82 of 1987, the triplets were born, and the Registrar of Births, Marriages and Deaths decided to register them as the children of their genetic parents. Had the Children's Status Act been signed by the State President and published in the *Government Gazette*, they would have been registered as children of their genetic grandparents. Legally their birthmother and genetic grandmother would have been the same person (Strauss & Maré 2001:165; Fremgen 2002:194).

Family planning and sterilisation

Although some people disapprove of family-planning methods on the basis of religion or moral objections, such methods are fairly generally available for the prevention of unwanted pregnancies. Opponents of the application of family planning must debate the inevitable consequences of the population explosion worldwide. In the faces and bodies of millions who are starving and diseased, one can see the failure of individuals, families and communities to take responsibility for rearing children (Bandman & Bandman 2002:127; Strauss & Maré 2001:127).

If human reproductive freedom is to be a reality, poverty-stricken women should also have access to expensive long-term contraceptives. The question arises whether affluent countries should aid developing countries with population control or with food. Individual freedom to produce large numbers of children without being able to provide for them, and then expecting society to supply food, housing, clothing, health care and education, becomes a global ethical controversy (Bandman & Bandman 2002:128-129).

Voluntary sterilisation in the form of either a vasectomy or tubular ligation as a permanent family-planning method is being used by an increasing number of people. Although ethicists and theologians may frown upon such non-therapeutic interventions, it is accepted as a lawful principle in Western Europe, the USA and South Africa. In South Africa the Sterilisation Act 44 of 1998 governs sterilisation. No person who is capable of consent, and 18 years or older, is prohibited from having the procedure performed on him or her, and this includes an unmarried person. Previously, based on the premise that there was a mutual right to procreate within the normal marriage, it was necessary to obtain the consent of the other spouse before sterilisation could be performed. The current belief is that each spouse is autonomous with regard to his or her body. In the case of persons with severe mental disability who cannot consent, sterilisation may be performed only at the request of a parent, spouse, guardian or curator of the patient (Strauss & Maré 2001:127-130).

Antenatal care

The pregnant woman and her foetus are regarded as two separate patients. Technological progress in the field of perinatal medicine and surgery make it possible to undertake both diagnostic procedures and treatment of the foetus *in utero*. The decision to allow foetal treatment is based on the pregnant woman's rights to her own body and her view of what is in the best interests of the foetus. Moral conflict can arise, particularly when the pregnant woman's health is endangered and a decision must be made as to whether the risk to the mother is greater than that to the foetus (Bandman & Bandman 2002:130-131).

Abortion

Throughout the world, abortion is one of the most contentious ethical issues. A pregnant woman makes the decision to produce a new life or to terminate it if the pregnancy is unwanted. Responsibility based on moral justification is inherent in such a decision. The idea that decision-makers possess power over life and death is probably the reason why all bioethical problems repeatedly come back to abortion. The moral principles that are supposed to accommodate decision-making on the termination of life, do not always work. Abortion therefore remains a problem (Bandman & Bandman 2002:141).

In South Africa abortions were prohibited in terms of the Abortion and Sterilization Act 2 of 1975. The Act defined abortion as the expulsion of a live foetus (which included an embryo and a foetus) of a woman with intent to kill it. The position here has since become much more lenient. The 1975 Act was repealed when the Choice of Termination of Pregnancy Act 92 of 1996 was put into effect on 1 February 1997. Termination of pregnancy refers to the separation and expulsion, by medical or surgical means, of the contents of the uterus of a pregnant woman (South Africa 1996:4). The legality of abortion or, for all one knows, the limits within which abortion ought to be lawful, remains one of the most controversial issues of the 21st century (Strauss & Maré 2001:142-143).

Emotion-laden arguments in political, social, legal, religious and moral circles are passionately set in motion by the ongoing abortion debate. Between the extremes of pro-life and pro-choice arguments lies a spectrum of other views. Based on religious principles, the pro-life supporters view abortion as unjustifiable murder. The proponents of pro-choice view that the woman is autonomous with regard to her body, and that the embryo or foetus is part of her body with which she can do as she wishes. Thus simplified, both extreme viewpoints have either the foetus or the woman to be viewed as an object. Either side poses a dilemma (Strauss & Maré 2001:142; Burkhardt & Nathaniel 2002:223-224; Bandman & Bandman 2002:156).

In the 1998 court case of the *Christian Lawyers Association of South Africa v Minister of Health*, the court upheld the constitutional validity of the Act. The plaintiffs referred to section 11 of the Bill of Rights that provides that everyone has the right to life. The court held that the inclusion of an unborn child under the word 'everyone' does not depend on medical or scientific evidence about when a human life commences (Strauss & Maré 2001:143). The age of the foetus or the gestational period is of vital importance for determining when a pregnancy may be terminated. During the first 12 weeks a pregnancy may be terminated on request. A medical practitioner or a registered midwife who has completed the prescribed course may perform the procedure. From 13 to 20 weeks a medical practitioner may perform termination after consultation with the woman and when at least one of the following indications is present:

- the continued pregnancy poses a risk to the woman's physical or mental health
- a substantial risk exists that the foetus would suffer from severe physical or mental abnormality
- the pregnancy resulted from rape (including statutory rape, that is sexual intercourse with a girl below the age of 16 or with a female imbecile) or incest
- the continued pregnancy will significantly affect the social or economic circumstances of the woman (South Africa 1996:4).

After the twentieth week a medical practitioner may carry out the termination only after consultation with another doctor or a midwife if the continued pregnancy endangers the woman's life, or would result in severe malformation of the foetus, or pose a risk of injury to the foetus (South Africa 1996:4).

The Act imposes a duty upon the State to promote the provision of non-mandatory and non-directive counselling, before and after the termination of a pregnancy (section 4).

The Act further imposes a positive duty on the doctor or midwife whom a woman requests to terminate a pregnancy, to inform her of her rights under the Act (section 6). Failure to do so is not *per se* a criminal offence under section 10 ("Offences and penalties") of the Act. Section 10 does, however, make it a criminal offence to prevent the lawful termination of a pregnancy or to obstruct access to a facility for the termination of a pregnancy; such prevention or obstruction may attract a penalty or a fine or imprisonment for up to 10 years (Strauss & Maré 2001:146.

Strauss and Maré (2001:146-147) further argue that preventing or obstructing the lawful termination of a pregnancy requires positive conduct that goes beyond a mere omission or refusal by a doctor or midwife to inform the woman of her rights. They propound that, if such an omission or refusal is interpreted as preventing or obstructing, it could be seen as an offence against the Constitutional rights of freedom of speech and conscience. The Act does not provide the legal grounds to interpret refusal to perform termination of pregnancy as criminal conduct. This is possibly the reason why the Act does not embody a conscience clause. The Act does not impose a duty on a doctor to refer a woman who requests an abortion to another doctor or facility, and it goes no further than to inform her of her rights under the Act. Thus the constitutionality of section 6 of the Act may be questionable in view of the Constitutional guarantee of freedom of religion, belief, opinion and expression.

No consent other than that of the pregnant woman is required for the termination of a pregnancy. In the case of a pregnant minor, section 5(3) of the Act imposes a duty upon the doctor or midwife to advise the minor first to consult with parents, guardian, family members or friends. Should such a minor choose not to consult them, provision of the termination shall not be denied (South Africa 1996:5-6).

A person who is not a doctor or midwife but who terminates a pregnancy shall be guilty of a serious offence and liable on conviction to a fine or a maximum sentence of 10 years imprisonment (South Africa 1996:8). Between February 1997, when the Termination of Pregnancy Act came into effect, and July 1998, an estimated 39 460 legal abortions were carried out in South Africa. Little provision was made in the infrastructure of the health-care delivery system to absorb the enormous impact of such a large number of abortions. Facilities where termination takes place need well-prepared professionals, clinics and finances. The consequences of this legislation place enormous strain on the nursing profession, because large numbers of nurses refuse to be involved with abortions (Poggenpoel, Myburgh & Gmeiner 1998:3).

Nurses feel offended because they were not consulted about their beliefs on legalised abortion. Contemporary nurses are very familiar with political issues in the legislative arena. Of particular interest to the nursing profession worldwide are political issues that involve moral values, professional regulation, the health of individuals in society and the distributing of justice. Nurses base their positions on these issues on, amongst other things, personal experience, ethical and cultural orientation, and religion. Needless to say the nursing profession provides a healthy diversity of viewpoints that can influence the outcome of political issues (Burkhardt & Nathaniel 2002:272). Many South African nurses prefer not to be involved in termination of pregnancy procedures or to nurse a woman who has had a pregnancy terminated. The Democratic Nursing Association of South Africa (DENOSA) states that nurses have the freedom of conscience and may not be discriminated against if they choose not to participate in termination of pregnancy. Furthermore, nurses who have been trained to save lives at all costs, and who associate themselves with nursing's ethical code, will need training to provide counselling to women who request termination (Poggenpoel *et al* 1998:6).

Paediatric care

The ethical issues concerning the care of children, from the newborn infant to the twelve-year-old child, are often compounded by the vulnerability of the child. Children are virtually universally regarded as the future of a nation and are traditionally protected in most cultures. Throughout the world, however, there are neglected, abused and illiterate children in dire need of health care. Nursing ethics endorses the preservation of life and the protection of the vulnerable, and nurses who care for children act as advocates for them. In practice, parents and nurses concerning the welfare of children may hold conflicting points of view, so that ethical conduct has to be maintained under great pressure.

Premature and low birth-mass neonates

Technological progress and neonatal intensive care units have considerably improved the viability of premature and neonatal babies with a low birth mass. A newborn infant with a mass of approximately 500 grams and a gestation period of as little as 24 weeks, and any neonate, for that matter, who makes an effort to breathe, is resuscitated and admitted to an intensive care unit. Specialist nurses with the aid of sophisticated machinery and small-format apparatus care for high-risk babies. Most vital functions can be sustained, for at least some time, by equipment that is constantly refined to measure every conceivable parameter. The question arises whether machinery in intensive care use has become more sophisticated than the codes of law and ethics that govern its use. Approximately 35% of neonates weighing between 500 and 750 grams survive, and about 60% of gestations between 24 and 26 weeks. Ethical issues arise in relation to the admission criteria of increasingly smaller babies, the commencement and continuation of treatment (which entails months of hospitalization), the chances of survival and the ultimate physical and intellectual outcome of survivors (Townshend 1990:38; Frith & Draper 2004:127, 130-131).

One of the most devastating events that can happen to a parent is the loss of a neonate. End-of-life care starts during pregnancy for parents with high-risk pregnancies. Parents should be informed before delivery, staff should be sensitive and involve the parents in care and decision-making (Frith & Draper 2004:131; Lundqvist, Nilstun & Dykes 2003:197 + 201).

Newborn infants with congenital abnormalities

There are no easy solutions to the ethical implications of infants born with abnormalities such as anencephalia, microcephalia and severe spina bifida. Besides having to deal with the tragedy of having a handicapped baby, both parents and medical staff must make a sensitive and difficult decision because the treatment options, under which are classed infanticide, passive infanticide and internal or surgical treatment with a prognosis of poor quality of life, are limited. The naturalistic approach of providing basic solace until nature has run its course is usually the only acceptable course of action.

After prenatal diagnosis, the parents - who experience disappointment, sadness, fear and unbelief - have to choose between carrying the pregnancy to term or to terminate it. They will always remember that choosing the lesser of two evils, whether desiring a child or avoiding pain, in reality left them with no choice. Confrontation with a real ethical dilemma implies that a choice will always compromise or negate certain values. One cannot 'not choose', or refuse to decide. In particular circumstances selected abortion seems justifiable, but it does not remove the moral evil of destroying unborn life. In real ethical choices, humanity can never be fully realised and people have to learn to live with the unsatisfactory and temporary. Irrespective of the parents' decision they will need holistic care (Gastmans 2002:82-83, 93).

Neonatal euthanasia

In South Africa neonatal euthanasia is regarded as infanticide and the nursing profession has a clearly defined position against this practice. The natural life expectancy of weak and disabled newborn infants is so poor that they do not live for long and no nurse would leave such babies to their own fate (Searle & Pera 1992:112; Strauss & Maré 2001:92).

Moral implications in the nursing of children

Cot death

The tragic occurrence of cot death is a specific health risk for babies and children under two years. The problem with the prevention of cot death lies in the fact that it usually takes place in the parental home and nurses are not directly involved. All nurses who work with children have a responsibility to inform parents about the potential danger of cot death.

A study in New Zealand has identified three risk factors that contribute towards the incidence of cot death. These factors are babies who lie on their stomachs, mothers who smoke, and a lack of breast-feeding. It has come to light that these factors apparently caused 80% of the cases of cot death (Aley & Mitchell 1991:22).

In the United Kingdom the Department of Health launched a campaign to persuade parents to get their babies to sleep face upwards. The occurrence of cot death declined by 60%. Prior to the campaign, for 20 years health workers had encouraged parents to have their babies sleep on their stomachs, and made the recommendations in accordance with government guidelines. The lesson which everyone learned from this is applicable to all health workers throughout the world. Nurses must be aware of new research that can alter the most basic established practices (Ogden 1993:18).

Child abuse

The growing number of cases of baby and child abuse, which includes sexual abuse, is alarming, particularly when one takes into account that official statistics do not represent all cases. Although the Child Care Act, 1983 (Act 74 of 1983) places a duty on health and social workers to report such incidences, this does not ensure the reporting of all abused children. Less conspicuous forms of physical abuse, such as sexual molestation, less serious physical injuries that do not require medical attention, and emotional abuse make the tracing of such cases difficult (Oosthuizen 1993:44; Redelinghuys & Mazarakis 1994:10).

With human rights currently in the foreground throughout the world, modern societies, which are characterised by materialism and the breakdown of traditional support structures, are once again being shocked into giving attention to moral and ethical standards. Nurses have an important role to play in the prevention of abuse and the identification and care of abused children. Nurses are at the forefront of the entire spectrum of health services available in the community and can give guidance at clinics, maternity sections, child and intensive care units (Oosthuizen 1993:44-45).

Nurses' ethical duty to act as advocates for children is by no means an easy task, but nothing is worse for the abused child than for the signs of his abuse not to be noticed and reported. Nurses have a moral and legal duty towards the child and the parents to offer expert professional care and to make use of available resources (Oosthuizen 1993:45-46; Redelinghuys & Mazarakis 1994:13).

Nursing care for adolescents

It is a challenge for nurses to work with adolescents since the developmental phase, from childhood to young adulthood from the ages of 12 to 20 years, is known not only by strong peer group identification but also by its peculiar teenage culture. Nursing care for adolescents is interspersed with moral implications. Adolescents lay claim to adult rights, but are not yet able to accept the responsibilities and duties that such rights entail. Serious health-related issues, such as irresponsible sexual activity, addiction and suicide among teenagers, have ethical and moral implications.

Sexual activity

Contraceptive practices

In South Africa a particularly large segment of the population consists of youths between the ages of 12 and 20 years. Contemporary adolescents reach sexual maturity and are often sexually active at an earlier age than in the past. The Department of National Health's family planning policy represents the views of all social groups. The Amendment Act, 1991 (Act 86 of 1991), to the Child Care Act of 1983 allows for persons above the age of 14 years to receive contraceptive devices, provided the supplier gives guidance and support (Strydom 1993:29-30).

Adolescents who request contraceptive devices have, as a rule, been sexually active for a considerable period of time. It is more difficult to alter already established patterns of behaviour, but a nurse will always try to establish a confidential relationship so that the youthful client can decide for him or herself (Strydom 1993:30-31; Bartter 2001:19).

Sexually active Black adolescents are not well informed on contraceptive devices and even those who are do not use contraception for fear of their parents' strong opposition should they find out. There is a definite need for sex counselling in black schools, and because numerous sexually active teenagers are still in primary school, the target group cannot be high schools only (Setiloane 1990:46-47; Mogotlane 1993:13). Sex counselling in Black clinics is impractical because the nursing staff are so overburdened that they cannot meet the requirements of such a service. Since sex counselling requires a multidisciplinary approach, the nurse's role can be supplemented by peer groups, popular theatre and role-play, as well as educational strategies to enlighten Black South African teenagers (Schoeman 1990:13).

Teenage pregnancy

In South Africa there are roughly 17 000 babies born every year to mothers under the age of 16. Teenage pregnancies are a problem for parents, educationists and society in general.

Adolescent childbirth is taxing for the health of a girl who, during the bodily changes of puberty, has to bear the change of pregnancy as well. The psychological and emotional burden of coming to terms with bodily change, of maintaining relations with the peer group, of becoming independent of parents, of preparing for a career and a marriage as well as acting in a socially responsible manner, all these things are difficult enough for any teenager without the additional responsibility of pregnancy. The likelihood of resorting to prostitution to ease financial privation poses a high risk to adolescent mothers in South Africa with its high rate of HIV/AIDS infection (Mogotlane 1993:1; Ehlers 2003:14).

Feminist researchers and theorists see human sexuality as a social activity, rather than a biological one. Issues like abortion, contraception and teenage pregnancy have been artificially separated and it would be more accurate to understand the hysteria over them as a distillation of a much larger issue, namely women's sexuality. Worldwide, increasing female independence is challenging traditional social norms and expectations about appropriate behaviour for women. Adolescents often receive a two-faced message about sexuality when responsible reproduction is encouraged while sexuality is used as a marketing strategy in the media (Spradley & Allender 1997:415).

An important component of holistic and sensitive care is paying attention to the sexual needs of women across the life span. Nurses can educate adolescents to claim their rights by making informed decisions about sexuality and productivity. Women in South Africa can use existing legislation to access contraceptive or termination of pregnancy services to improve their quality of life (Ehlers 2003:23).

AIDS

It is reported that South Africa has the largest number of people living with HIV/AIDS that is mainly transmitted through heterosexual means. Evidence suggests that most HIV infections occur during adolescence and early adulthood (Simbayi, Chauveau & Shisana 2004:605). As if adolescents did not already have enough problems in coming to terms with their sexuality within the social and cultural framework, they now have to contend with the spectre of AIDS as an additional, frightening dimension (Brooks-Gunn & Furstenberg 1990:59).

In a nationwide survey conducted in 2002, behavioural data obtained from South African youths aged 15-24 years clearly indicate positive responses to the HIV/AIDS epidemic. The median age of sexual debut for both sexes was 16.5 years, with the highest incidence of sexual activity among Blacks living in informal urban areas. Partner turnover was low but multiple partners were more common among Black males in informal urban areas. Frequency of sexual activity was relatively low among sexually active adolescents and the phenomenon of secondary abstinence, where sex is discontinued for periods of time after initial sexual activity, was observed. A number of self-reported virgins was found especially among White and Indian girls and in some rural areas. Condom use was high and the majority of youths had discussed HIV prevention with their partners. Thus it seems that South African youths are taking notice of their country's HIV/AIDS prevention programme in trying to abstain, be faithful and use a condom (Simbayi, Chauveau & Shisana 2004:613-616).

A recent study undertaken by the University of Witwatersrand's Reproductive Health Research Unit (RHRU) confirms that in spite of the high prevalence of HIV among youths, it looks as if the epidemic is stabilising in this age group. From this study, in which 11 904 people were interviewed, it has become evident that the brunt of the HIV/AIDS epidemic is borne by young women in South Africa with nearly one in four women aged 20 to 24 testing HIV positive compared to one in 14 men of the same age. It was found that most young people reported that they knew how to avoid HIV infection, but persisted in risky sexual behaviour. With sexual partners on average four years older, many young girls are coerced into having sex, while sexually active young women placed themselves at greater risk of exposure to infection, because they admitted to be having more sex than their male counterparts (Ndaki 2004: 52-53).

Health-care practitioners must still be aware of the urgent need to support all HIV/AIDS prevention programmes for current youths and especially new entrants to this risky age group.

Alcohol and drug addiction

The serious effects of alcohol and other drugs on developing children and youths have far-reaching physical, psychosocial and developmental consequences. Youths with a drug dependency are more vulnerable to life-threatening accidents and injuries, physical complications, sexually transmitted diseases, memory loss and impairment of the cognitive and motor abilities, and are more prone to impulsive and hazardous behaviour and illegal activities. In addition, psychoactive agents have a detrimental effect on the emotional development of young people with the result that they are unable to address the important developmental challenges of adolescence and later adulthood (Czechowiczh 1988:189-190).

Teenage suicide

The tragic occurrence of suicide among adolescents and even younger children puts pressure on parents, communities and health-care workers to address the problem. It is generally accepted that problems associated with teenage suicide are based on the family environment, social environment and self-image. The most general characteristic among teenagers with suicidal tendencies is the occurrence of depression, which is seldom linked to a single event in the teenager's life but rather manifests itself as the culmination of a longer history. Problems dating from childhood intensify during the teens until they overwhelm the trials of adolescence (White *et al* 1990:655-656).

It is fairly generally accepted that suicidal behaviour among adolescents corresponds in many respects with that of adults. But there are important differences, such as the development of cognitive processes and the formation of identity, which distinguish adolescents from adults (Barr-Joseph & Tzuriel 1990:215). All adults have a moral duty to respect the self-image and thought processes of adolescents so that they can develop to full maturity. In the light of tempestuous behaviour and a teenage culture which excludes adults, it is a difficult to reach teenagers. A young nurse would probably find it more difficult to work with rebellious teenagers than her more experienced colleague would.

Concluding remarks

Ethical issues surrounding reproduction, antenatal care, paediatrics and adolescence compel every nurse to stay abreast of national and international events which affect nursing practice.

Critical thinking activities

1. Name the different ethical issues relating to reproduction and antenatal care.
2. Discuss reproductive technology and infertility as an ethical concern, and refer to the legal implications.
3. Discuss the ethical implications of abortion and indicate how this issue relates to political, social, religious and legal institutions throughout the world.
4. Write short notes on the moral implications of nursing minors.

Nursing and health-care issues from the beginning of adulthood to the end of life

Miemie Groenewald

Outcomes

Studying this chapter will enable you to:
- discuss the ethical issues relating to adulthood
- identify and discuss legislation affecting the nursing care of adults
- identify problems in the care of the aged in the family and in the community
- discuss the ethical issues relating to the end of life.

Introduction

From young adulthood to old age, people are in a state of continuous physical, emotional, economic and social change. Health-care issues that affect adults are legion and vary from one community to the next and from one person to another. During the 20th century an unprecedented and silent revolution in longevity has taken place. The increasing number of aged persons demands the attention of professionals in diverse fields like science, ethics, care-giving, economics, medicine, architecture and urban planning. Socioeconomic policies and social ethics are interwoven in respect the allocation of resources and the responsibilities of the government. Challenging issues concerning the autonomy, rights and quality of life of the aged have to be faced. Funds are needed for health care and social assistance to deal effectively with the frail and bedridden and to advance long-term care programmes for all ages and conditions. The time has come to rethink retirement age and end-of-life decisions. Questions about dying, euthanasia, assisted suicide, the living will, as well as suffering, terminal and machine-dependent patients, need to be reconsidered.

Sexual freedom

The adult's right to sexual freedom is proclaimed in liberal and permissive terms in the media throughout the world. Appeals are made for society's recognition and acceptance of and respect for the emancipation of women, the rights of minority groups, and homosexual and lesbian communities. These appeals may, of course, be offensive to communities with a predominantly traditional conservative view of sexual activity. Irrespective of a person's individual preference and morality in general, adult sexual activity can hold a health risk and contentious arguments must be approached from a health perspective. Various issues, such as sex-change surgery, castration and the danger of AIDS, are directly related to sexual freedom and give rise to moral, ethical, political, social and legal problems.

Adult sexual activity

Sexuality as a basic human need is an integral part of health care. Health-care practitioners work with adults in a variety of clinical situations in which patients' sexuality is affected. In addition to matters associated with reproduction, sexuality is of concern to postoperative patients who have undergone procedures such as mastectomy, hysterectomy, colostomy and other radical surgery (Waterhouse & Metcalfe 1991:1048-1049).

Although it is generally accepted that sexuality has to be taken into account in nursing situations, investigations have revealed a degree of ignorance and anxiety about sexual matters among nurses. Frith and Draper (2004:110-123) explore the relationship between the midwife, the reproductive continuum and sexuality. The proponents of natural childbirth argue that it is not merely an isolated occurrence at one end of a woman's body, but forms part of her whole psychosexual life. Natural childbirth focuses on the power of the woman and the home birth. On the other hand, the scientific, medical model, with its technological procedures, takes childbirth out of women's hands into the powerful, male-dominated hospital setting. There are three discourses of motherhood, namely the natural, in which the midwife is seen as the earth mother; the medical, which portrays the midwife as a coy maiden; and old wives' tales. Midwives need to recognize and acknowledge the sexual nature of childbirth in order to be able to support the woman who is seeking professional assistance.

Sex-change surgery

Sexual identity or psychological sexual identity is the individual's self-concept of being male or female (Gupta 1990:283). Transsexualism is the desire of a biologically normal person of one sex to function as a person of the opposite sex (Benjamin in Chong 1990:88).

Two types of transsexualism are distinguishable, namely primary transsexualism, which begins in childhood and persists throughout the patient's life, and secondary transsexualism in which the condition does not occur during sexual awakening but rather manifests itself after childhood (Stoller in Chong 1990:88). Homosexual and transvestite transsexualism are two types of secondary transsexualism (Chong 1990:88). Hermaphroditism is a congenital abnormality. A hermaphrodite is a person who is born bisexual with characteristics of both sexes. A medical examination must be conducted to determine the sex of such a person. Sex-change surgery on a hermaphrodite is undoubtedly legally permissible, provided the required consent has been granted for the intervention. Surgery is aimed at enabling a person to bring his or her outer appearance in line with the sex concerned (Strauss & Maré 2001:175).

In South Africa, the amendment of sexual description has been legally recognised for identification purposes. With the necessary medical reports and the recommendation of the Director-General of National Health and Population Development, a person can, after undergoing sex-change surgery, have the necessary amendment entered in the register of births by the Director-General of Home Affairs in terms of the Births, Marriages and Deaths Registration Act, 1963 (Act 81 of 1963), section 7B, inserted in the Act by Act 51 of 1974. This section 7B arrangement has been repealed in the new Births, Marriages and Deaths Registration Act, 1992 (Act 51 of 1992) (Strauss & Maré 2001:172).

Legal problems arise when a married person wishes to undergo a sex-change operation, because this would affect the essence of the marriage. The courts tend not to regard the surgery as unlawful, but postoperatively such persons are not allowed to marry. South African law regards a marriage between an adjusted transsexual and a person of the same somatic sex as null and void (Strauss & Maré 2001:175).

Castration

Castration, or emasculation, involves the surgical removal of the male reproductive organs (scrotectomy or testectomy). This is an extremely sensitive therapeutic intervention applied in a life-saving situation to prevent the spread of cancer. Nursing understanding and compassion are of the utmost importance during postoperative care because for most men the loss of manhood and the inability to reproduce are traumatic.

In some countries non-therapeutic castration, which is applied surgically or chemically with the aid of drugs, is used to curb the abnormal sexual urges of sex offenders. Medicinal castration in the area of forensic psychiatry is, however, unacceptable on social and ethical grounds because the drugs apparently contain a high potency that can alter the essential composition of the person's personality (Tancredi & Weisstub 1986:257). In South Africa non-therapeutic castration is regarded as decidedly unlawful (Strauss & Maré 2001:126).

Acquired immune deficiency syndrome (AIDS)

After over a decade of increasing but mainly latent HIV prevalence, the HIV/AIDS epidemic in South Africa is now causing loss of life on a large scale. With 11-20 percent of South African adults HIV infected, 600 000 children orphaned by AIDS, and around 1600 new HIV infections daily in 2002, the projected impact of the disease will account for 75 percent of premature mortalities by the year 2010, compared to 39 percent in 2000. The impact by 2010 will be the greatest on females (Kalichman & Simbayi 2004:572; Bradshaw *et al* 2003:26).

It was estimated that worldwide, by the end of 2003, 34-46 million adults and children would be living with HIV/AIDS. Between 25-28,2 million of these people live in sub-Saharan Africa. The joint United Nations Programme on HIV/AIDS (UNAIDS) and the World Health Organisation (WHO) publish model-based estimates of HIV prevalence, AIDS mortality and orphan numbers for all countries of the world, and these projections form the cornerstone of policy-making on prevention and care. In order to assess the validity of these estimates, a large-scale household survey was undertaken in 2003 to provide an independent source of data for comparison with the published projections. In most sub-Saharan African countries the estimates were found to be lower, but one should not be misled because there is a great lack of reliable statistics. In Zimbabwe and South Africa, where independent estimates of adult mortality from vital registration exist, it was found that these estimates are in close agreement with the published ones (Grassly *et al* 2004:207, 214-216).

In spite of South Africa's efforts to curb the epidemic, the HIV infection rate increased significantly between 1994 and 1998. In July 1999 a meeting was held with representatives of various sectors to review the HIV prevention, treatment and care efforts in South Africa. The HIV/AIDS/STD Strategic Plan for South Africa 2000-2005 was completed in January 2000. This plan focuses mainly on prevention. In 2004, Dr Peter Piot, UNAIDS Executive Director, warned that only widespread access to antiretroviral treatment would substantially mitigate the devastating impact of HIV/AIDS. He also stressed that the focus on treatment should not overshadow the equally important issue of prevention. The Director-General of WHO, Dr Lee Jong-Wook, said that delivery of antiretroviral treatment to the millions who needed it demanded change in the way people think. He said that business as usual would not work because it would mean watching thousands of people die every single day (WHO 2004:24-25).

Since it is a public health crisis with deep social roots, AIDS is unique and presents serious challenges to society. There are no simple choices, easy solutions or quick-fix models. AIDS policies are too weighty to leave in the hands of technocrats (Nattrass 2004:89). It seems that the discussion on AIDS policy has been formally treated on technicalities of affordability and sustainability without knowing what the public wants. Curtailing the size of a national treatment programme suppresses the social values of addressing the AIDS pandemic. South Africans want their government to supply large-scale treatment that will reach all who need it (Nattrass 2004:17). Recently a South African pharmaceutical firm obtained permission from an American one to produce more affordable generic antiretroviral medicines.

In some segments of South African society, AIDS-related stigmas are pervasive. They disrupt the promotion of voluntary counseling, testing and other prevention efforts of the disease. In a recent study it was found that many people would not be willing to share a meal or a room with a person living with AIDS. Some even indicated that they would not talk to a person if they knew he/she had AIDS. The common belief in many traditional African cultures that illness can be attributed to spirits and supernatural forces, like witchcraft, is related to the stigmatising of afflicted persons. Even well-informed and educated professionals have been shown to harbour AIDS stigmas. These believers are all too willing to endorse social sanctions against HIV/AIDS sufferers (Kalichman & Simbayi 2004:572-573, 576).

In the developing world where stigma ensures the survival of the group, at the expense of the individual, the AIDS-related stigma is getting worse. Otherwise rational people express fear and anger through stigmatisation of people living with AIDS. The roots of stigma lie in the logic of basic survival, not the logic of compassion. When people have sufficient resources, they feel compassionate towards the sick, dying, elderly and disadvantaged members of society, but when tough times arrive, they see them as a burden. Humans may be prepared to sacrifice the afflicted ones to ensure survival of the group. To argue that AIDS equals death is to focus on fear instead of on a desired future. Life will be valued, protected and respected when people living with AIDS have a reason to live and contribute to society. The term 'Living with HIV/AIDS' is more positive than 'AIDS victim', and inspires a person to engage in a productive life which will in turn reduce stigma. Emphasis on quantity of life will enhance quality of life and has more benefits for everyone than stigma-based behaviour (Orr & Patient 2004:10-12).

A recent study in the Free State province indicated that HIV/AIDS in South Africa has now reached a stage of rapidly increasing morbidity and mortality. Against the background of widespread poverty and inequality, most people living with AIDS are dependent on government health services. The study looked at income and expenditure on food, education, health care, transport, monthly payments of debt and clothing, as well as remittances made to persons not living with the household. The vicious cycle of AIDS and poverty in poor communities and households was clearly demonstrated. For people living with HIV/AIDS, their families and neighbours need more support than just health care (Bachmann & Booysen 2004:817-826).

For nurses, the ethical implications of AIDS persist. Not only are matters such as professional confidentiality, social stigma and the person's right to health care continually being addressed by the nursing profession, but the time has also arrived to take an introspective look at AIDS-related ethics (Groenewald 1993:22-23).

Euthanasia and adults

In South Africa a nurse may under no circumstances participate in any act which is aimed at the deliberate termination of a patient's life. Such an act is not only unlawful, but also unethical in accordance with the rules of the Nursing Council in South Africa, which provide that nurses shall at all times safeguard human life (Searle & Pera 1992:289).

In a recent international survey on nurses' attitudes towards active euthanasia, the majority of respondents from the seven countries which took part in the survey found no ethical justification for active euthanasia. Some nurses, however, viewed the administering of morphine as a means to control pain as active euthanasia. The majority of respondents were convinced that it would still be unethical for a professional health worker, particularly a nurse, to apply active euthanasia, even if her country had legalised this. The survey also brought to light the fact that religious convictions and the extent to which nurses were involved in their religious practices made no difference to the view of the majority (Davis *et al* 1993:302, 307-309).

A survey in Australia indicated that most nurses were in favour of active euthanasia and wanted legislation which would allow doctors to let a patient die under certain circumstances. Many of the respondents had co-operated with doctors in active euthanasia and a few nurses had applied active euthanasia of their own accord, without consulting a doctor. The researchers concluded that nurses ought not to take matters into their own hands and regarded the present practice of the secret application of euthanasia as undesirable. In the case of incurably ill or terminal patients who prefer death, euthanasia is permissible, according to Kuhse & Singer (1993:321), but such decision-making should take place openly, with adequate opportunities for public investigation and control, something that is not possible under current Australian legislation.

Nurses should incisively investigate ethical and legal problems relating to euthanasia. Opportunities for open discussion among nurses could add to existing knowledge, avoid possible conflict situations and promote personal ethical decision-making (Wilkes, White & Tolley 1993:101). In countries in which euthanasia may possibly be legalised in the future, professional health workers will probably be allowed, as in the case of abortion, to refuse to participate in the procedures on the basis of personal belief or ethical and moral convictions (Ringerman & Koniak-Griffin 1992:8).

Abuse of women

Domestic violence is a common social problem in communities worldwide today. Some believers in some of the world's religions support patriarchy and consider women to be inferior to men (Burkhardt & Nathaniel 2002:305, 308-309).

In cultures in which males are dominant one of the first signs of spouse abuse is when the husband speaks for the wife. In many cultures in Asia, the Middle East and Latin America this is seen as a way of protecting the wife from the outside world. Health professionals should not, however, jump to hasty conclusions based on this evidence only. A more reliable indicator is when there are discrepancies between the location of injuries and the explanation given for them (Galanti 2004:104-105).

In America nurses have investigated abuse in various health-care and community institutions. Research results have led nurses to conduct an assessment of possible abuse as part of their routine assessment of women's health status (Parker & Ulrich 1990:248). In view of nursing's holistic perspective, nursing research can add its unique outlook to the development of knowledge in this field. Given that nurses care for both victims and perpetrators of violence in all health-care settings, they can use their knowledge to provide leadership in health-care policy changes (Spradley & Allender 1997:45-47)

Women of all socio-economic, racial and ethnic groups are abused. They all end up with health complications that range from acute traumatic injuries to chronic physical and emotional impairment. Deliberate physical violence during pregnancy, when they are especially vulnerable, is particularly detrimental to a woman's health and to poor pregnancy outcomes (Burkhardt & Nathaniel 2002:309).

Women who are abused avoid medical help because they are ashamed and fear retribution, or because their husbands do not allow them to consult a doctor. Many women who do make their way to doctors, hospitals or clinics fabricate stories to explain their injuries. Even when health personnel suspect abuse, the women are seldom questioned directly or privately. Health personnel are also sometimes under the impression that it is a private affair or they do not have sufficient time or knowledge to support the abused women. On countless occasions abused women receive a prescription for sedatives or analgesics and simply return to their homes and the violence. Health systems that minimise abuse very often lack proper referral systems, and fail to admit that abuse is the evildoer. Such systems add insult to the abused woman's injuries (Bohn 1991:95; Burkhardt & Nathaniel 2002:309).

Community resources such as shelters for abused women are scarce. Family and friends usually offer only temporary relief and in many instances they do not want to become involved in the problem. Sometimes the abused women fear that their husbands will cause harm to the persons who offer them help (Bohn 1991:93).

Continual abuse of women always has the underlying danger of loss of life. Men may murder their wives under the influence of alcohol or drugs, or in a moment of blind rage. Family murders do occur. Women are in danger of viewing suicide as their only way out and many abused women become so desperate that they murder the perpetrator of the violence.

Abused women who have murdered their husbands appeal for mitigating circumstances on the grounds of self-defence or provocation (incitement to crime). Jurists who defend abused women in the courts are often faced with a jury that displays the traditional social response of denying family violence and the abuse of women, thereby having a negative influence on the administration of justice. The effect of cumulative provocation, fear, anxiety, ensnarement, long-term trauma and the desire for self-preservation are relevant facts in the ultimate conduct of an abused woman (Edwards 1990:1392).

The public outcry against violence and the abuse of women and children is currently under the spotlight of South Africans. Nurses can address this sensitive matter by assessing and identifying the problem, and through advocacy for the patient and co-operation with the multidisciplinary team that has been set up to break the vicious cycle.

Economic-ethical issues

The ideal of 'Health for all by the year 2010' has been proposed by the World Health Organization (WHO), and the Western world endorses this humanitarian philosophy. The question is whether it is realistic to expect the realisation of the WHO's ideal in the current economic, political and social climate. The most important economic-ethical issues lie in the distribution of scarce medical resources, access to health services for all citizens and continually rising costs of medical services. What would a health policy that provides adequate care at an affordable amount look like? The answer is subject to a network of interrelated problems.

Obstacles which reformers of health services have to contend with are the belief in the individual's right to unlimited medical care, the traditional acceptance of the maximalistic approach among doctors, and the belief that the individual should be insulated from feeling the cost of treatment.

Proponents of the individual's right to health care support the unique doctor-patient relationship. On the other side of the debate are policy makers and health economists who have to contend with budget claims that rise faster than any other public spending. As health policy makers decentralise their budgets, constraints enter the consulting rooms of doctors. Concerns like long waiting lists and insufficient care become political issues and patients are suing health-care facilities.

Nursing care for the elderly

Aging is an inevitable process that sets in after adulthood has been attained. Aging is distinct from disease because it takes place even in otherwise healthy people. Senescence is the medical term for the deleterious aspects of aging that contribute to death. Certain diseases are age-related because of their increased incidence in the aged and are believed to be the clinical manifestation of underlying senescence (Butler & Jasmin 2000:62-63).

The aging individual in the longevity revolution

Around the world, nations are experiencing a spectacular increase in longevity of their populations, and five-generation families will soon become the norm. At the end of the 18th century, life expectancy was about 28, whereas at the end of the 20th century a sixty-year old person could expect to live another 20 years, which may extend to 40 years in the 21st century. It is estimated that by the year 2050, the population over the age of 65 will constitute between 20-25 percent of populations in Western Europe, North America and Japan, and more than 15 percent of populations in developing countries.

With regard to the revolution in longevity, there are nowadays four outstanding events that need to be mentioned, namely the:

- extension of human life to 80 or 90 years
- extension of life expectancy without incapacity, even if it varies between different countries or societies
- confirmed difference between the sexes, with most aged societies consisting of female members
- extreme diversity of outcome, in which life's inequity is neither fortune, riches nor poverty, nor gifts or talents, but the last 20 or 30 years of life (Butler & Jasmin 2000:277).

The spectre of loneliness and existential misery that is the lot of many old people is so serious that people under the age of 65 often cannot envisage a long-term future, even when many persons over the age of 85 have proven that octogenarians can have a healthy and productive life. No one can ignore the pathos of progressive isolation and impoverishment, the pain of increasing dependence and repeated incidents of mourning, the feelings of worthlessness, the disruption through hospitalisation and institutio-nalisation, and the increasing vulnerability to family, societal and political changes. As they grow older, the meaningfulness of the lives of aged persons is very much determined by the norms, values and ethical-professional conduct of those who care for them and of those younger than themselves. Nurses can enrich the lives of the aged by caring for them in a holistic manner and treating them with respect, understanding, patience and wisdom.

The older person as a family member

No institution compares with the family when it comes to caring for the elderly.

In current health-care models in the United States of America, it is recommended that the frail elderly will be cared for at home by family and friends to alleviate strain on the health-care system. Family members may, however, actually be unable to provide such care because they have other personal responsibilities or they are geographically separated from their aged family member. Caregivers of the elderly experience financial and emotional strain. The age revolution also implies that the caregivers are often aged as well and in need for assistance (Burkhardt & Nathaniel 2002:310-311). The additional, often permanent and uninterrupted, care of old and dependent family members often aggravates physical, emotional and financial stress to such a degree that the dependent person is regarded as a burden or a nuisance. Reluctance, unwillingness and resentment at their obligation, together with a sense of guilt, further complicate the task of caring and may even lead to the neglect and abuse of the dependent person.

There has been an enormous change in the structure of households across the globe. There is a trend away from three or even two-generation households towards the one-generation household. In 1995 Germany introduced a care insurance which pays family members to provide care in private households. Many family members have since been motivated to assume the difficult responsibility of full-time care of their elders (Butler & Jasmin 2000:246).

The social arrangements of traditional Africa were based on the extended family system that can be seen as a type of social welfare system. Economic development during the colonial period simply viewed traditional arrangements as a barrier to economic and social progress. The concentration of government investment in the urban areas of most countries of tropical Africa, resulted in substantial rural-urban migration. The aftermath of such cultural blindness and demographic pressures was family disintegration. The traditional practice in rural Africa of support for the elderly in kind has now changed in the urban context to support requiring cash (Butler & Jasmin 2000:276-277.

There is a general consensus that low-income countries lack resources in the public sector to care for their elderly populations. Policy makers need to explore the opposition between family care and public service delivery. The prospects for mutual support and opportunities, which are concealed by the tendency to view the aged simply as recipients of care and services, are no model for Africa. Aged Africans should be empowered to exercise maximum autonomy, but lack of education has to be addressed first. The assumption that classrooms are for children must be resisted to give older persons a chance to gain literacy.

With their legacy of generational skills, like traditional craft and cultural history, the elderly can enhance the educational process.

In the face of modern lifestyles, economic pressures and the longevity revolution, the ideal of family caring for the aged becomes more and more difficult to attain. Many health systems have day or periodic care centres, or professional home-care services, to support families who care for their elders at home, as well as for aged people who live on their own.

Care of the aged within the family requires attention to their safety and privacy. Resources such as wheelchairs and walking aids, which the family can seldom afford, facilitate home care. Methods of acquiring the necessary resources and of periodically releasing the home-caregiver and the particular family from a never-ending obligation must be found urgently, if necessary even at political level.

The older person in the community

In many instances the aged no longer enjoy the respect they did in the past. The Constitution of the Republic of South Africa contains a Bill of Rights which specifically prohibits the state from unfairly discriminating against anyone on one or more grounds, including, among others, age; but in practice there is still discrimination against the elderly. This is known as ageism, and if society and individuals want to prevent it, it needs to be honestly acknowledged (Jenkins 2002:67).

Policies on aging reflect the society as a whole. A welcoming, community-oriented society, which respects its members, will tend to practise the same morality regarding its elders, while an individualistic society in which corporate interests dominate, will tend to treat its aged in a less caring manner. The question arises whether individuals are really ready to live longer, and whether society is prepared to make this prolonged life worthwhile. The tendency to view working life as a relatively short-term necessity and retirement as exclusion from society needs a turnabout. Re-integration of the aged into society will probably be supported by a minority, because of deeply held views on the place of retired people in society. Policies should not be determined only by questions of what can be done for the elderly, but also by considerations of what the aged can do for society (Butler & Jasmine 2000:15, 19, 254).

Certain economic discussions give the impression that longevity is a bad thing because it affects the rising costs of health care and pensions. However, given the scientific effort that has gone into prolonging human life, increased life expectancy should be a cause for joy and not only a financial liability (Butler & Jasmin 2000:255).

The lack of research on aging by national and international bodies for geriatric studies, and the indifference of authorities to the age revolution, are unethical (Butler & Jasmin 2000:280).

Retirement

In military terms, retirement refers to retreat and defeat. Retirement can be seen as a horrible experience in civilian life too, especially when people are forced to retire and then excluded by society. Retired persons may feel isolated, useless, expendable and victims of a system of perpetual humiliation. They end up feeling ashamed for not being young and guilty for still being alive. The elderly were previously respected, obeyed, admired and appreciated, for old age was synonymous with wisdom. In ancient civilisations the older men were leaders, and the Bible also teaches respect for the elderly. Today the paradox exists that, on the one hand, medical science is determined to extend human life, and on the other, people are often prevented from enjoying it. The challenge is to adjust the traditional ways of providing for retirement and, since people live longer, to raise the age of retirement (Butler & Jasmin 2000:191, 284).

Quality of life

Technology enables medical science to keep people alive and physically functioning, but its unforeseen consequence is how it impacts on the quality of life. What makes life worth living means different things to different people and cultures. Each individual has a personal perspective on quality of life and, therefore, health-care professionals must take care not to judge the quality of somebody else's life on the basis of their own values. The aged and people with debilitating health disorders may still consider the quality of their lives in a positive light (Butler & Jasmin 2000:179).

Although it is possible to analyse and measure some physical, psychological and social determinants that are relevant to the quality of life, the notion remains difficult to define. Quality of life is an obvious factor in deciding on treatment for conditions such as senility and dementia. However, since a reliable qualitative measure of a patient's experience is impossible, caution must be exercised when deciding whether or not a person's life has quality (Monagle & Thomasma 1994:170).

The quality of life of the aged population poses a challenge to medicine and nursing not to view the elderly in materialistic or mechanical terms, as the recipients of more and more sophisticated technology. The older person remains a human being with feelings, experiences and a specific life project. Caregivers should always be in the service of the person. To ensure quality of life the emotional intelligence of the patient should be taken into account (Butler & Jasmin 2000:156-157).

People from all walks of life and cultures agree that dignity is of cardinal importance to the individual and society. Dignity refers to a person's self-importance (internal), and to the state or quality of being worthy of honour (external). The violation of dignity can be divided into four broad categories: not acknowledging a person, group-categorising an individual, violating personal space and humiliating a person by separating him/her from the group (Butler & Jasmin 2000:149-151).

When the aged are still strong and active, they command respect, but family members and caregivers often mistreat dependent old people. Elderly persons with diminished faculties, and partly or greatly reduced abilities, are still entitled to unqualified respect for what is human in each individual (Butler & Jasmin 2000:279).

Growing old implies deterioration and decrepitude, an inevitable decline that moves to a predestined end. The modern trend is to grow old without looking old, because nobody likes old age in a society that focuses on youth. Frankly speaking, there is a cult of youth worship which views young people as gods. No wonder old age is referred to as the golden age in America, and the third age in France (Butler & Jasmin 2000:283).

Institutional and long-term care

It is the functional status of an aged person, rather than a particular illness or disability, that will determine the need for long-term care. Functional status is generally measured in terms of the person's ability to perform five activities of independent daily living, namely bathing, ambulating from a bed or a chair, dressing, eating and going to the toilet. Most older persons need assistance with at least one of these activities (Monagle & Thomasma 1994:159).

The autonomy of the elderly living in nursing homes poses an urgent challenge for ethicists and others. In spite of the guarantee of legal rights, residents' rights can be violated. The tendency of many nursing home staff members to treat the elders as infantile complicates the situation. Based on the medical model of governance, nursing home management is often inclined to emphasise its obligation to ensure the safety of residents, but in fact end up curbing the free movement of the aged. Elderly people who receive attentive treatment from staff are often willing to accept a subservient role in exchange for it (Monagle & Thomasma 1994:179-182).

Palliative care

Palliative care is the active, comprehensive and interdisciplinary care of patients with an advanced, progressive and incurable disease. Palliative care affirms life and regards dying as a natural process. It focuses on the comfort and support of patients and families. There are three precepts of palliative caring, namely utilising the strength of interdisciplinary resources, acknowledging and addressing caregiver concerns, and building systems and mechanisms of support (Butler & Jasmin 2000:184-185; Miteff 2001:1; Burkhardt & Nathaniel 2002:193-194).

Nationally and internationally there is a growing awareness of the need to improve the care of the dying. Owing to the prevalence of chronic and progressive disease, and technological intervention, the experience of dying has changed over the past decades with many people enduring prolonged death. The efforts to improve the needless suffering of dying patients are often frustrated by deficient caring models, lack of education and inadequate knowledge about the course, treatment and outcomes of caring for dying patients and their families. In the 1990s the Project on Death in America (PDIA) was initiated to address the issue of death and dying. Palliative care has become a medical speciality in the United Kingdom and Australia (Butler & Jasmin 2000:181, 185).

The philosophy of palliative care is underpinned by two principles: the inclusion of the patient and family as the unit of care, and the palliation of total suffering. The subjectivity of the term 'suffering', that is what one person may consider unbearable and another may find tolerable, often leads to ethical arguments in which the goal of care and acceptable courses of action are debated. In critical situations, conflict may arise between the dying patient, family, doctor and nurses.

In this age of technological advances nurses still act ethically in providing end-of-life care. The two primary obligations to dying patients are comfort and company. Co-ordinated and continuous service in the home, hospice and hospital is needed. Palliative care does not intend to hasten death or to prolong life, but to ensure comfort, dignity and quality of life as understood by both patient and caregiver. Good nursing is the backbone of palliative care. Apart from providing measures to relieve pain and other distressing symptoms, nurses give continuous care that supports the emotional and existential concerns of patients and their loved ones. Nurses co-ordinate palliative care team-members to explain and negotiate care decisions. They are willing to allow time for families to decide whether or not to withhold further interventions in favour of palliative care. In a caring environment, nurses help the patient to maintain a sense of well-being and to experience a dignified and peaceful closure to life. They support families near the end of life, at the moment of death, and in bereavement (Burkhardt & Nathaniel 2002:193-194; Miteff 2001:3; Pang 2003:237).

The ethical issue of withholding or withdrawing artificial nutrition and hydration from dying and permanently unconscious patients has become a grave problem because thousands of patients are on tube feeding. Discontinuing artificial feeding is more difficult to apply than stopping antibiotic treatment, because there is a uniquely symbolic significance attached to nourishment. Yet, there are sound ethical grounds for discontinuing artificial feeding to permit death to occur from natural causes. There is no medical, nursing or ethical justification for ceasing to provide care to a dying patient. The question is whether artificial feeding is a basic care procedure or part of medical treatment (Monagle & Thomasma 1994:217-218; Miteff 2001:4).

Artificial feeding is profoundly problematic because a basic instinct of survival and human caring is now linked to a medical procedure. This evokes the fear of becoming imprisoned as a living dead person. Considered as a low technology, or so-called care replacement, artificial feeding is often left to the jurisdiction of nurses. How it fits in with the caring/treatment debate is not clear and adds to uncertainty about its use. Older people themselves have different viewpoints on medical treatment during end-of-life care. Some are against aggressive treatment, while others are willing to accept higher mortality risks associated with intervention, even if possible survival may reduce their quality of life. To predict patients' reactions in this regard would be unwise. There is in any case still no consensus on the advantages or disadvantages of artificial nutritional support for dying older people. Inextricably linked to appropriate use of artificial feeding are the concepts of care, natural death, personhood, family and clinical obligation (Gastmans 2002:171-173, 189).

Depending on the etiology of the condition, the age at which dementia most likely manifests is 85+ years. The effects of tube feeding in patients with advanced dementia were previously regarded as nearly risk free and the treatment, therefore, beneficial. But now evidence shows that the risks are exceeding the rather illusory benefits. People who support tube feeding argue that it is a moral duty to provide nourishment and to relieve thirst. They see liquid as a symbol of life, administration of food and fluids as an expression of concern and compassion, while withdrawal is viewed as systematic killing. Supporters of stopping tube feeding believe that withdrawal is more comfortable for the terminal patient with dementia, and therefore it is the patient's moral right not to be fed. They recommend close contact with the patient and maximum comfort instead. Continued feeding may in fact be a way of refusing to accept an inevitable death. There seems to be consensus among medical practitioners and ethicists on withholding tube feeding for patients with advanced dementia in the terminal phase. Difficulty with eating indicates that the final stage of this fatal disorder has been entered, and the inability to swallow is unfortunately part of dying naturally in this patient group (Gastmans 2002:198, 200, 201, 214).

The use of sedation in palliative care has its therapeutic value to prevent a known and unforeseen harm, like pain relief and relief of emotional distress, but in the context of palliative care, sedation can also be interpreted adversely as slow euthanasia. Depending on the clinical situation, palliative sedation can be properly used. Sedation for the relief of a refractory symptom or severe mental distress is a humane act. Refractory or obstinate symptoms are symptoms that cannot be adequately controlled despite aggressive efforts to identify a tolerable therapy that does not compromise consciousness. Breathlessness or anxiety can cause mental distress when the feeling of suffocation or loss of control persists. A patient who faces the last few days or hours of life in a state of cognitive impairment and pain is a frequent occurrence. The time frame for decision-making collapses and the symptoms become refractory because there is no time for treatment other than sedation. The required reduction of consciousness is obtained by superficial or deep sedation. Consent must be obtained from the next of kin because at this point the patient's consent is usually unavailable, unless the palliative team has discussed such issues with the patient and family in advance. Palliative caregivers should bear in mind that the clinical outcome of sedation is the calmness of patients, and not their lives or deaths (Gastmans 2002:220-223).

Death and dying

Dying and death are the culmination of life. Death is the one certain event that does not make an exception of anyone. For most human beings dying is a terrifying experience. Notwithstanding religious beliefs that are consciously held, the mystery of death is obscured by fear. In some ancient cultures and according to some contemporary healing techniques, death is seen as a transition from one state of consciousness to another. Some bioethical enquirers find it impossible to accommodate such beliefs in their intellectual and scientific framework (Cohen 2003:262, 265-267).

In a society where youth, health and fitness are emphasised, there is a tendency to deny or disregard the subject of death. Frequently the dying relative, friend or neighbour is quarantined in a retirement complex, an old-age home, nursing home or hospital. This enables people to avoid confrontation with death and it becomes the enemy instead of the natural culmination of life. Modern medicine is often hailed for its imagined unlimited capacity to reverse dying and death (Devine 2000:208-209). The death of an aged person is often a source of embarrassment to professional and other health workers, particularly those who have not achieved a full understanding of their own approach to life and death. In order to deal with the suffering, dying and death of the aged with empathy and compassion, nurses have to have overcome the fear of their own mortality.

Death is a fact, an event that has occurred, and a life that has ended. Dying refers to the process of passing from life to death. It may be swift, unexpected and instantaneous, or slow, painful, extending over weeks, months and even years. No matter how death occurs, it gives rise to many medical, legal and moral questions (Devine 2000:195).

Traditionally the irreversible cessation of all cardiopulmonary function indicates death, or cardiac death. However, now that machines that can take over the functioning of heart and lungs, it has become impossible to ascertain whether all spontaneous cardiopulmonary functions have ceased permanently (Devine 2000:197-198; Fremgen 2002:213). The problem with the traditional definition is that a person who has suffered a cardiac arrest may be successfully resuscitated with CPR, even if the person was clinically dead. Another problem associated with cardiac death involves organ transplantation. Waiting for a donor's cardiac death will render the donated organs useless for transplantation. Changing the definition of death to increase the availability of the number of organs for transplantation is obviously unethical. However, many people agree that a cardiac-orientated definition of death is no longer adequate (Fremgen 2002:214).

Brain death is a condition of irreversible coma that describes the characteristics of a permanently nonfunctioning brain. The four criteria that indicate that all cerebral and brain-stem function has ceased, are: unreceptiveness and unresponsiveness to externally applied stimuli; no spontaneous muscular movements or voluntary breathing; no reflexes; and a flat electro-encephalogram (Devine 2000:198-199; Fremgen 2002:214).

The fact of death is legally significant because the individual is legally no longer a person, and all rights cease. All that remains is the need for a respectful interment to be arranged by the family. Other legal consequences of the fact of death are payment of insurance, the passing of assets to heirs, and the changed marital status of the spouse. Finally, the state requires that a death certificate be issued indicating that life has ended due to natural causes, or by accident, or through criminal intent (Devine 2000:203).

Euthanasia

Euthanasia, painless death or mercy killing poses serious problems. There are two main categories, namely active and passive euthanasia.

Active euthanasia occurs where the doctor, or health worker, both provides the means of death and administers it. Euthanasia always involves someone else, other than the individual who dies. In South Africa, the causing of death by a positive action is unlawful. There is no legal defence in South African law for consent to homicide. When a doctor merely facilitates the death of a patient by providing the necessary means required to enable the patient to end his/her life, it is called physician-assisted suicide.

In accordance with South African law, to hasten death is in fact to cause it. A doctor who is sincerely and reasonably attempting to relieve a patient's pain, and indirectly hastens the death of the patient, is not guilty of murder, because the conduct was not unlawful. When the administration of a pain-alleviating method can be qualified as an act with double effect, it must not be defined according to its side-effect, the unavoidable shortening of life, but according to its main aim, which is to combat pain (Burkhardt & Nathaniel 2002:225; Devine 2000:219, 221; Strauss & Maré 2001:91-94).

Whenever a mentally competent person, who possesses all the necessary information and who has voluntarily refused certain treatment (e.g. chemotherapy) and/or agreed to only selected treatment (e.g. repeated administering of an increasing dose of analgesics and sedation to remain pain-free), is allowed to die, this is usually regarded as passive euthanasia. As requested by the Roman Catholic Church, and others, the term 'passive euthanasia' is being replaced by the phrase 'allow to die' (Fremgen 2002:217).

Related to passive euthanasia is the debate on the right to die. One can rightfully ask whether a right to die exists, and whether anyone could claim such a right. Is a person who is in a dying mode or irreversibly dying, or who is gravely ill or disabled but clearly not dying, competent to exercise such a right? Incompetent people like elderly, senile persons in a permanent vegetative state, the mentally ill, those who have lost competence or who have never been competent, may need proxies to exercise such a right. In spite of people's fears of living too long, with no purpose or meaning to life, of being dependent on others and becoming senile and losing control over life and destiny, there is still no philosophical or legal foundation for a right to die, or for suicide or assistance from another to die. The basis of all human rights is the right to life (Devine 2000:207).

Advanced directives are written statements in which people state the type and amount of care they wish to receive during a terminal illness. If these documents, such as a living will, durable power of attorney for health care, Anatomical Gift Act, or 'do not resuscitate' (DNR) order, have to be drawn up after a patient has entered a facility, then they should be done so in a non-stressful manner. These documents not only allow a person to plan for the management of health care and/or financial affairs in the event of incapacity, but they can also contain a patient's written request to ask for maximum care and treatment for as long as possible. Although the South African Law Commission published a report in the late 1990s to recommend statutory recognition of living wills, it has not yet resulted in legislation (Fremgen 2002:221-222; Lindberg, Hunter & Kruszewski 1998:369; Strauss & Maré 2001:103).

One of the disadvantages of advanced directives is that they usually do not apply to mentally incompetent persons and minors. There are also several drawbacks to living wills. There is no guidance in unanticipated situations if a person has given specific instructions. Alternatively, if a person tries to give general guidelines, applicable to any situation, there is ambiguity, leading different people to different interpretations of the person's wishes. Additional defects in living wills are the failure to anticipate unwanted medical interventions, and the possibility of ending lives in ways people never intended, years earlier than natural death. Policies that often seem pretty obvious and simple, are in fact extremely complicated (Lindberg et al 1998:369; Hall, Bobinski & Orentlicher 2003:552; Smith 1996:204-205).

From a nursing point of view there are many vague and troubling issues in relation to euthanasia. Nurses, who traditionally support patients and families with the idea of natural death as being the best and most loving choice, now have to deal with a situation where the patient indicates that life has become intolerable and asks for euthanasia. Under all circumstances the nurse has to do her best and, together with the family, remains closely involved with the dying person, continuing to provide empathic and compassionate care up to the last moment (Burkhardt & Nathaniel 2002:226).

Concluding remarks

The ethical issues affecting adults and the elderly until the very end of life cover the entire spectrum of human rights and place particular emphasis on the freedom, privacy, autonomy and human dignity of the individual. The longevity revolution is changing the demographic composition of societies and professional health workers, who attach particular value to their confidential relationships on which their services are based, will have to take note of the growing elderly population's needs. Nurses act as advocates of the patient's interests and rights, especially of the vulnerable aged patient, and handle sensitive matters with circumspection.

Critical thinking activities

1. Discuss the rights of adults to sexual freedom as an ethical issue for nurses.
2. Write concise notes on nursing ethics relating to the following:
   - sex-change surgery
   - castration
   - the abuse of women
   - economic-ethical issues.
3. Describe the impact of longevity on families, communities and health services.
4. Discuss the issues related to euthanasia.
5. Make a list of the various Acts with which nurses who work with adults and the elderly come into contact.

11

Management ethics

Anne-Mart Oosthuizen

Outcomes

Studying this chapter will enable you to:

■ recognise possible ethical violations in the management of health-care organisations
■ critically discuss the role played by management in promoting ethical conduct in the health care organisation
■ identify the common ethical issues that arise at the workplace.

Introduction

What do business and ethics have in common? The answer to this question is neither straightforward nor without controversy. Paine in Donaldson, Werhane and Cording (2002:586) argues that many managers think of ethics as a personal matter between individuals and their consciences. These managers describe any wrongdoing by employees as isolated incidents and the work of bad employees. They do not consider the possibility that the company might bear any responsibility for an individual's misdeeds because they believe that ethics has nothing to do with management. The author asserts, however, that, in fact, ethics has everything to do with management. Ethics is as much an organisational as a personal issue. Managers have to provide proper leadership and institute systems that facilitate ethical conduct. If they don't, they share responsibility with those who execute and benefit from corporate misdeeds. Ethical behaviour in the health-care industry is essential and setting ethical standards is vital. Wells & Spinks (1996(b):21) indicate that administrators of health care institutions and health care providers should work together to establish codes of ethics that define boundaries for ethical behaviour in the health-care industry.

Organisational ethics defined

'Business ethics... has to do with the authenticity and integrity of the enterprise' (McCoy (1997) in Tappen 2001:417). Within health-care organisations, the focus on ethical issues usually has to do with the care and protection of individual patients. Continuous change, rising costs and the increasing demand for quality health-care services have contributed to changes in the way that managers in health-care organisations view ethical issues. The possibility of fraud in medical aid schemes, the introduction of managed care and other issues such as sexual harassment have contributed to the introduction of a new concept: namely organisational ethics. According to Spencer, Mills, Rorty and Werhane (2000) in

Groenewald (2001:35), organisational ethics is the articulation, application and evaluation of the consistent values and moral positions of an organisation by which it is defined, both internally and externally. Organisation ethics consists of ways of addressing ethical issues associated with the business, financial and management areas of health-care organisations, as well as with professional, educational and contractual relationships affecting the operation of the health-care organisation. The aim of an organisational ethics programme is to create a positive ethical climate for an organisation's activities.

Core values for making ethical decisions in the workplace

Tappen (2001:417) lists the following core values underlying ethics in the workplace:

- honesty
- integrity
- fairness
- trustworthiness
- respect
- responsibility
- accountability
- good citizenship.

The author points out that in health-care settings, patient welfare and excellence in the delivery of health care are additional core values.

The role of management in ethical business practices in health-care organisations

Most institutions and organisations want to portray an image of integrity and ethical behaviour. Consequently, social responsibility programmes and codes of ethics are developed to reassure employees that company leadership is committed to ethical conduct. The code of ethics, as well as management's support of the code, must be communicated clearly to all persons in the organisation (Wells & Spinks 1996(a):28). Managers must acknowledge their role in shaping organisational ethics and seize the opportunity to create a climate that can strengthen the factors on which their organisation's success depends (Donaldson *et al* 2002:587). The leaders/managers in an organisation should set an example. According to George S. May International Company (2004(a):5) the most important leadership trait is setting an example of the behaviour you expect from others. Regardless of what is written in the code of conduct of an organisation, the behaviour of the managers/leaders sets the standard that employees will follow. A standard of ethical behaviour will reduce pressure on employees to compromise ethical standards and improve trust and respect at all levels. It will increase pride, professionalism and productivity and enhance an organisation's ability to attract and retain high-quality and diverse employees.

All organisations should develop a policy on ethics. Ethics is part of corporate culture. Swansburg and Swansburg (2002:246) assert that ethical organisations try to satisfy all of their stockholders, are dedicated, committed to learning and try to be the best in whatever they do. Leaders of ethical organisations have the moral courage to change direction, hire brilliant subordinates, encourage innovation and stick to values. Management can encourage ethical behaviour by introducing internal workshops or conferences on ethics while welcoming contributions of clinical nursing and health-care staff. Ethics can be built into orientation programmes, management development courses and participative management policies and procedures. George S. May International Company (2004(b):3) found that only a limited number of organisations are taking positive steps to improve and enforce ethical operation. The author concludes that the ethical focus must come from the top of any organisation, but should not remain only at the top. It needs to be instilled by example and by training through all levels of an organisation.

Administrators of health-care institutions and providers of health care should investigate all aspects of ethical behaviour in their operations. Differences between ethical and unethical practices should be identified and sanctions placed against unethical practices. The identification of ethical and unethical practices is not always easy. In today's highly complex health-care industry even ethical health-care providers find it difficult to determine exactly what actions are ethical and what actions are not (Wells & Spinks 1996(b):22). This is sometimes because the definition of 'ethical' may differ from one individual to another.

An overview of stakeholders in the health-care industry affected by ethical management

Management plays a special role in the contemporary health care organisation. Freeman in Donaldson *et al* (2002:44) points out that, on the one hand, management's stake is like that of employees, while on the other hand, management has a duty to safeguard the welfare of the abstract entity, the organisation or corporation. Management must look after the well-being of the corporation and this involves balancing the multiple claims of conflicting stakeholders. Owners and investors want higher financial returns, clients want more money spent on development and services, while employees want higher wages and better benefits. It is the task of management to keep the relationship among stakeholders in balance.

Ethics in the management of a health-care institution can be examined from various perspectives. The question of ethical versus unethical management in the case of investors, employees and patients in a health-care organisation (Wells & Spinks 1996(b):22) will now be addressed.

Investors

Most health-care institutions share characteristics of other business corporations where investors have entrusted their money to the management teams of those companies. These investors play no role in the administration of the companies and usually know little about their operations. There are many opportunities for unethical practice that could harm these investors. A controversial area in health-care ethics is the responsibility of administrators to remain ethical while returning profits to their investors. Some actions in pursuit of profits, such as using medicines that have passed their expiry date or denying treatment to critically ill people who may not have adequate funds or medical aids, seem clearly unethical and even illegal. However, grey areas are common. For example, how often should safety precautions be performed in an institution? The frequency with which certain precautions are performed could result in lower profits for investors or cost increases for patients. On the other hand, if the measures are performed less frequently than necessary, it could endanger employees and patients. The allocation of nursing staff can also pose ethical questions. Too few nurses in attendance would be unethical; however, more nurses per shift take away profits from investors and increase costs to patients (Wells & Spinks 1996:23).

Employees

Unethical business practices can arise in the areas of equal employment opportunities, pay, gender, disabled employees, employee safety, sexual harassment and other forms of discrimination. Although much has been done in South Africa to end discriminatory practices in the workplace with regard to gender and pay, unethical behaviour in the areas of the rights of disabled people to equal opportunities and sexual harassment still exist. Employee safety is another concern related to ethics in health-care institutions. Shindul-Rothschild, Berry and Long-Middleton (1996:25-39) report that some nurses are at risk of work-related injuries or violent acts against them. This also applies to other health-care professionals. It is suggested that understaffing in health-care settings may put health-care practitioners at even greater risks for injury from violent assaults. Health-care practitioners working in hospitals in South Africa in areas with very high crime rates and gang related crimes are vulnerable and their personal safety is at risk. According to Geyer (2004:36) South Africa is one of the countries with the highest prevalence of violence in the workplace of health care, with patients and their families being the biggest perpetrators. The question according to Wells & Spinks (1996b:25) is how much safety is necessary for ethical treatment of employees and how much safety is an unnecessary waste of investor's money and an unnecessary increase in patients' costs.

Patients

Wells and Spinks (1996(b):26) assert that a major area of ethical concern in health care is the area of relationships between health-care institutions and patients. When a patient uses the services of a health-care provider, a main concern is safety. It can be assumed that adequate safety measures will be taken to protect the patient against infection, improper procedures and medication errors. However, more safety measures erode the profits for investors and/or increase costs to patients.

Patient safety is also at stake in hospital settings that are understaffed and lacking resources. Expecting nursing personnel to work long hours without enough staff to provide safe nursing care or adequate resources to provide for the health needs of patients, raises questions regarding the ethical management of the institution. Certainly, adequate safety measures should be taken. But, how many safety measures are enough and how many would be a waste of investors' and patients' money?

Management of resources

The allocation of resources is another ethical issue affecting patient care. Llewellyn, Eden and Lay (1999:7) argue that the priorities and interests of providers, rather than patients, drive the allocation of resources in health care. The authors maintain that the medical profession is in a strong position in health-care organisations and there are potential risks for an abuse of their power. There has been an assumption that medical practitioners rely purely on ethical codes when making decisions about patient care and that the principles of autonomy, beneficence, non-maleficence and justice form the basis for ethical decision making in health care. The problem with these principles is that they do not provide any definitive guide for the management of resources in health-care organisations. Since medical ethics does not provide clear answers, the opportunity for financial and professional incentives to drive decision-making is created.

Social responsibility programmes and codes of ethics

The growing demand for social responsibility and ethical behaviour in business has resulted in the development of social responsibility programmes. Wells and Spinks (1996(a):29) assert that the effectiveness of these programmes differs widely from company to company. In order for these programmes and their supporting codes of ethics to be effective, upper-level management must develop and communicate them throughout the organisation.

Most companies that wish to improve their ethical behaviour develop codes of ethics for their organisations. A code of ethics informs everyone in the organisation that management is committed to ethical behaviour and that it expects ethical behaviour from every employee. It provides a set of written guidelines for each employee to follow. The attitude of management towards the company's code of ethics sets the tone for lower-level employees. Schlegelmilch and Houston (1989:10) have found that the mere existence of a code of ethics can raise the ethical level of business behaviour because it clarifies what is meant by ethical conduct. In their analysis of the contents of the ethical codes of companies, the authors found that employee conduct was the most widely covered topic. Following in importance were the community and environment and, lastly, the customers.

Development of an organisational code of ethics

A committee representing all groups and levels of employees and managers should develop the code of ethics for the organisation and also develop a plan for implementing all aspects of the code. If necessary, outside communication consultants and ethics experts should be called in to assist in the development of a viable plan for implementing the code (Wells & Spinks 1996(a):29). How the code is developed, and why the code is developed, is as important as the code itself. According to Von Baeyer (2004:1) the focus of a code, whether it points the way for employees to do business with integrity or just sets out some prohibitions, is also crucial.

Implementing a code of ethics

The company's social responsibility programme is a programme that must be handled competently if the company's social responsibility objectives are to be met successfully. Wells and Spinks (1996:30) explain that the development of the programme and the adoption of a code of ethics involves not only providing for ethical behaviour, but also structuring and writing the programme and the code in a language that will be easily understood and successfully implemented by the employees in an organisation. The authors explain that implementing a code of ethics involves communicating:

- the code to everyone in the organisation in a way that can be understood
- support of management for the code
- ways in which the code should be implemented by each individual in the organisation
- the code to the public
- ways in which the code should not be violated.

However, the authors warn that listing every possible example of unethical behaviour is impossible and, therefore, management must exercise care. Many employees might conclude that anything not on the list is considered a legitimate, ethical action. The major focus of the code of ethics should, therefore, be positive, by emphasising the demonstration of ethical behaviour instead of emphasising unethical behaviour. In order to ensure the approval and support from everyone in an organisation, the value of such a code should be communicated to all employees. Without every employee's support a code of ethics will not be successful.

Once a code of ethics has been implemented it should be used to address dilemmas in the workplace or organisation. Recognising workplace dilemmas is the first step in making the code of ethics a living document. Resolving a dilemma involves gathering the facts and working through the code of ethics. The ethical options and implications should then be discussed with colleagues. If these steps are followed, there will be consistent, sound decision-making in the organisation (Von Baeyer 2004:1).

Guidelines for promoting ethical conduct

The greatest leadership responsibility is setting an ethical example. George S. May International Company (2004(a):3) provides the following guidelines to managers to assist with ethical management in their organisations:

- Provide employees with all the relevant policies and guidelines, thus eliminating ignorance of the rules.
- Involve employees in identifying core values in the organisation and use them to guide and evaluate decisions and conduct.
- Ensure highly competent employees by providing opportunities to improve skills, knowledge of job requirements and information about the organisation.
- Make 'ethics' a regular topic of conversation in the organisation.
- Identify people within the organisation to whom employees could turn for guidance and help with ethical issues and for reporting suspected ethics violations.
- Ensure that employees face no negative consequences for doing what they feel is right, for questioning the decisions and actions of others, including those of management.
- Recruit, employ and promote people who have demonstrated a commitment to business ethics. Make it known that to work and advance in your organisation, you have to perform with the highest integrity.
- Respond quickly and thoroughly to all unethical behaviour that come to your knowledge. Demonstrate zero tolerance for ethics violations.

Ethical issues in the health-care organisation

For Tappen (2001:420) the most common unethical business practices are covering up incidents, lying about sick leave, deceiving customers, lying to supervisors and doing inferior work (cutting corners). The author, however, adds some ethical concerns that are specific to the health-care setting. These relate to:

■ receiving gifts – the effect of receiving a gift on quality of care
■ theft and property damage – costs are raised when damaged or lost equipment has to be replaced
■ cover-ups – individuals are sometimes expected to change information to protect someone
■ leaking confidential information – revealing confidential information can harm the organisation, patients or employees
■ inappropriate assignments – nurses should reject an assignment that puts patients and/or themselves in serious jeopardy
■ reporting fraud (whistle-blowing) – padding costs, submitting bills for services not rendered, offering kickbacks for referring patients, are some of the types of fraud that occur in health care
■ protecting patients – inadequate staff, incompetent practitioners, unavailability of services and human error can put individuals' lives in jeopardy.

Concluding remarks

Ethical behaviour in the management of health-care organisations is essential and in the best interest of the patients, employees and the organisation and its shareholders. It is, however, not always easy to determine what behaviour is ethical and what is unethical. It is, therefore, necessary that organisations develop ethical codes to provide guidelines for those who are responsible for managing the organisation and for promoting ethical behaviour among employees. This chapter concludes with a warning from George S. May International Company (2004(b):3) that '[c]odes of ethics and ethics departments are good. However, these should be viewed as means to an end, not the end in themselves. Acting ethically is the responsibility of every person in a company. That is the only practical way to stop the ethical problems confronting businesses today'.

Critical thinking activities

1. Explain the role of management in ethical business practices in the health-care organisation.
2. Describe a situation where you were confronted by possible ethics violations in the management of the health-care institution where you work.
3. Discuss guidelines to promote ethical conduct by employees in the organisation where you work.

Ethics in research

Dirk van der Wal

Outcomes

Studying this chapter will enable you to:

- design an ethics evaluation matrix for your research
- question whether a research project is ethical
- indicate how you would alleviate vulnerability of research participants during a research project
- indicate how ethics relate to research and the research process.

Introduction

In this chapter we pay attention to the application of ethics in research. This application requires some proficiency with the terminology (fundamental concepts, theories and principles) of both ethics and research, so that researchers and members of research and ethics committees are in a better position to anticipate and identify possible ethical (and legal) problems resulting from research.

Key definition

For the purpose of this chapter, the term *participant* refers to all human data sources and includes the terms *informants* (qualitative research), *respondents* (positivist and quantitative research) and *subjects* (quantitative and experimental designs), but excludes the terms *researcher* and *fieldworker*.

The ethical intention of health research

The primary aim of research into health-related issues, namely the improvement of the quality of life of individuals and groups, situates research within the realm of the ethical: doing what is *good* and *right*. Moreover, the ethical component of a research project constitutes the *caring* component of that research: 'There is no doubt about the fact that research is an ethically significant activity, and any research project must be pursued in an ethically reflective manner' (Ashcroft 2002:278).

The potential ethical dilemma in health research

The inherent ethical dimension of health-related research does not, however, guarantee that the actual research process will comply with sound ethical practices and standards. Research calls for scientific objectivity and detachment, thus creating the potential for a divided loyalty between the obligation towards science, on the one hand, and humanity, on the other. Reconciling these two conflicting loyalties is often extremely difficult. This situation is aggravated in cases where researchers and participants were previously involved in a close, though professional, therapeutic relationship. Although research in the human sciences bridges inevitable scientific detachment via *qualitative* research techniques, it is not necessarily the case that the respondent's vulnerability will be alleviated by the associated involvement, dialogue and listening on the part of the researcher. It might be exactly these interactive features that enhance the informant's vulnerability, his/her psychological trauma, mental suffering, and general sense of unease.

In addition to research in the health sciences often being conducted on groups, such as patients and clients, who have already been defined as *vulnerable*, certain research interventions (e.g. experimental drug testing and interviews on sensitive issues) undeniably create vulnerability in participants. Nonetheless, it is often the mundane issues in research that go unnoticed, only to be picked up at a later stage, often by someone other than the researcher. This can cast serious doubt on the ethical and scientific integrity of the researcher and the overall trustworthiness of the research results.

Participating in health-care research

In the light of the current increase in health research, it is highly likely that health professionals will become either directly or indirectly involved in some kind of research. In both instances there are certain ethical issues that need to be considered.

As a health-care professional one could be asked - because of one's professional, privileged access to the field of research and to data sources - to act as a *research fieldworker*, to assist researchers in gathering data. In this instance, health-care professionals might see their role as involving responsibility but not *accountability*; in other words, that one merely has to collect data and do so on time, whereas ethical accountability rests with the principal researcher. However, by committing oneself to something, albeit as mechanical and as detached as collecting data, one often finds oneself in the frontline of creating situations of *vulnerability*. Health-care professionals, who serve as fieldworkers, need, therefore, to acquaint themselves with the ethical implications of the research project. These need to be clarified with the principal researcher.

As a supervisor or manager in a specific field in health care, one could be approached for permission to do research in that specific area. When this happens, the primary ethical principle will still be responsibility and concern for patients and clients (Ashcroft 2002:278). Professionals in supervisory positions are accountable for the well-being of their clients and patients, especially when these individuals are subjected to research interventions. Supervisors remain accountable, liable and culpable.

Should a supervisor receive a request for research to be conducted in the area overseen by him/her, he/she must insist on serving on the Research and Ethics Committee that is considering the research proposal. The health professional should insist on the following information: firstly, the complete research protocol, including measures relating to participants' personal protection (informed consent forms, privacy, anonymity), and psychological and physiological protection (especially if experiments with certain interventions are going to be conducted); secondly, the maintenance of participant autonomy; thirdly, the way in which the research might encroach upon medical and nursing care; fourthly, the expectations of the supervisor during the research; and, finally, issues relating to financial remuneration (Brink 2001:52).

Yet another way in which the health professional can become involved in research is by being asked to participate in a research project as a *respondent* or *informant*. In such instances, it is important that the health professional is informed about the ethics of research, his/her rights as a participant in the research and the liability relating to information provided by him/her.

The moral obligation to do health research

It is the moral obligation of each health-care professional to contribute to the advancement of the body of knowledge of the profession and the scientific discipline supporting that profession. The maintenance and survival of individual professions within the field of health care reside in the body of unique knowledge or science these professions develop. Professional organisations and bodies cannot alone fight the battle for professional standing and survival. All efforts in this regard are meaningless if health professions cannot give evidence of a body of scientifically generated and tested knowledge that improves the quality of life of people. It is, furthermore, a professional and moral obligation to do research that is evidence- based. Evidence-based practice eliminates some of the fallacies health-care practice is often plagued with, such as appeals to misplaced authority and tradition, hasty generalisations, and the like (Bandman and Bandman 1995:125-137). These fallacies embody deceptive thinking and give rise to professional dishonesty.

Both newly acquired scientific knowledge and existing traditional practices need to be tested and evaluated. Traditional practices need to be assessed and understood in terms of science in order to determine if they are effective or not. These traditional practices reside within certain scientifically grounded practices within the health-care profession as well as in traditional cultural practices imported into the profession.

Vulnerable participants in health-research

Though health-care professionals are alert to vulnerability, some groups of potential research respondents and informants may feel particularly vulnerable when pressure is put on them to participate in health research. Both vulnerability and the potential for exploitation increase when *autonomy* is diminished, as in the case of a child or someone who is mentally incapacitated. But circumstances also render individuals who are otherwise quite competent vulnerable. Vulnerable communities are characterised by one or more of the following:

- limited economic development
- inadequate protection of human rights
- discrimination on the basis of health status
- inadequate understanding of scientific research
- limited availability of health care and treatment options
- impaired ability of individuals in the community to provide informed consent.

(The South African Medical Research Council's [MRC] ethics guideline on medical research MRC, 10-04-2004.)

The MRC (MRC, 10-04-2004) also identifies 'special groups'. Among these special groups are pregnant women, children, prisoners, people with mental impairment, the elderly, students and people in dependent relations. Readers are strongly advised to obtain the MRC guidelines on basic research ethics.

There are, in addition to the special groups mentioned by the MRC, people who, for political and social reasons, are displaced, who find themselves in refugee camps or are prisoners of war detained in either special prison camps or in existing correctional facilities. These people too need to be treated as special groups. The autonomy of these people may in one way or another be diminished, their vulnerability enhanced and they, therefore, may be easily coerced into participating in research. If no specific reasons exist for the inclusion of members of vulnerable or special groups in a research project, they should rather be excluded.

Bioethics: a unifying and divisive ethic in health research

When thinking about ethics in both practical and research contexts, *bioethics*, as a field of applied ethics, is perhaps the word that most often comes to mind. According to Kuhse and Singer (1999:1) the term bioethics originally referred to an ethic that would incorporate our obligations to the biosphere as a whole. The ecological tone underlying the original definition of the term makes it appealing to an all-inclusive field of human endeavour such as the health sciences.

The original meaning of the term bioethics has, however, changed and has come to refer more pertinently to the study of ethical issues arising from the biological and medical sciences (Kuhse and Singer 1999:1). Given the continuing dominance of medicine and the medical and biological sciences in the field of health care, bioethics - under its contemporary definition - has come to dominate the ethical thinking of health professionals. (In this regard see Chapter 15 on the ethics involved in HIV/AIDS.) Bioethics has become *the* ethic of the health sciences to the extent that whenever research is conducted in the health sciences and it does not involve biological and biomedical research interventions (clinical research), it is either considered not 'genuine' research, or as not having any ethical implications. Both these ways of thinking about ethics and research in health care are fallacious; they push health research towards the natural sciences, thereby marginalising the human aspect involved in health care.

Sources of ethics for research

The aspiring health researcher needs to acquaint him/herself with the sources of research ethics. However, according to Fox, 'there is a relative absence of specific legal rules regulating research' (2002:251). Most of the codes of conduct pertaining to research are based on international declarations, such as the World Health Organisation's update on the Declaration of Helsinki (Fox 2002:254). In general, sources of ethics in health care and research include the following:

Legislation, law, and policy statements, and charters: In this regard the following Internet addresses might be useful for research in health care, though this is not a complete list of resources on the Internet.

■ *Government Gazette* can be downloaded from http://www.doh.gov.za/docs/index.html.
■ Helsinki Declaration: http://www.wma.net/e/policy/pdf/17c.pdf
■ South African Medical Council Guidelines on Ethics for Medical Research: General
■ Principles: http://www.sahealthinfo.org/ethics/ethicsbook1.pdf
■ National Health Act (Act 61 of 2003) http://www.doh.gov.za/docs/index.html
■ Patient Rights Charter: http://www.doh.gov.za/docs/legislation/patientsright/chartere.html
■ Health Research Policy in South Africa 2001: http://www.doh.gov.za/search/index.html
■ Guidelines for Good Practice in the Conduct of Clinical Trials in Human Participants in South Africa. http://www.doh.gov.za/docs/index.html

Professional codes of conduct: Within the health professions the oath of Hippocrates is an obvious example. In the nursing profession the Nurses' Pledge unambiguously states: 'The total health of my patients will be my first consideration … I will maintain the utmost respect for human life' (Muller 2001:4). Other health profession are also guided by specific codes of conduct.

Fundamental moral principles: Notwithstanding the ongoing debate about the relative or absolute nature of values, most traditional religions and many philosophical schools of thought have maintained that certain values and ethical principles are innately human. According to this view, people have an inherent knowledge of what is right and wrong, good and bad, in relation to the four fundamental ethical principles of autonomy, beneficence, non-maleficence, and justice.

The application of ethical concepts, principles and theory to research

When applying ethical principles to research, it is helpful to bear the following three considerations in mind:
■ the participant
■ the institution (consent, research ethics committees)
■ the scientific integrity of the researcher (research process).

In addition, the basic ethical principles of autonomy, beneficence, non-maleficence and justice must at all times be endorsed.

The participant

The research participant is always the researcher's first concern. All measures towards practising ethically sound science and research are directed towards maintaining the *self-respect* and *dignity* of participants. From a caring ethical point of view, the participants' involvement in research must also be an opportunity for *growth*. Advocacy during research can become problematic especially when the advocacy role of health researchers involves advocating for, on the one hand, patients and clients and, on the other, the research project and its outcomes (Fox 2002:285). The relevant ethical principles are: autonomy, confidentiality and anonymity, informed consent, permission and veracity, non-coercion and non-exploitation, and the maintenance of the scientific integrity of the researcher.

■ Permission

Permission to use personal data should be sought, regardless of its source, but within the moral framework of maintaining autonomy, confidentiality and anonymity; providing informed consent; telling the truth; and guaranteeing the non-coercion and non-exploitation of the individuals concerned. If patient and client records are used, at the very least the permission of the institution holding these records must be obtained (Brink 2001:52). Where the contact details of personal records are available, the individuals concerned should be contacted and their permission to use the data be obtained. All aspects relating to informed consent apply. If permission is not obtained, privacy is transgressed and civil law suits might follow.

■ Autonomy

Autonomy, as the right to self-determination, is respected in health research just as it is in clinical practice. Individuals have the freedom to conduct their lives as autonomous agents, without external control, coercion or exploitation, especially when they are asked to participate in research. Autonomous individuals are capable of being informed about the implications of a proposed study and this allows them voluntarily to accept or decline an invitation to participate. This, however, is not the case with persons who have diminished autonomy. In the case of groups of vulnerable people, although individuals in these groups might readily understand the implications of participating in a research project, they might not feel free to choose not to participate in the research. These groups are generally more prone to being coerced into participating in research and are more easily exploited because of their perceived restrained position, where they feel that they have little choice in the matter or where their position leaves them open to retaliation, discrimination and retribution on the part of the researcher and fieldworkers. It is the researcher's responsibility to respect the autonomy of vulnerable individuals and individuals with diminished autonomy and, where necessary, locate the legal guardians or suitably responsible persons from whom consent to include these individuals in research could be obtained (Brink 2001:52).

Autonomy also implies that individuals have the right to withdraw from research at any point in time (Burns and Grove 2001:196). Neither the participant nor the researcher must see the signing of a consent form as an irrevocable commitment on the part of the participant.

■ Informed consent

Informed consent is supported by the ethical principles of *autonomy* and *liberty*. As a general rule, these must be upheld by the principal researcher, and informed consent must be obtained from participants by the principal researcher or the person who is going to intervene in the lives of the participants via study treatment, control measures, and the like (Ashcroft 2002:284).

Information given to the candidate must be pitched at the intellectual level of the candidate. The language used must be clear and unambiguous, and the researcher must avoid using scientific jargon. *Veracity* must be upheld consistently in the sense that the truth, the whole truth and nothing but the truth about the research should be told. Skewing information entails manipulation and eventual encroachment upon the candidate's informed status. It involves deceit and dishonesty and relegates the candidate to a position of vulnerability. In no way should the candidate be coerced into consent by having certain aspects of the research subtly emphasised or by omitting others. In this sense the researcher advocates for the prospective participant. However, advocating for the prospective candidate in this manner can result in advocating *against* the research quest for objectivity in that certain information provided to the participant might eventually lead the participant to act and to give information that is in line with what the researcher wants - the so-called *halo-effect* in research. At this point the researcher walks a very tight rope, especially if the candidate is a patient, client or student of the researcher since the candidate may not always be able to distinguish between the researcher's role as caregiver and as researcher. A candidate might in other words feel that his/her loyalty to the caregiver dictates that he/she must participate in the research. Patients and clients need to be reassured that their care will not be compromised if they refuse to participate in research (Ashcroft 2002:284).

The things that candidates must be fully informed about include the purpose of the research; the method and procedure to be followed; the duration of the study; the nature of the participation expected of the participants; the way in which the results will be used and disseminated; the identity of the researcher(s) and fieldworkers; possible side-effects and detrimental aspects; the risk-benefit ratio; the manner in which confidentiality and privacy will be secured; and the financial implications - whether or not the candidate will be remunerated (Brink 2001:52). The latter is a very sensitive point. Remuneration, especially in the case of certain vulnerable groups, might coerce individuals from these groups into participation. In some way or another the principal researcher needs to reciprocate; however, paying participants for participation and information can be interpreted as buying information, and this can in fact skew the final results and undermine the trustworthiness of the research results.

The final agreement between the researcher and candidates should be mutually contractual. In addition to the candidates' acknowledgment that they have been adequately informed, the contract should also pertinently mention:

- The nature of involvement of the participant. Participant involvement in research does not entail only a face-to-face presence during data collection. Involvement also includes the use of information (records) about the patient as well as the use of any anatomical parts of a person, including body fluids and normal and abnormal tissue that have been obtained by whatever means (Brink 2001:52). It must therefore be clearly stated whether and to what extent involvement implies *invasion*.

- The fact that the researcher is willing to answer truthfully all questions that might arise during the research. Information should be made available to candidates about whom to contact in this regard.

- A non-coercive disclaimer that states that participation is voluntary and that refusal to participate will involve no penalty or loss of benefits that the participant is otherwise entitled to (Burns and Grove 2001: 208). In practice this means that once a patient, client, student, or any other person in a professional relationship with the researcher has been approached to participate in a research project, and then turns down the request, such a disclaimer should be issued.

- In the 'option to withdraw' statement, it must be stated clearly that the candidate has the autonomy to decide at any point to withdraw from the research. In this regard it must also be stated clearly whether the data collected up to that point will be used by the researcher, how the reciprocation agreed upon between the candidate and the researcher will be affected, under what circumstances the researcher is entitled to discontinue participation and under what circumstances the entire project might be terminated (Burns and Grove 2001:208).

■ Confidentiality and anonymity

While preparing candidates to give informed consent, the researcher must indicate how *confidentiality* and *anonymity* will be secured.

Confidentiality means that no information provided by a candidate should be divulged in any way except for research purposes. This is, however, not possible if it is not coupled with anonymity. Measures should be devised to avoid linking information (data) to any individual participant. However, complete anonymity is seldom attainable (Brink 2001:51). In cases where areas and institutions at which data have been collected are reported, the possibility of individuals being identified becomes stronger. It is imperative that, in order to secure the anonymity of participants, the anonymity of the institutions at which the research was conducted is maintained.

The researcher should uphold the promise to confidentiality and anonymity throughout the research project; however, this promise should in no way be used to coerce candidates into participating in a research project.

■ Privacy

In research, the privacy of participants is assured once confidentiality and anonymity, and the nature and degree of invasion, have been secured. Privacy is further assured if the participant is informed and has given voluntary informed consent to share private information (Burns and Grove 2001:199) and the following aspects have been clarified: the extent of disclosure and the general circumstances under which personal (private) information will be shared. Privacy can be transgressed in several ways during research. If 'research' questions do not relate to the research objective, they are bound to be inquisitive and a transgression of privacy.

The institution

Whenever research is undertaken in the field of health care, permission for such research must be obtained from the authority in charge of that field or service point (Brink 2001:52) at which the research will be conducted. This also applies to health professionals who wish to conduct research in the area in which they are working. It is imperative that the institution be treated as a *person* by the researcher. The ethics that apply to the individual participant also apply to the institution.

■ Matters relating to institutional autonomy and permission

The *autonomy* of the institution or governing body should be respected. In addition to the information participants are furnished with - which should also be made available to the institution at which the research will be conducted - the following information needs to be made available to the authorities: the data collection instrument; the sample (means of selection and size); the principal researcher's qualification and expertise (Brink 2001:51); the perceived ethical issues that might be encountered; and a statement of approval of the research proposal or protocol by the institution under whose auspices the research will be conducted. Only by being aware of this information can the authority, usually via a Research Ethics Committee, arrive at an *informed* decision either to grant, or to refuse, permission for the research to be conducted at the institution. The *ethics clearance* that a Research and Ethics Committees might request ensures a double check. For instance, where a student conducts research towards an advanced academic qualification, the university's Research Ethics Committee should first approve the research proposal or protocol before it is submitted to the institution at which the research will be conducted.

With regard to *anonymity*, the institution should be protected by ensuring that it is not possible to relate particular data to a particular person in an institution or to the institution itself (Brink 2001:51). It should be clearly stated that statements made by participants or the researcher represent these individuals' personal opinion and not necessarily that of the institution at which the research was conducted.

Matters of privacy are closely related to matters of anonymity and the granting of permission for the research to be conducted. These entail time, resource and facilities management, and often interfere with health-care delivery and the day-to-day operations of the facility or institution. These issues are often ignored in a research protocol; even by the person or committee granting permission. Most of the time research involves staff time and the use of basic equipment and resources, and as such involves 'opportunity cost' (Ashcroft 2002:281). On the other hand, research often offers some benefit to participants in terms of access to new treatment, increased access to nursing or other health services, or financial and other inducements (Ashcroft 2002:281).

■ Research Ethics Committees

Research ethics committees are essential to protect individual patients and clients as well as the public's health. These committees appraise the scientific and ethical contents of both research and practice as researchers should not be the sole judges of whether their research conforms to generally acknowledged ethical codes (MRC par 9.5.2; Tschudin 2001:146).

In South Africa, research and ethics committees in the field of health care are a legal requirement (National Health Act, Act 61 of 2003; par 73) (http://www.doh.gov.za/docs/index.html).

Membership of a Research Ethics Committee should be based on the individual's proficiency in the following:

- *Ethical assessment skills*, including the ability to identify the ethical implications, assess social and interpersonal dynamics, and clarify and critically evaluate a research proposal.
- *Process skills*, including the expertise to facilitate formal and informal meetings, identify key decision-makers, set ground rules, create rapport and navigate competing moral views.
- *Interpersonal skills*, including the capacity to listen well, communicate respect, and support all involved parties, including committee members; to convey the views of involved parties to others; and to help all involved parties communicate effectively (Garattini, Bertele and Li-Bassi 2003:1199).

The **composition** of Research Ethics Committees should reflect the multi-disciplinary nature of the field of health research. In addition, clergy, legal representatives and community members, as well as representatives of disadvantaged communities when research is conducted in such communities, should serve on such committees. Both sexes and members of different race groups should be represented on Research Ethics Committees (MRC par 9.9.2; Muller 2001:74).

The **terms of reference** and scope of activity of Research Ethics Committees extend to:

■ informing the appointing authority of the Research Ethics Committee about all aspects relevant to the ethics of research in progress

■ reviewing research proposals and protocols for research on humans in the area under the appointing authority's management

■ giving frequent account of research in progress to the appointing authority

■ monitoring the progress of research with special emphasis on ethical problems that might be experienced

■ attending to any allegations of misconduct in research in the area of authority of the appointing authority (MRC, par 9.8.3)

■ developing and co-ordinating institutional resources and developing formal training programmes for members of staff under the appointing authority's jurisdiction (Siegler 1999:583).

The **objectives** of a Research Ethics Committee are implied by its terms of reference and relate to three main areas: applications for research, matters pertaining to research in progress and clinical practice.

Objectives regarding the evaluation of **applications** for research must:

■ consider research protocol and proposals with regard to their relevance and feasibility (by evaluating the extent to which scientific quality, design and conduct meet with set standards); the possibility of harm coming to participants; the risk/benefit ratio of the research; and issues relating to consent

■ determine the researcher's expertise in relation to the proposed research

■ determine whether the objectives of research are directed towards justifiable advancement in knowledge and are compatible with prevailing community interests and priorities. In addition to the definition of health research provided by the National Health Act (Act 61 of 2003), the aims of research in health care are broadly outlined in paragraph 1.5 of the Health Research Policy in South Africa 2001 (Health research policy, 16-12-2004) as: promoting competitiveness and employment creation; enhancing the quality of life; developing human resources; working towards environmental sustainability and promoting an information society.

■ ensure that proposed research interventions are justified in terms of the stated objectives

■ ascertain whether, with regard to participants, data and the institution, privacy, confidentiality, autonomy and anonymity have been secured

■ ascertain whether a satisfactory, relevant preliminary literature review has been conducted (MRC par 9.6.2-9.8.1).

Objectives with regard to **research in progress** should endorse all the above by:

■ probing allegations of scientific misconduct and conveying findings to an appropriate body to act on this (MRC par 9.7.1)

■ overseeing research in progress with a view to maintaining ethical standards of practice in research; protecting participants and researchers from harm and exploitation; preserving the participants' rights; ensuring that participants are adequately informed about the research aims, objectives, consequences and risks relating to their involvement; ensuring that informed consent is obtained with due regard to related ethical issues; securing confidentiality of data; upholding participant autonomy by securing their liberty to air their views and to withdraw from the research at any point in time they may choose (MRC par 9.6.2 – 9.7.1).

As a condition for granting permission for research to be done in a certain area or within a certain institution, the Research Ethics Committee should stipulate that some publication(s) should flow from the research. The Research Ethics Committee should specifically assist in minimising the non-publication of negative research results (Garattini, Bertele and Li-Bassi 2003:1199). This should be done with due caution (Tschudin 2001:149). Finally, the Research Ethics Committee should reassure the community (both scientific and public) that all the above are constantly being observed (MRC par 9.6.1).

With regard to objectives relating to clinical practice, ethics committees, through their close observation of research in practice, can also give advice about the ethical aspects of health care and support the ethical aspects of decisions in individual cases (Tschudin 2001:146). In some institutions Research and Ethics Committees fulfil the dual role of watchdog over both research and practice. However, such a dual perspective often poses problems as research and ethics committees could become caught up in the advocacy dilemma previously discussed.

Whatever the case, Research Ethics Committees should **not** trespass on, or cast any doubt on, the researcher's professional autonomy, the relationship of patient/client and health professional, and the integrity of health professionals. Research Ethics Committees can cause interference by:

■ developing regulations and endorsing institutional decisions that limit the prudential clinical-ethical discretion that would normally be exercised by the responsible health-care professional or researcher

■ reviewing retrospectively the decisions of health care professionals and researchers (presumably for the purpose of disapproving of a decision)

■ consulting on aspects of research in operation and by having the committee's opinion carry the authority of the institution

■ serving as a quasi-judicial body that makes decisions and takes the authority away from health-professionals and researchers

■ influencing health professionals and researchers to make the 'right' decisions through moral suasion and group power (Siegler 1999:584).

The scientific integrity of the researcher

'Bad science is bad ethics' (Ashcroft 2002:280). The scientific integrity of the researcher must be indisputable and incontrovertible. However, expertise does not guarantee ethical conduct in research and science. Often the opposite is true. Misconduct in research can figure in a number of ways, including the fabrication and falsification of data through inappropriate techniques of analysis, plagiarism, and the dishonest manipulation of the design or methods (Burns and Grove 2001:191) as well as irrelevant, exploitative, unoriginal, incompetently and fraudulently performed research (Ashcroft 2002:278).

The competence of the researcher

The scientific integrity and competence of the researcher are relevant to the whole research process. As indicated earlier, a substantial amount of research is presently being conducted in the field of health care, part of which primarily aims at furthering the educational qualifications of individual professionals. The question thus arises as to whether 'student research' should be judged according to the same high standards as those of 'real research' or research primarily aimed at advancing scientific knowledge (Ashcroft 2002:282). Research undertaken for educational purposes usually aims at developing and improving the researcher's (students') research skills. Consequently these research projects have to meet *different*, though not *lower*, standards from those applicable to 'good' or 'real' research (Ashcroft 2002:280). Research undertaken for educational purposes should be assessed in the same way as would any other educational project. Above all, it should be assessed in terms of whether or not the student researcher has mastered the relevant research methods and, indeed, whether or not basic ethical principles have been adhered to. A way of reconciling 'student research' with 'real research' is to provide for a study of limited scope, limited in *scope* but not necessarily in *depth*. For instance, the number of research objectives could be limited by making the research less intricate. This may in some instances lead to ethical issues becoming less obscure, thus making it easier for the student researcher to comply with the ethics of research.

From a point of view of competence and negligence, there is a clear obligation for the research undertaken to lie within the capability of the principal investigator or the investigating team. Such competence refers to both professional health care and research competence. In the case of research conducted for educational purposes, the required competence is often supplemented by the input of research supervisors and promoters. Clear guidelines regarding accountability and responsibility need to be set in this instance. A formal contract between the student researcher and the supervisor or promoter is indispensable. In addition to the involvement of supervisors and promoters in the student researchers' projects, both the pilot study and peer reviews can serve as an extended supervisory mechanism.

With regard to the research problem or topic, the relevance and importance (Streubert, Speziale and Carpenter 2004:312) of the research must be of primary concern. However, no matter how important and how relevant the topic is, research should not be undertaken if it is technically, philosophically or financially beyond the abilities of the researcher (Brink 2001:51). Research involves exposing participants – clients, patients and colleagues – to certain risks and, if the research is unlikely to produce reliable and relevant results, it might be argued that the participants will be subjected to risk without there being any benefit in it for them (Ashcroft 2002:280).

Notwithstanding the inherently ethical nature of research and its intended good for the greater part of society, it can nevertheless be pursued unethically and selfishly. When deciding on a research topic, the researcher must consider the number of people who would benefit from the research. Often, lack of research in an area affecting a small number of people outweighs the importance of doing good to a greater number of people (see the debate about utilitarianism in Chapter 3). Furthermore, when research is conducted for the sole purpose of benefiting the researcher, the debate about *altruism* versus *egoism* comes to the fore. When too much pressure is put on the researcher to do research according to the priority lists of the institution or granting authority, the researcher becomes caught up in a situation of *paternalism* versus *libertarianism*. Throughout the research process, in respect of every aspect of the research, the researcher needs to question his/her actions, attitudes and position as far as these alternative models of morality are concerned as well as the position of participants within these models.

With regards to the **purpose of the study**, all aspects concerning the choice of a research topic apply, as does the inherent ethical nature of health research. The latter should not be compromised by the educational purpose of a research project.

As far as the **literature review** is concerned, it must be noted that no research is so original or unique that it does not build in some way on the results of previously developed research methods and designs (Ashcroft 2002:281). Any claim to the contrary unquestionably indicates the necessity for an in-depth review of the literature.

The literature should be approach with an open mind; arguments both for and against the research problem, purpose, design, and the like, need to be mentioned (Brink 2001:51). Skewing arguments in favour of the researcher's point of view or in support of 'proving the research problem' constitutes *deception*. No matter how remote from the research topic certain sources may be, all ideas taken from other authors and researchers, in whatever form, *must* be acknowledged. Failing to do so constitutes a serious offence: *plagiarism*. At a more personal level it is simply dishonest.

In the light of the development of information technology, and especially the Internet, the opportunity for committing plagiarism has been greatly advanced. Cutting and pasting information from web sites and claiming it as one's own original work has been termed 'cyberplagiarism' or 'web-napping' (Eysenbach 2000). Closely related to this are copying and pasting from other electronic documents, such as those produced by word processing packages, and the ease with which most documents in hard copy format can be scanned and converted into re-workable electronic text. Clearly, this is an emerging phenomenon and it is a cause for great concern in research and publishing ethics.

With regard to problems of *plagiarism* and *cyberplagiarism* , the conduct implied by the following terminology should be upheld:

Plagiarism: the Oxford Concise English Dictionary defines plagiarism as 'to take and use another person's (thoughts, writings, inventions) as one's own.' Plagiarism is therefore a form of intellectual theft.

Cyberplagiarism : the act of plagiarising in cyberspace; the downloading, cutting and pasting of parts of, or entire, articles from the Internet or the Web. Several electronic engines or programs have been developed to check for *cyberplagiarism*. In South Africa too, several universities have engaged in the development of such software. Such software is becoming more readily available to teaching staff and editors of journals and is available on the Internet at some financial cost. The interested reader can access the following web sites: http://www.plagiarism.org and http://www.turnitin.com

Attribution: crediting an author, artist or scientist with a particular work or an idea.

Citation: the precise rewriting (quoting), or attributing 'intellectual credit' to another person's scholarly or artistic creations. Quotes must appear in 'quotation marks'. It is, in some circles, customary to *italicise* direct quotations.

Copyright: the legal entitlement an author, artist or scientist and publisher or distributor has to exclusive financial benefit from a work. Copying *any* items under copyright, such as cutting and pasting sections from literature, or copying music CDs or DVDs, constitutes illegal and unethical conduct. Exceptions are made with regard to educational institutions (with the necessary consent, citation and acknowledgement) that need to access materials protected by copyright.

Common knowledge: information known to a large number of people. Common knowledge facts need not be cited.

Infringement: the act of using the work of authors, artists and scientists without the necessary authorisation; *plagiarising*.

Paraphrasing: unlike the act of *citation*, paraphrasing involves the rewording of a passage of text. This is often done to clarify the meaning contained in the text. Quotation marks are not necessary, but the source must be acknowledged through a completed reference.

Intellectual property: the original creative outcome of the artistic and scientific ventures of individuals 'that can be protected through a copyright, trademark, patent, industrial design or integrated circuit topography' (University of Alberta, http://www.library.ualberta.ca/guides/plagiarism/terminology/index.cfm Accessed 17 December 2004). Also see MRC par 10.4.1.

Referencing: the way in which authors and other sources of information are acknowledged. The detail contained in a reference and the format of listing sources in a bibliography accompanying a research report or article depend on the institution through which the research is conducted (such as a university or a health professions body) or the journal in which it is published. In addition to crediting and acknowledging authors, sources must be referred to in such a manner that the reader can easily access them.

During the **sampling and recruiting** of participants, a particularly difficult situation arises when patients and clients know the researcher. All the ethical issues surrounding vulnerability and diminished autonomy again become important, as do issues of equality and justice. Although equality as *equal opportunity* is secured in random sampling in quantitative survey research, it is not upheld to the same extent in qualitative research. Furthermore, though the selection of participants to an experimental design and the allocation of such participants to a control and an experimental group might reflect *equality*, the intended difference in treatment of these groups during the research may raise concerns about *justice* and *fairness*, especially if possible *risk* and *benefit* differences between the two groups exist.

The **pilot study** epitomises the researcher's ethical intent. It is at this point that the principles of science and ethics for the first time converge in practice. Though the number of participants affected by ethical problems may be fewer than during a full-scale project, the intensity of the experience is not less. Researchers who are aware of ethical issues in their research design should not use the pilot study to 'test' for participants' sensitivity to these issues.

Researchers must be honest about the outcome of the pilot study. Changes that need to be made on the basis of the results of the pilot study must be implemented. If necessary, a follow-up pilot study should be conducted. The changes that the researcher has brought about must also be reported in the research report. Truth-telling in this instance not only pertains to ethicality, but also to good science and good character.

Data obtained during the pilot study should not be used during the final data analysis, especially not if changes have been made to data collection instruments or intervention schedules. Using data from the pilot study may compromise the trustworthiness and validity of the final research results and may have grave implications when put into practice.

Data collection is a minefield of ethical concerns. The ethical issues are different for qualitative and quantitative research, and for the different research designs and methods within these two research paradigms. During the data collection phase of the research, participants are most actively involved: interviews are conducted, questionnaires completed, interventions are imposed, and actions and reactions under experimental conditions are observed. It is also during this phase that the participants are most vulnerable. Vulnerability impacts on participant autonomy, dignity, anonymity, privacy, advocacy, and the like.

Although the promotion of *beneficence* is a fundamental research principle, certain actions in health care and research do cause harm, pain, and stress (for example, venepuncture, experimental drug trials, sensitive interviews) but are justified because they are carried out with beneficent *intentions* (to make a diagnosis or to provide pain relief). Where it is not possible to eliminate harm or trauma completely, Brink (2001:53) suggests the following guidelines:

- 'Temporary discomfort, anxiety or physical pain that is no more than that which could have been experienced in daily life and that would ease once the research has been completed is acceptable, provided that it has been communicated to the respondents and informants and that consent thereto has been obtained.

- 'Exceptionally high levels of pain, discomfort and anxiety that will continue after the research has been completed are only acceptable if the benefits outweigh the negative effects and if the treatment upon completion of the research will relieve the side-effects experienced by the subjects' (Brink 2001:53).

In face-to-face research the possibility exists that the researcher might manipulate participants to give information (data) the researcher wants, resulting in skewed data and raising ethical questions about the *validity* of the data. In the case of poorly constructed questionnaires, the *reliability* of the instrument and, ultimately, the validity of the data become ethical issues. Vis-à-vis (face-to-face) research can further compromise participants' *privacy*. The immediate nature of the interview and the opportunity for probing might lead the researcher to gather information merely for the sake of inquisitiveness. The researcher may also dwell on aspects that the participant may feel uncomfortable with. *Privacy* is also compromised in covert observational studies. Observing people without their knowing it constitutes *deceit* and an *infringement* on privacy. Whatever the case, the rule is to collect data that is pertinently related to the research objectives and not to collect more data than is necessary to attain the objectives.

As indicated in the section on sampling, collecting data via experimental designs and clinical trials can pose grave ethical issues relating to beneficence, non-maleficence, justice, equity, and equality and fairness.

During **data analysis** and **interpretation** *truth* and *truth-telling* (veracity) are central ethical concepts. Under no circumstances should the research in any way fabricate or falsify data. In addition to the fabrication of raw data (e.g. completing questionnaires on behalf of non-existing participants), the application of statistical analysis procedures that do not match the level and type of data collected can lead to the distortion of results and, ultimately, to the results becoming a transgression of the principles of beneficence and non-maleficence.

In qualitative research, where the analysis of data is founded on 'interpretation', *bracketing* (the bringing into mind of what one knows about the phenomenon in order to interrogate each and every piece of data for its meaning within a specific context rather than within the frame of reference of the researcher) has become the *ethical dictum*.

In data analysis, the whole issue of whether the research is conducted for educational purposes or whether it is conducted as 'real' or 'genuine' research becomes important again. With regard to quantitative research, although the researcher may make use of the assistance of a statistician, it can be expected, as part of the researcher's expertise, that he/she at least knows which statistical analysis procedures are appropriate, and why specific procedures should be used in analysing numerical data. In the case of qualitative research, the use of co-coders is often suggested. The ethical issue at hand is the extent to which the final result reflects the insight of the student. Is the final result authentically the intellectual property of the student?

During the **communication of research findings**, science and research become what they really are: public knowledge (Ashcroft 2002:280). Research results which are kept secret or go unreported breach the requirement that science is a collective enterprise, that it is to benefit all of human kind, including the scientific community. The issue of selfishly clinging to findings of good research as opposed to sharing it with the broader scientific community incorporates the alternative models of morality of egoism and altruism. The ethic of reciprocity is at issue.

'Underreporting' (Eysenbach 2000), not publishing research results or not giving a complete report constitutes *scientific misconduct*. Both positive and negative findings must be published. Hypotheses that have been refuted are as valuable a research finding as those that have been endorsed. Reviewers and policy makers need a complete picture of the research results. Biased publications jeopardise future literature reviews and research guided by these reviews.

The communication of research findings requires excellence in writing and language proficiency. Arguments must be clear, unambiguous and open only to the interpretation the actual research findings lend to it. Again, readers should not be misled or deceived by jargon. Nonetheless, well-defined scientific terminology is essential for ensuring a more or less uniform interpretation by readers.

Concluding remarks

Ethical issues often figure extremely subtly in research. The issues addressed in this chapter represent only the tip of potential ethical issues in research. It is trusted that the above introduction will alert the reader to ethical issues inherently involved in research and also to ethical issues that may result from specific research topics and designs. With the contents on ethics proper contained in this book in mind, the reader is advised to rethink the whole research process.

Critical thinking activities

1. Construct a two-dimensional matrix which, in the first left hand column, exhibits the general phases and steps of the research process. In the upper top line, enter different ethical principles and concepts. In the cells that are formed, enter the ways in which the listed ethical concepts and principles may figure in relation to the matching step in the research process.

RESEARCH PROCESS	ETHICAL PRINCIPLES AND CONCEPTS			
	Autonomy	Beneficence	Advocacy	etc.
Problem				
Objectives				
Sampling				
etc.				

2. Repeat the above activity choosing a specific research design either from the qualitative or the quantitative paradigm.
3. Again, repeat the exercise detailing aspects relating to the participant, the institution and the researcher.

part 5

Perspectives on transcultural issues in health-care practice

Knowledge of the religious obligations demanded by various world religions may, together with other theoretical knowledge, be acquired from textbooks. However, the comfort, understanding and empathy some patients demand from nurses require an individual and humane approach which cannot be learnt from books. Such an approach can only come from the nurse herself and her identity as a human being. A nurse who has no understanding of, or who is not in touch with her own spiritual values, will not be capable of empathizing with the spiritual values of the patient in her care

(McGilloway & Myco 1985:3).

Dealing with cultural differences

Anne-Mart Oosthuizen

Outcomes

Studying this chapter will enable you to:

■ explain why it is necessary for the nurse to develop cultural awareness
■ identify and discuss obstacles in the path of culture-sensitive care
■ list specific categories of stressors that are involved in culture shock
■ give examples of how the nurse can achieve the objective of culturally congruous care.

Introduction

In Chapter 6 it clearly emerged that the nurse-patient relationship formed the basis of nursing. It is in the interests of both nurses and patients to have good relations. Substantial cultural differences between nurse and patient can, however, have both positive and negative consequences for the patient.

The presence of patients from multicultural and multi-ethnic backgrounds gives rise to numerous issues in nursing. Nursing care across cultural boundaries is, however, a reality today and the key to successful relations lies in an understanding of the cultural differences between patients and between patients and nurses.

Culture in the broad sense may be viewed as the way of life of a group of people. Culture is defined as the values, beliefs, norms and customs of a specific group. These are acquired and are shared by the group. These characteristics govern ideas, decisions and conduct in a specific manner (Burkhardt & Nathaniel 2002:339). Cultural groups are distinguished by many characteristics, such as the way their members dress, language, values, rules of conduct, legal and social control, eating habits and health care. The maintenance of health, the prevention of disease, the causes of ill-health, treatment, caring and death are part of the health component of each culture (Boyle & Andrews 1999:7).

There are clear cultural differences, as well as some similarities, in the way nurses provide care and in the way patients expect it to be provided. Leininger (1985) in Oermann (1997: 83) contends that care as a phenomenon is common across all cultures, but the way in which people express care varies from one culture to another. The provision of holistic patient care in a multicultural society is an ideal that must be pursued.

Holistic patient care in transcultural/multicultural nursing

Cultural competence: an essential component in delivering holistic patient care

Cultural competence includes cultural awareness and cultural sensitivity. Burkhardt and Nathaniel (2002:338) explain that cultural awareness is the knowledge about the values, beliefs and behaviours of cultures other than one's own, while cultural sensitivity is the ability to incorporate the patient's cultural perspective into nursing assessments and to adapt nursing care so that it agrees as much as possible with the patient's cultural perspective.

Holistic patient care will remain an ideal and will not become a reality until everyone who is responsible for caring for patients receives adequate education and gains cultural competence in nursing patients of cultures other than their own. Since a nurse works very closely with her patient, a lack of sensitivity on her part could have disastrous consequences for the patient. In other words, whether a nurse works in a state or private hospital, a community health clinic, a doctor's surgery or in industry, her patients will most likely represent different ethnic groups, social classes, ages, sexes and religious backgrounds.

The presence of patients from multicultural and multi-ethnic backgrounds is a source of potential problems. The main causes of the problems are language and cultural differences. To be sensitive to other cultures does not mean to be culture-free or indifferent. Health-care practitioners should accept the values, beliefs and attitudes that identify their subgroup. Patients and nurses are different, but even more basic than this is the fact that people are different. It would be counterproductive to treat all patients alike. All people share certain characteristics, such as the basic need for food and protection, and some people share certain characteristics with others, such as language and culture. Certain characteristics are unique to only one group by virtue of their unique racial or ethnic heritage. The secret of effective nursing and health care lies in knowledge of the similarities and the differences between groups (Henderson & Primeaux 1981:196-198). The nurse must develop cultural awareness. It is not realistic to expect a patient to dissociate him/herself from his/her own cultural background and to identify with the norms of the dominant group of nurses in whose care he/she is. On the contrary, it is more reasonable to expect the nurse to learn to understand cultural differences in order to provide optimal care. Holistic patient care will become a reality only if patients are approached within the framework of their individual cultural patterns (Henderson & Primeaux 1981:30).

Obstacles to culture-sensitive care

It is impossible for one individual to know all the rules and norms of communication for all subcultures. Culture sensitive care requires effective intercultural communication. It requires people from different cultures to create shared meanings. Various obstacles and barriers can prevent meaningful relationships in transcultural nursing. Lindeman and McAthie (1999:170) list five common barriers to intercultural communication, namely:

- anxiety which tends to make a person focus on the feelings that inhibit communication
- the assumption that all cultures are the same instead of being open to differences
- ethnocentrism
- stereotyping which includes making negative or positive judgments about an individual based on observable or assumed group membership

- prejudice, such as irrational suspicion or hatred of a particular group, race, religion or sexual orientation.

Cultural values and beliefs

It is important that nurses should be secure in their own values and beliefs. Even though a nurse may feel strongly about her values and beliefs and would obviously wish to retain them, it is important not to lose sight of the fact that values differ from one culture to another and that a patient's values may often be entirely contrary to her own. Sullivan (1999:323) cites DeSantis (1988) who states that nurses must temporarily step out of their own cultural traditions and look at situations from a patient's perspective and then strive to incorporate these perceptions into a mutually agreed upon plan of care. What a person believes is reflected in what he/she says and does, and by listening to the patient sensitively, the nurse can often draw a conclusion about the value system that the person subscribes to. When the values of nurse and patient coincide, this strengthens the treatment—but when they are in direct conflict, it is the responsibility of the nurse to adapt her actions towards the patient. Conflicts arising in a transcultural environment are not the result of interpersonal conflict only, but may be the result of conflicts arising from the socialisation process. Every person has been brought up in a particular culture with particular values and beliefs conveyed to him/her by parents, teachers and peer group. Adults are shaped by these influences and may adhere to them or rebel against them by behaving contrary to expectations. Individuals continue to be affected by their cultural heritage (Sullivan 1999:323).

A nurse may classify certain patients as moral or immoral. An unpopular patient who is regarded as immoral may consequently receive inferior care. Such situations may occur, for example, when the patient is a prostitute, is in police custody, or has used physical violence. In other words, when a patient's behaviour or conduct conflicts with the nurse's value system, the person is viewed as immoral and unpopular. These negative sentiments about unpopular patients may lead to hostility on the part of the nurse, who may resort to turning a deaf ear to call-bells and ignore the basic psychosocial needs of the patient by being indifferent and cool instead of warm and sensitive. Such behaviour would undoubtedly be detrimental to the patient, as well as to the nurse, who may later grapple with feelings of guilt. The nurse should examine her motives and make a decision to change her negative behaviour towards so-called unpopular patients. After all, all people are entitled to respect, care and compassion, irrespective of their circumstances in life and conduct (Kus in McCloskey & Grace 1990:554-558).

Ethical conduct requires that nurses respect each patient irrespective of his/her cultural values and beliefs. Without respect for a patient's values and beliefs, caring in the nurse-patient relationship will remain merely an ideal.

Communication

An important obstacle to culture-sensitive care is communication. This does not apply to verbal communication only. Communication encompasses the entire sphere of human interaction and behaviour. All behaviour, whether it is verbal or non-verbal, in the presence of another person is communication (Giger & Davidhizar 2004:22). A nurse receives both verbal and non-verbal messages from her patients. Although both nurse and patient may have full command of a language, different cultures attach different meanings to certain expressions.

When neither patient nor nurse makes an effort to understand each other, or even worse, if neither is aware that they are not communicating with each other, the gap between them simply becomes wider and wider. A communication gap is something more than the mere difference in languages. Non-verbal expressions within each culture are critical for mutual understanding. Language differences refer only to language problems, whilst differences in cultural expression are far greater and encompass various non-verbal customs, values and beliefs (Andrews & Boyle 1999: 27-37).

In order to communicate effectively, nurses should therefore be aware of racial, cultural and social factors that make people what they are and influence their behaviour. Furthermore, nurses should be aware of communication patterns and the relationship between communication and behaviour, feelings and attitudes. For this reason it is important for nurses to take note of differences in dialect, style, volume of sound or even silences during a conversation, the use of touch, emotional overtones, as well as gestures and eye movements (Giger & Davidhizar 1990:199; Haynes, Boese & Butcher 2004:220).

A nurse can promote effective communication by working within the individual's cultural frame of reference. Recognition of cultural differences in language use, orientation in respect of time, distance and health-care preferences affords the nurse an opportunity to respond so that individual needs are taken into account in a personal manner. Communication, whether it is verbal, non-verbal or written, is always important. It may be necessary for the nurse to make use of other people, such as interpreters, to ensure clear communication. Whenever a nurse is not familiar with the cultural conventions of a group, it may be necessary for her to consult experts on the culture concerned and its implications on nursing care. Cultural misunderstandings can give rise to litigation (Burkhardt & Nathaniel 2002:347).

Communication problems give rise to various ethical issues, such as the rights of patients to informed consent and to make decisions about their own health.

Although it is the doctor's responsibility to give the patient information about surgical interventions or other medical procedures, a nurse has to explain nursing procedures to patients in a clear, comprehensible manner. Because a nurse spends more time with patients, she should be aware of communication problems that are the result of differences in cultural background. If a patient does not have command of the language in which the nurse communicates, it is not possible to obtain informed consent. An ethical issue arises when a nurse is aware of communication problems but neglects to ensure that no intervention is carried out before informed consent has been obtained.

Ethnocentrism, cultural imposition and prejudice

Differences between the cultural values, beliefs and conventions of a patient and those of the health-care personnel may have unexpected consequences. A person who regards his own culture as superior and all other cultures as inferior or second-class is ethnocentric. This includes an inability to understand the values and beliefs of another culture. Ethnocentrism may be a result of lack of exposure to or knowledge of other cultures. Most people are gradually exposed to the beliefs, conventions and values of their own culture over a lengthy period that begins as early as birth. This acculturation process is known as socialisation. The ability to understand alternative points of view and to respect the beliefs of other cultures, even if they differ from one's own, is described as ethno-relativity. The principle of relativism informs us that we should refrain from judging the way of life of others in terms of the culture of the persons concerned (Tjale & De Villiers 2004:69). The problem does not lie in the conviction that one's own culture is the best, but in the danger that one person may try to impose his/her values on another. Cultural imposition refers to attempts by an outsider, be they subtle or less subtle attempts, to impose his/her own cultural values, beliefs and practices on other individuals while disregarding their cultural beliefs and practices (Andrews & Boyle 1999:4-5).

Cultural imposition is the tendency for health personnel to impose their beliefs, practices and values on people of other cultures because they believe that their ideas are superior to those of another person or group. This phenomenon has serious ethical and professional implications, since the patient has both a human right and a cultural right to have his/her cultural values and way of life taken into consideration in nursing practice. Nurses must recognise this right and work with the patient, not against him/her.

Another consequence of ethnocentrism is prejudice. Prejudice may be based on a strong sense of ethnocentrism, or it may be the result of ignorance, incorrect information, experiences in the past, or fear, and it manifests itself in many interrelated forms. Examples of these are, *inter alia*, racism, which refers to negative attitudes towards people of a different skin colour; and sexism, which refers to negative attitudes typically towards the female sex. Whenever prejudice is the result of ignorance or incorrect information, the negative attitudes can easily be overcome by education. However, prejudice which is deeply rooted in the socialisation process is far more difficult to overcome (Eliason 1993:226). All people have prejudices. The danger arises when health-care practitioners allow their prejudices to influence their relationship with culturally different patients.

Culture shock

The last obstacle to be discussed in this chapter is culture shock. This is a phenomenon that can occur on the part of both health-care practitioner and patient because it is not only patients who are suddenly exposed to nurses and other health-care practitioners of different cultures – health-care practitioners are also exposed to patients of other cultures.

The basic stressor involved in culture shock is the sudden transition from a familiar to an unfamiliar environment. This sudden transition involves many great and smaller differences ranging, for example, from the water tasting strange to an inability to speak the language. Andrews and Boyle (1999:530) assert that culture shock is often accompanied by feelings of alienation and homesickness and a temporary dislike of the host culture.

Specific categories of stressors in development of culture shock:
■ **Communication**

It would appear that the primary stressor is a change in the communication system, both verbal and non-verbal. Although the person still hears and sees, little significance is attached to verbal and non-verbal messages. Although the language is familiar to a certain extent, there may still be factors, such as differences in tone and the vernacular, which obscure the meaning of words.

■ **Mechanical differences**

Significant progress in hospital technology has made it necessary for both patient and nurse to learn to use the technology. Patients have to learn where to press the button in order to move the bed up and down, how to call the nurse in the nursing service station and how to meet their basic needs, for example when in plaster or traction and during intravenous transfusions. Learning to manipulate the mechanical environment requires time and effort and could lead to frustration.

■ **Isolation**

Apart from the isolation patients experience because of communication problems, a measure of isolation is inherent in any situation where a person is exposed to total strangers. Patients are separated from family, friends and colleagues for virtually the entire day. Furthermore, visiting hours and regulations also limit contact with family and friends. Hospitalisation is a lonely experience.

■ **Habits**

This stressor is directly related to the communication system. The entire social structure must be understood to determine where the person fits into the framework. Becoming a patient for the first time requires learning a new role. This new role requires the patient to act according to the standards set by the hospital personnel. Thus it may be expected of the patient to remain in bed even if he feels well, to wear pyjamas even if it is the middle of the day and to reorganise his daily schedule to adapt to the hospital schedule.

■ **Attitudes and beliefs**

The attitudes, beliefs and values that govern people's lives and behaviour distinguish one cultural group from another. Nurses and doctors often proceed from a conviction that the patient does not have to be informed of his diagnosis, treatment or prognosis. The attitude that the doctor 'knows what is in the best interests of the patient' leaves little opportunity for decision-making by a patient (Brink 1990:127-135). To deny a patient's right to information about his/her state of illness, or not to involve him/her in decision-making has far-reaching ethical implications.

Each stressor brings about changes in a familiar series of activities of life and each change means that a patient has to adapt to it to a certain extent. When all five categories are present at the same time, the impact is so much greater, which could give rise to the condition of culture shock (Brink 1990:129-135).

A nurse should ask herself whether a demanding and difficult patient is not perhaps experiencing culture shock. A patient who is angry and dissatisfied with the staff and for the most part does not co-operate, may be reacting to all five stressors. Hospitals with limited visiting hours may reinforce the sense of loneliness and rejection. Anxiety and fear of the unexpected and the unknown, as well as frustration with the service, delays and a lack of information, may increase. All these feelings can contribute towards culture shock.

A nurse who knows that these stressors exist can try, through personal contact with the patient, to reduce the stressors, or the policy for patient care could be changed to reduce the intensity of environmental stressors.

The scope of knowledge and skills which nurses must possess in order to provide culturally congruous care

The nursing profession has a duty to train practitioners to provide care that is meaningful and sensitive to the needs of patients of all cultures. It is important that a nurse who works with patients of other cultures should carefully consider the following aspects:

- recognition of her own cultural orientation
- understanding of the importance of the patient's perspective
- development of communication skills in order to examine the patient's perspective
- identification of issues which influence providing care to people of other cultures.

Recognition of own cultural orientation

All people have specific views on health and illness that are unique to them. These views are partly formed by cultural beliefs and values, which in turn are determined by the social context in which a person lives. A person's attitudes and values influence his/her behaviour towards people whom he/she sees as different. There is a real need for nurses to analyse their own beliefs, which may influence their willingness to care for some people.

Understanding the importance of the patient's perspective

It is important that a nurse should try to understand the patient's perspective. The effectiveness of this approach is that it enables the nurse to identify differences and then to find ways of working with such differences.

Development of communication skills

The nurse practitioner cannot identify a patient's perspective or involve the patient in a discussion if for some reason he/she is unable to communicate effectively. Furthermore, her attitude influences the extent of her success in gathering cultural data. The patient will express few of his/her true feelings to a nurse who is prejudiced and displays a lack of respect. Nurses are often guilty of ethnocentrism and must learn to build a relationship with patients of different cultures.

Identification of issues that influence caring

Nurses should try to gain knowledge of the circumstances under which patients of other cultural origins live. Many cultures have specific customs relating to the death of a family member or a member of the community. These could give the nurse an indication of how they spend their time with a dying person, the care of the body after death and the patterns of mourning. Many cultures also have specific customs relating to childbirth. If a nurse who is nursing a patient with specific cultural customs is sensitive to these customs, it will be of great value to the patient (Lynam 1992:151-156).

Concluding remarks

A nurse cannot be a walking encyclopedia about the ethnic and social backgrounds of her patients. She can, however, develop cultural awareness. A nurse who has developed cultural awareness will be better equipped to understand why a so-called difficult patient is not co-operating. She will realise that he/she may be suffering from culture shock and will regard the situation as a challenge to offer the patient better care. This does not require the knowledge of an anthropologist, merely the recognition that differences occur on the part of patients in their value orientations and their attitudes towards illness and hospitalisation (Brink 1990:42-43).

South Africa is a country in which people of many cultures live together. If caring and quality nursing are to be pursued actively by the nursing profession, it is essential for its members to develop cultural awareness. Without a good understanding of this concept it could be all too easy to lapse into a habit of dividing areas of difference into compartments. Such compartmentalisation poses a threat to the pursuit of holistic nursing care in a multicultural society.

Critical thinking activities

1. Describe a situation in which you had to nurse a patient with cultural values and beliefs different from your own. What problems did you experience?
2. Would you, through knowledge of the patient's cultural background, have been in a position to provide better nursing care?
3. What do you understand by culture shock? Which categories of stressors are involved in culture shock?

Religious and cultural forces in transcultural nursing

Sally van Tonder

Outcomes

Studying this chapter will enable you to:

- incorporate the religious and cultural preferences of patients in the drafting of a nursing-care plan
- describe the diversity of people groups, religions and cultures with which a nurse has to deal
- identify the influence of the diversity of people groups, religions and cultures on nursing
- assess the influence of different religious and cultural conventions on the health and illnesses of the community
- describe the principles of faith healing
- explain the vocation and role of spiritual and traditional healers
- identify the influence traditional healing practices and medicine have on Western healing practices and medicine
- evaluate possible co-operation between Western and traditional healers in the health services.

Introduction

In Chapter 13 it became clear that the maintenance of health, the prevention and causes of illness and death, treatment and nursing all form an important part of the health component of every culture. In this chapter we look at various religious and cultural forces that influence the nursing of the sick and the dying.

It is impossible to know everything about every culture or religion with which South African nurses come into contact. As far as the universality and diversity of cultures are concerned, it is important that nurses should be sensitive and flexible in their approach to those who are ill or dying. In caring for their patients, health care practitioners should exercise caution in their own assumptions of what would be helpful to a patient. Sensitivity and dialogue often prevent cultural conflict. It is important to take note of any specific needs or requirements patients or their families may have. Sherr (1989:37) points out that families usually appreciate the interest nurses take in their culture and religion and in their awareness that patients may have specific religious needs.

In their daily dealings with patients and clients, health-care practitioners are exposed to many religions. Nurses may identify with some of these religions and cultures, but when they are confronted with an unfamiliar culture or religion, or with views that are at variance with their personal religious beliefs, they should have some knowledge of these religions in order to understand fully and nurse their patients.

Connection between religion and health

Religion is an all-inclusive value system which governs a person's existence in the world and, indeed, in the universe. According to Vanderpool (1990:10), central to religion is a belief in a supernatural being or beings. Each religion is traditionally viewed by the adherent of the religion as the only or most important reality, and each religion is characterised by rituals and often also by constant internal debate. In religious traditions humanity searches for meaning in life, for protection against the uncertainties of life and for strength to cope with its drives, frustrations and limitations. Through these traditions humanity also strives for peace, meaning, pleasure and strength.

The World Health Organization's definition of health is accepted in most countries, namely that health is a state of optimum physical, psychological and social welfare, and not merely the absence of illness or ill-health. Dreyer *et al* (1993:7) assert that most literature indicates that health is the well-being of the body, the psyche and the spirit, and that it includes the harmonious integration of a person with himself/herself, the community and the environment. Factors such as culture, development, literacy, socio-economic status and philosophy of life influence a person's view of health and methods of preventing ill health. Health should therefore be viewed within the specific community's sociopolitical, cultural, religious and interactive framework, and never in isolation. Health is a dynamic that encompasses the promotion of optimal physical, psychological and spiritual functioning.

Connection between religion and health service

In the practice of religion a distinction is often drawn between good and evil, and between what is acceptable in life and what is forbidden. Religion fills a person's life with specific emotions, motivations and integrity.

A health service may be viewed as the science and art of understanding and treating physical and psychological illness. It is committed to relieving suffering, restoring health and prolonging life, and its application of science is guided by definitions of health, illness and deficiency, as well as by aetiological theories about the causes of physical and psychological illness and the application of scientific knowledge and techniques for therapeutic purposes.

It is expected of both religion and health care that they are based on certain fundamental principles or truths. These truths deal with the meaning of life and the nature of and interplay between body and spirit.

In both religion and health care special attention is paid to aspects such as a person's sexual development, suffering, illness, injury, disfigurement and death. Religious explanations of physical suffering are generally less verifiable than scientifically based medical explanations. Both explanations, however, deal with the primary reality of the meaning of a person's life in relation to the harshness of nature (Vanderpool 1990:11).

Religious principles are influenced by the discoveries and technical capabilities of the highly developed science of medicine. Modern medicine contradicts, revises or confirms existing assumptions about life, the body and the psyche by describing the assumptions in a comprehensible and workable manner. Religion, in turn, influences health practices. A case in point is the value the Judeo-Christian religion attaches to the worth of the individual, the sanctity of life and the malevolence of death. Vanderpool (1990:12) asserts that health care is supported or inhibited by religion, regardless of whether religion is recognised or practised in health care.

Religion and health care present prescriptions or prohibitions about what may or may not be done in respect of life, the body and emotions. Religion and the health care are, therefore, continuously engaged in the process of describing and evaluating what is right and wrong. In religion the ethical principles of what is virtuous and sinful are clear (explicit). Ethical aspects in health care are both explicit and implicit. Examples of explicit ethical aspects are what is considered to be right or wrong in medical procedures, the relationship between health personnel and patients/clients, and the manner in which health services are organised and presented. Implicit ethical aspects are found in controversial procedures such as the manipulation of the body (organ transplants, cosmetic and transsexual surgery), human reproduction (abortions, test tube fertilisation, surrogate motherhood, birth control), the use of drugs (LSD in psychotherapy) and the care of the dying (prolonging of life, active or passive euthanasia).

Vanderpool (1990:12) believes that the ordinary person expects both religion and health care to provide guidance, education and moral norms. Throughout history healing has been accomplished by a variety of religious and medical treatments. Many treatments fall within the medical field (nursing), while others are of a more religious nature (prayers, rituals).

If health personnel understand religion better, religion can be utilised to provide better care, especially in situations where religious practices have a detrimental effect on health care. At the same time religious leaders can contribute towards the health, comfort and decision-making of believing patients. Because the course of illness and other forms of human suffering is uncertain, informed interaction between health-service personnel and religious leaders in providing care can only be to the advantage of the patient/client.

Cultural and religious traditions and nursing

Cultural anthropologists assert that if a human being is a historical being, a basic understanding of a person's place in the world is impossible if he/she is viewed separately from the culture in which he/she finds him/herself. This means that a person is 'culturally biased' and, to a degree, 'culturally determined' (Brock 1990:286).

Cultural formation begins with the relationship between a mother and her baby. The foundation for cultural development is laid in the emotional and physical needs of the baby and the mother's responses to these.

Within cultural traditions, specific rituals or ceremonies are found which are peculiar to the community that practises them. To the community concerned these rituals/ceremonies may mean nothing more than the way they do things. These ceremonies clearly emerge in religious practice.

Differing slightly in definition from Vanderpool, Jonker (in Hodgson 1989:12) defines religion as humanity's pervading orientation to life as it is expressed in its thoughts, emotions and actions. A person's orientation may be towards one god, as in the case of Judaism,

Christianity and Islam. In other instances the orientation may be towards many gods, as for example in Hinduism, and forms of Buddhism. The orientation may be atheistic as, for example, in Communism or Dialectical Materialism, or it may glorify the state as in, for example, Fascism.

Be that as it may, the fact remains that humans are religious beings, and have, since the earliest times, displayed an irresistible need to worship. Human beings must have some kind of religion (De Ridder 1961:162).

Judaism

Judaism is the oldest of the world's three great monotheistic religions. It is the father of both Christianity and Islam. The central concept of Judaism is that there is only one God, the Creator and Ruler of the entire world. He is transcendental and eternal and He sees and knows everything. He made His Law (Torah) known to the Jews and chose them to be the light of the world and an example to all people (Harley in Beaver *et al* 1982:272).

The Law of God is recorded in the first five books of the Bible. The Torah contains the revelation of God to Moses on Mount Sinai. Harley (in Beaver *et al* 1982:273) points out that it contains 613 commands that cover the entire spectrum of daily life, from civil law to personal hygiene and diet. These instructions are summed up in the Ten Commandments. Many of the world's legal codes are based on the Ten Commandments. Some Jews try to apply the regulations of the Torah to their lives today. Others, in turn, give preference to certain regulations with which they wish to comply. The extent to which a Jew complies with the rules of the Torah rests on his/her own conscience (Harley in Beaver *et al* 1982:273-274).

View on illness

According to Rosner (1986:316), Judaism attaches great importance to human life. Jews believe that life is a gift from God that must be preserved. Nurses should realise that a Jew is obliged to care for his/her health and life. Only God gives life and it is, moreover, only God who can take away life. A human being is not totally in possession of his/her body or life. It has been lent to him/her to use and not to abuse. A human being is obliged to preserve, honour and sanctify his/her life. Jewish law requires a health care practitioner to use every means at his/her disposal to prolong a life but prohibits the use of measures that will prolong the process of death (Rosner 1986:316).

During illness the religious needs of a patient are very important. The general observance of the religious prescriptions and objections of a patient can speed his recovery. Aspects such as the kosher diet, the observance of the Jewish Sabbath and other Holy days are important to a patient. Nurses should be sensitive to these needs and should remember that religious prescriptions and practices still apply when a patient is admitted to a hospital (Rosner 1986:318).

The Jewish dietary laws regulate not only the type of food that they may eat, but also the method of preparation. These regulations apply to the daily routine in the household environment but are as valid in the hospital environment.

The Jewish Sabbath begins at sundown on a Friday and ends after dark on a Saturday evening. During this time the activities of a working day or creative procedures are forbidden to Jews. When a Jewish patient is admitted to hospital on the Sabbath or any other Holy Day, the nurse should be receptive to his/her commitment to his/her religious prescriptions. At the end of the Sabbath a candle is lit and the coming week is blessed. It may mean a great deal to a Jewish patient in hospital if he/she can light a candle at the beginning or end of the Sabbath or other religious days (Sherr 1989:40).

When a member of a Jewish family becomes ill, the whole family feels the suffering. It is normal for a Jew to talk about his/her discomfort and pain. Nurses may find this burdensome, but they must remember that it is part of Jewish culture. Jewish patients should preferably be nursed in the same ward as this will not only help the nurse but also create a safe environment in which the patients can recover.

The patient must consult a rabbi before a decision can be made on procedures that may have religious implications. The following procedures are at issue here: abortion, sterilisation, prostate operation, prevention of pregnancy, artificial insemination, circumcision, euthanasia, postmortem examination, the cessation of life-supporting treatment or devices, and any other dangerous procedures which could have religious implications. The rabbi should form an integral part of the medical team.

View on death

According to Rosner (1986:322), the Jewish tradition provides that information about a terminal illness may be withheld from the patient if the slightest possibility exists that such knowledge would have a detrimental effect on the patient's physical or psychological condition. The patient must, however, be made aware of the seriousness of the illness to enable him/her to make whatever arrangements are necessary. A doctor should preferably not predict a maximum lifespan, because this could reduce the morale and the defensive ability of the patient and his family. Nurses should remember that the word 'death' should be avoided as far as possible, because it could undermine the will of the patient to live (Rosner 1986:322-323). A critical ill patient may never be left alone. Family members will take turns to sit by the patient and will encourage the patient to recite the Jewish confession or affirmation. If the patient is too sick to fulfil this commandment, the family member will do it for him/her (Newman *et al* 1999:520).

Active euthanasia is viewed in the Jewish religion as brutal murder. Even if it is clear that the patient is dying and approaching the end of his/her life, any form of active euthanasia is forbidden. If mechanical devices do not help to prolong life but merely delay death, these devices may not be put into operation and may be switched off if in use (Newman *et al* 1999:519). Judaism teaches that the human being is created in the image of God and that the human body must be regarded as worthy in life and in death. For this reason the body is regarded as inviolate. Jewish law allows postmortem examinations in exceptional cases, however. Note that the rabbi's consent is required for a postmortem examination. Consent for a postmortem examination is given only if:

■ it is legally required
■ the information so obtained will help other patients
■ the family can benefit by this information e.g. hereditary illness.

According to Jewish laws all body organs and fluids must be buried with the body (Newman *et al* 1999:520).

Health care professionals should remember that the body must be treated with respect and that disfigurement of the body is not permissible. Orthodox Jews may not grant consent for organs to be removed for transplant, but where an organ transplant can save the life of another person, it may be done only when the dying patient suffers total brainstem death.

Upon death, a son of the nearest relative will close the eyes and mouth of the patient or the nurse must simply close the eyes, straighten the limbs, wrap the body in a sheet and send it to the mortuary. The body is not washed. The Jews themselves will wash the body in a special way and prepare it for the funeral (Sherr 1989:41). According to McGilloway & Myco (1985:105), in the case of a progressive Jew the body may be laid out in the normal manner after the family and rabbi have been consulted. A non-Jewish nurse must, however, wear disposable gloves to ensure that she does not touch the body.

Islam

The Muslim faith has followers throughout the world. The language of a Muslim depends on his country of origin. Those who adhere to the Islamic religion are called Muslims, never Mohammedans or Moslems.

Mohammed was born in Mecca in approximately AD 570. In AD 610 he began to believe that he was the messenger of God. He had to convey the messages that he received to his fellow men in Mecca. These messages and revelations are recorded in the Koran. The messages confirm that there is only one God (Allah), that he is merciful and powerful and controls the course of events. On the Last Day man will be judged in accordance with his deeds and be sent to heaven or hell (Beaver *et al* 1982:305).

Muslims believe that every individual is a worshipper and a slave of God. There is no difference between worship and the wholeness of human life. Kerr (in Beaver *et al* 1982:317) asserts that every created thing may exist in dependence on God and in obedience to his creative and supportive power. The word 'Muslim' means 'someone who lives his life in accordance with the will of God'. 'Islam' means 'subject to God' (Beaver *et al* 1982:317).

According to Kerr (in Beaver *et al* 1982:317), the Islamic religion rests on five pillars. The first pillar is confession of religion in the one God, and in Mohammed as the apostle of God. Prayer is the second pillar of Islam, and specific prayer times are stipulated. The giving of alms is the third pillar. The fourth pillar concerns the fasting period during Ramadan, when no water or food is taken between sunrise and sunset for a full month. The fifth pillar refers to the pilgrimage to Mecca, which, if possible, occurs at least once in a lifetime (Beaver *et al* 1982:318).

View on illness

Many cultural groups in the Islamic world, and indeed beyond in the subcontinent of India, Latin America and China, divide all foods into two main groups, namely 'hot' and 'cold'. This binding classification system includes not only food, but also medicine, illnesses, mental and physical conditions, and natural and supernatural forces. Hot and cold do not signify actual temperatures, but are symbolic values attached to each category of food. Because health, according to Helman (1990:35), is defined as a balance between these categories, illness is treated with hot or cold food, or medicines, in order to restore the balance.

Nurses should bear in mind that there are various dietary restrictions in the Islamic religion, such as abstinence from alcohol and pork products. Only the meat of ruminating and cloven-hooved animals may be eaten. These animals must be slaughtered in accordance with the 'halaal' or ritual slaughter. Only fish with fins and scales may be eaten. Shellfish and eels, for example, are forbidden (Helman 1990:34).

It is sometimes believed in the Islamic world that spirits cause illness. The 'jinn' or 'ginn' are omnipresent mercurial spirits. Helman (1990:109) asserts that these spirits, which also cause illnesses, are more semi-human than supernatural beings.

The Muslims' fasting period, Ramadan, takes place during the ninth month of the year of the moon. During this time no food or liquid may be taken between sunrise and sunset. Of importance to nurses is the possibility of health problems occurring during the month of Ramadan, for example, in the case of a diabetic patient. The health counselling and control therapy of diabetes are not merely dependent on the person's belief in the potential advantages of the treatment; they must also be reconcilable with his/her cultural environment and religion. During the feast of Ramadan a diabetic patient is therefore compelled to bridge the effect of the fast by, for example, amending his food intake and the frequencies of his mealtimes (Hodgson 1989:132).

To some Hindu and Muslim women, medical examinations are potential areas of conflict because their health condition compels them to act in a manner contrary to their value system (Hodgson 1989:129). Female patients accordingly prefer female doctors to examine them.

Many Muslims are vegetarians. Because they feel strongly about the type of food they eat, patients may prefer their food to be brought from home. Nurses should remember that it is sometimes necessary for a Muslim patient to gain consent to eat food that is contrary to his/her religious convictions. Special diets should be carefully explained to both the patient and his family. According to Burnard and Chapman (1993:87), Muslims use their right hand to prepare and eat food, while the left hand is used for ablutions. When a patient can no longer perform ablutions, owing to illness or injuries, the nurse should solve the problem through advice and discussion with the patient.

To a dedicated Muslim the washing of hands before and after meals and the rinsing of the mouth are important. According to McGilloway & Myco (1985:122), this washing of hands may be more of a cultural act than a religious act. A Muslim patient who is bedridden might want to wash his/her hands in running water before prayers and after having a motion or urinating. By pouring water from a jug, the nurse can comply with the patient's wish (Sherr 1989:42).

View on death

The Muslim confession of faith is the first words whispered into the ear of a newborn baby. These are also the last words that a dying Muslim will say on his deathbed. The confession of religion is the light on the road of life and the hope of God's mercy for the life after death (Beaver *et al* 1982:317). Remember that it is the greatest wish of a dying person to continue with his/her normal prayer patterns as long as possible. An Imam is not required at the deathbed because the families perform the necessary ceremonies, prayers and scripture readings. Nurses should take note that the body may not be touched or washed by a non-Muslim. The head is turned towards the right shoulder so that the face will be turned to Mecca when he/she is buried. The limbs are straightened and the body is wrapped in a clean sheet. The funeral should preferably take place within 24 hours after death. Consent for a postmortem examination is not normally given. If a postmortem examination must be carried out, the family may request that all organs be replaced for the funeral (Sherr 1989:42).

Islamic leaders have not yet stated their point of view on euthanasia. However, McGilloway & Myco (1985:140) refer to Islamic doctrines as proof of the fact that Islam does not approve of euthanasia. A person's birth and death are predetermined and any form of euthanasia may be viewed as intervention in the divine plan.

Muslim communities are sometimes inclined to consult Muslim 'hakims' when they fall ill because these healers have a better understanding of their culture and faith. Adequate knowledge of the Islamic religion and practices can assist nurses to make a nursing diagnosis, to plan nursing intervention and to guard against cultural misunderstandings.

The Christian religion

The Christian religion arises directly out of the Jewish religion. The Christian believes that the awaited Messiah of the Jews was fulfilled in Jesus. The Christian therefore believes that a start has already been made on the fulfilment of God's plan and the promises of the Old Testament. God's dominion has been established in a new way (Beaver *et al* 1982:249). The crucifixion and death of Jesus atoned for the sins of humanity and brought reconciliation between God and humankind.

The various branches of Christianity, as they are known today, can be ascribed to two historic movements. The first movement, in approximately 1054, was the great schism between the East and the West. The second movement took place during the sixteenth century, and from this the Reformation and Protestantism arose. Eastern Orthodox Christianity includes the Greeks, Russians, Syrians, Armenians and the Coptic peoples. Western Christianity includes the Roman Catholic and Protestant churches, the latter of which embraces many denominations including, for example, Lutheran, Reformed, Presbyterian, Pentecostal, Anglican/Episcopal, Baptist, Methodist, as well as several independent churches (Beaver *et al* 1982:354).

Medicine and nursing are key characteristics of the Christian life in poor sectors of the world (Beaver *et al* 1982:382). The Christian demonstrates his/her love for God by rendering loving service to his/her fellow man.

As in the case of Judaism and Islam, Christians also have a scripture, the Bible, with reference to which a Christian directs his/her life. All Christians accept the Bible as imperative, both in terms of guidance for their activities and as a basis for their faith (Beaver *et al* 1982:366). The Bible consists of an Old and a New Testament. The Old Testament consists of the Hebrew (Aramaic) scriptures for the Judaic religion. It gives the history and religious conceptions of God up to the coming of the Jewish Messiah. Christians view themselves as the rightful heirs to the ancient Israelite religion and accept the Old Testament in full. Without the Old Testament it would be difficult to comprehend the specific Christian scriptures (Beaver *et al* 1982:364). Owing to Christianity's origins in the Jewish religion, Christians have also inherited the Law of Moses (Beaver *et al* 1982:375). To Christians, the Ten Commandments are the yardstick for their way of life. Nurses should remember that sick Christians like to read from the Bible and if they are no longer able to do so, they would greatly appreciate the nurse doing it for them.

View on illness

A Christian believes that God is the creator of humanity. Nurses should remember that the entire person, not only the soul, belongs to God. A human being is the image-bearer of Christ and His representative here on earth (Koekemoer 1989:3). In the Old Testament one finds that God sometimes uses sickness and death as punitive measures against sin. Individuals, and even peoples, were punished with sicknesses and death.

In the New Testament it is asserted that Christ died for the sins of humanity. Humanity was freed from the bonds of sin and in Christ there came forgiveness of sins. In helping a patient it is necessary to know that Christians no longer experience illness and death as punishment, because they believe in the forgiveness of sins. Christians may believe that the Lord afflicts humanity with illness and adversity to test them and to bring them closer to their Creator. Nurses should bear in mind that illness and adversity, with a view to the hereafter, may therefore be a testing or purification process to the Christian.

View on death

Christians believe that at the second coming all believers will be roused from death. According to Sherr (1989:38), Christians believe that humanity was reconciled to God through the death of Jesus. They also believe that death and evil were conquered through Christ's resurrection and that He gives new life to all who believe in Him. This new life extends beyond the grave (Sherr 1989:38).

It is difficult to express an opinion on active and passive euthanasia on behalf of all Christians. In the modern communities in which Christians live, even the fundamental value of a person's life is questioned. Cultural changes influence the view of suffering and death, all the more so because medical science has succeeded in curing illness and prolonging life under certain circumstances, which gives rise to further moral problems. People have begun to think of old age and a 'comfortable' death that will relieve suffering (Larue 1985:35). Leaders of several Christian denominations have expressed their total opposition to active euthanasia. Some leaders respond cautiously in respect of passive euthanasia. If it is clear that the patient is already dead and that mechanical devices are merely keeping the bodily functions going, life support systems may be switched off. It may be accepted that the decision in favour of passive euthanasia should be taken on an individual basis by a team consisting of the doctor, the patient, his family and the spiritual leader. Note that the family may request at the time of death that the minister be present to pray for the dying person, to give him/her over into God's care and to comfort the family.

Christians do not have any religious objections to a postmortem examination or the donation of organs for transplants (Sherr 1989:39). Owing to their religious convictions, most Christians are opposed to abortion.

Jehovah's Witnesses

Inasmuch as nurses often come into contact with patients in hospitals who are members of the Jehovah's Witnesses, it is important to devote attention to their religious preferences and commandments. According to Hewat (1967:12), the Jehovah's Witnesses were founded by Charles Russell in 1852, in Philadelphia, USA. Members of this religious denomination believe that they are Jehovah's earthly representatives and that they are Jehovah's earthly organisation. God uses the Watchtower Bible as His communication channel with humanity (Gruss 1975:137).

View on illness

It must be remembered that Jehovah's Witnesses believe that God's new dispensation will come even during the present generation. This new dispensation means that people will no longer become ill and those who have been afflicted with any illness will permanently recover (Larue 1985:117).

Although Jehovah's Witnesses do not forbid medical assistance during illness, they are opposed to blood transfusions from a donor. The 1 July 1945 edition of *The Watchtower* announced a prohibition on blood transfusions. The instruction was that all worshippers of Jehovah, who were desirous of eternal life in the new world of justice, should refrain from the transfusion of blood into the human body (Gruss 1975:85). It is important that nurses respect this instruction. The prohibition on blood transfusions is based on various biblical texts. In the magazine *Awake*, Jehovah's Witnesses assert that there are alternatives to blood transfusions. One of these alternatives is that the patient's own blood be recovered during the operation and recirculated into the patient's veins. The magazine also refers to bloodless expanders which could be used to stimulate the body to supplement its own red-blood cells. Another remedy that has been approved for limited use is recombined erythropoietin (*Awake* 1990:13). Despite the above-mentioned alternatives, scientists are still searching for an effective replacement for blood. According to Larue (1985:117), a person may donate his/her own blood, which is then frozen and can later be given back to him during a surgical intervention.

Initially Jehovah's Witnesses regarded inoculation against diseases as a direct injection of animal material into the bloodstream of man, and according to them this was a direct contravention of the law of Jehovah. This view was amended in 1952 and it was argued that the individual should decide for himself on inoculation (Gruss 1975:65). It would therefore appear that there is no longer any opposition to inoculations.

View on death

Jehovah's witnesses believe that a human being consists of dust and ground and the breath of life. When sinful patients who are not saved die, they will perish while the believers will enter the Kingdom of Joy and Happiness. They do not believe that there is a burning hell and eternal pain but that hell is merely a person's grave (Giger & Davidhizar 1999:81-82).

Larue (1985:116) points out that the opposition of the Jehovah's Witnesses to active euthanasia is based on three aspects, namely the commandment against murder, good conscience and obedience to a higher authority. They view active euthanasia as murder. Passive euthanasia is acceptable, provided there is clear proof that death is inevitable and unavoidable and that prolonging death would only bring about unnecessary suffering.

Hinduism

Hinduism originated in India between approximately 1000 and 800 BC and it is the religion adhered to by the majority of Indians. According to Hammer (in Beaver *et al* 1982:170), some people claim that Hinduism is more of a culture than a religion. Most Hindus believe in God in one form or another but, popularly speaking, it is true to say that Hinduism has many gods. The individual Hindu may worship one god, a few gods or no god (Beaver *et al* 1982:172).

Dolan (1978:30) identifies three gods that Hindus generally worship together or individually. The first one is Brahma', the source of life. Vishnu is the second, the preserver of life and Siva, the destroyer of life, is the third. The Ganges and Jumna rivers in India are regarded as sacred. The waters of these rivers are in themselves the symbol of never-ending life. Thousands of Hindus visit these rivers daily to perform their ritual washing away of sins, to drink of the life-giving water and to make sacrifices to the sun. Every twelve years, on certain days that are determined by astrologers, millions of Hindus come to the confluence of the Ganges and Jumna rivers to be cleansed of their sins.

View on illness

Hinduism believes that a person's body consists of five natural elements: earth (which is bone and muscle), water (which is phlegm), fire (which is gall), wind (which is breath) and space (which is hollow organs). Water, fire and wind are the three elements which must interact harmoniously to create good health. Illness develops when there is an excess or shortage of one of these three elements. To pray for health is the lowest form of prayer. It is better to accept illness than to pray for recovery (Giger& Davidhizar 1999:471).

Of importance to nurses are the Hindu concepts of reincarnation and transmigration. To the Hindus the flow of life passes through many existences. Hammer (in Beaver *et al* 1982:172) points out that the consequences of work and deeds in one existence influence the character of the next existence. In the Hindu community the Doctrine of Karma gives meaning and purpose to life. Karma means that all actions bring corresponding consequences. If a person, therefore, does good deeds, he/she will be rewarded with the good in life, but ill deeds lead to punishment. Karma constitutes a strongly juridical view of the universe. Cox (1989:18) asserts that an individual's illness and suffering are the result of actions in previous lives. Individuals are responsible for their deeds and they can blame no one for their illness or suffering. The Hindu hopes one day to be freed of the chain of life or the cycle of existence.

Health care professionals should remember that the Hindu views humanity as part of the cosmic whole and this includes respect for life in all its manifestations. According to Hammer (in Beaver *et al* 1982:175), an individualistic approach is viewed as constituting the disintegration of life and for this reason strict discipline and meditation (yoga) are required so that the individual can be reintegrated into the whole.

Dolan (1978:30) defines yoga as a method of charging an individual's soul with the Supreme Being. The mystical experience of spiritual detachment involves certain exercises. The physical purity obtained through ablution is followed by the purification of thought. The value of certain yoga positions, breathing exercises, breath control, concentration and relaxation has attracted the attention of health authorities in recent times. Health workers are studying and evaluating the effect of ancient Hindu meditation and relaxation procedures with a view to the improvement of health. Consideration is also being given to biofeedback techniques to relieve conditions of stress.

Nurses must realise that hygiene and purity are important aspects of the Hindu's life. Hindus believe that stagnant water cannot purify and prefer to wash in running water. Skill, honesty and confidentiality are expected of the practitioners of traditional medicine. Similarly high standards are imposed on those who practise Western medicine (Sherr 1989:41).

According to Sherr (1989:41), Hindus have no conscientious objections to blood transfusions or organ transplants.

View on death

Hindus believe that death is a transition to a next life. They believe that all creatures are in a spiritual evolution through unlimited cycles of time. Each life strives to climb in merits to a level of liberation from this earthly existence (Giger & Davidhizar 1999:473).

A dying Hindu's greatest desire is to be taken to Varanasi, the holy city on the banks of the confluence of the two sacred rivers, to be purified in the waters. After death the body is cremated and the ashes are strewn over the river of life to ensure the continuation of life (Beaver *et al* 1982:171).

Whenever a Hindu approaches death in hospital, the family may bring money and clothing so that the patient can touch them before they are distributed to the needy. If the family cannot be at the bedside of the dying patient, they are very grateful if the nurses can be there. Family members like to sit by the dying person and read from their book, the B*hagavadgita*. If the Hindu priest is present, he can help the dying person to accept the inevitable. The priest blesses the patient by tying a piece of cord around his neck or wrist and pouring water into his mouth. The patient may ask to lie on the ground, close to mother earth, to assist his incarnation into the next life (Sherr 1989:41).

Nurses should remember that after the patient has died, the family likes to wash the body themselves and put clean clothes on the deceased before the body is taken away. According to tradition, the eldest son of the deceased, irrespective of how young he is, must take the lead in performing the last minor tasks for the deceased (Sherr 1989:41).

Hinduism has not yet made any pronouncements on euthanasia. The decision is left to the individual. Approval for postmortem examination is not normally given. Remember that the body must be handed over as quickly as possible. Some families send the body to India for cremation so that the ashes may be strewn on the sacred river Ganges.

Buddhism

Just as Luther was a reformer of the Roman Catholic religion, Buddha (meaning 'Enlightened One') was a reformer of Hinduism. Just as Luther, a reformer, grappled with the problem of the forgiveness of sins, Gautama grappled with the problem of escaping from the wretchedness of endless rebirths. Although Buddha founded a new religion, Buddhism itself shares certain central ideas with Hinduism, such as reincarnation and the doctrine of Karma.

Hindus believe that Buddha is the ninth reincarnation of the Hindu god Vishnu. During the period from Buddha's death in 483 BC to AD 300 Buddhist influence in India was great, including in the field of health services. Hospitals for both people and animals, and medical schools were founded. Buddhist influence declined in India, but spread elsewhere into southeast Asia, China and Japan where it still flourishes.

Buddhists believe that a person has had innumerable lifetimes in the past and that innumerable lifetimes in the future still exist. Future lifetimes will continue until a certain level of Enlightenment has been achieved. According to Lecso (1986:52), there are six realms or areas of existence in the Buddhist's cosmology. These areas are the realm of hell, the hunger-spirit realm, the animal realm, the human realm, the *asura* realm, the realm of the demigod and the realm of god. A being does not only transmigrate through these realms here on earth, but also in other world systems in the universe (Lecso 1986:52). The realm of hell, the hunger-spirit realm and the animal realm are associated with intense suffering and reduced intellectual abilities. The realm of the demigod and the realm of god are associated with so much pleasure that they have a detrimental effect on the zeal for spiritual development. The human realm is regarded as the most beneficial of all the realms and to be reborn as a person is the most desirable. This is very difficult to achieve, however (Lecso 1986:52).

View on illness

The Buddhists' view on illness or happiness is very interesting and it is important that nurses should understand it. The causes of illnesses can be described with reference to the Buddhist doctrine of karma (destiny). The causes of suffering are negative karma or delusion. Negative actions lead to suffering and positive actions lead to happiness. Both positive and negative actions leave a karmic impression (or instinct) on the intellect. These instincts remain dormant until an appropriate condition arises which activates the instinct. If the matured instinct is positive, the person experiences happiness, but if it is negative, suffering ensues.

In Buddhism four noble truths are central to its teaching. The first truth is that the human condition is essentially one of suffering. The second is that craving causes suffering. The third truth is that craving can be stopped, and the fourth truth is that following a programme of action will stop craving.

Of the four virtuous truths of Buddha the first truth is of importance to nursing. According to Lecso (1986:53), this truth indicates that birth, illness, age and death are inevitable realities of all beings in the six realms of existence. In Buddhism illness and karma are, of necessity, connected. Illness is the result of sinful actions in the past.

The medical system of Tibet, which is based on Buddhist thought, defines the causes of illness as 'far' and 'near' types. It is impossible to describe the 'far' causes of illnesses because all illnesses have their origins in the intellect, or the karma of the past. Ignorance is a negative condition of the intellect which gives rise to a chain reaction of negative conditions, which ultimately result in physical and psychological illness. The 'near' causes of illness are improper diet, bad conduct and unfavourable environmental factors (Lecso 1986:54).

The Buddhist 'Road to Life' prescribes regulations for the ethical and spiritual well-being of every individual. It also urges compassion for all forms of life. Abortion is not allowed because helping others is the foundation of the Buddhist faith. However, blood transfusions and organ transplants are permissible. Most Buddhist patients are vegetarians and will request a vegetarian diet. Some Buddhists may also appreciate a place in hospital where they can meditate undisturbed (Sherr 1989:39).

View on death

Death (illness) is attributed to actions in the previous life, which manifest themselves in the present lifetime in the form of terminal illnesses. The nurse should understand that a terminally ill person represents the payment of a karmic debt. Because the intellect at death is the immediate cause of the continuation of life in the next lifetime, it is important to have a clear mind as death approaches. It does not matter what has happened in terms of good or bad in the present lifetime; what happens during the process of death is the most important factor. Nurses should remember that it is important that a patient be allowed to die peacefully. Excitement and nervousness should not be stimulated in a dying person.

Nurses and other health professionals should realise that the patient may refuse medication that might dull his/her consciousness and, therefore, the ability to meditate. Buddhists normally cremate the dead so that the soul can be freed from the body and can enter the next existence (Sherr 1989:39).

Buddhists are neither for nor against euthanasia. They merely assert that a person's suffering does not end with his physical death but that it goes on forever. A person's suffering can only end if the karma changes for the good. Death is not the final solution to suffering. Family members who cannot bear to have their loved ones suffer are merely relieving their own suffering by applying euthanasia (Larue 1985:137).

Atheism and agnosticism

Atheism

Although an atheist does not place any religious demands on the nurse and atheism does not have a religious basis, it is nevertheless important to be aware of the thinking of the atheist. An atheist is someone who denies the possible existence of a divinity and is usually referred to as an unbeliever. Burnard and Chapman (1993:63) point out that atheists' moral decisions on what is right or wrong are not based on religious considerations but on their own convictions. Believers are forgiven, but unbelievers must forgive themselves.

Because an atheist does not seek the meaning of life in a divinity, this does not mean that such a person does not have spiritual needs. According to Burnard and Chapman (1993:63), some atheists find meaning in secular humanism. Secular humanism means that a person as an individual is not only responsible for himself, but for others as well. There is no place for selfishness in secular humanism. The bases for morality and meaning is therefore vested in the rule of 'treat others as I wish to be treated' (Burnard & Chapman 1993:84).

Agnosticism

An agnostic is neither a believer nor a non-believer. Because the existence or non-existence of a divinity cannot be proved, agnostics prefer not to adopt a point of view on a divinity. To the agnostic, meaning in life is an intrinsic concept that is dependent on the individual's reasoning and perceptions, and on the significance they attach to their deeds.

Whether a health care professional is a believer or a non-believer, he/she should accept other believers or unbelievers and not disregard them. The nurse as caregiver is not expected to win patients over to belief or unbelief.

Spiritual healing and the nurse

Whenever one hears the words 'faith or spiritual healing', one involuntarily thinks of miracles. Christians usually perceive healers as people with a deep faith who receive their healing power from God. However, faith healing does not take place only through Christian faith healers. There are several hot-water springs throughout the world to which people attribute healing powers. Even certain wells and fountains are singled out for their healing powers. Healers are also found in Southern Africa. In certain South African communities there are prophets and diverse healers who have Christian associations, as well as so-called witches and soothsayers who have traditional roots (Steegman 1982:17).

Health care practitioners must remember that it is possible to make use of any method – medical, surgical, psychological – to regain health. It is important that nurses in South African hospitals should understand that many black Christians may use elements of their own culture in their worship, in the administration of the sacraments and in their church services. Traditional laws and taboos may still be very important to many black people. African religious concepts encompass mythology, the tribal concept of power and God, ancestors, the sacred and the unity of the natural and the supernatural. Religious leadership is found in the priest, prophet, medicine man/witchdoctor, rainmaker/medium, seer/ soothsayer and the reincarnation of the ancestors.

Faith healing

The term 'faith healing' generally refers to the numerous non-medical methods of healing illnesses. It is true that healing through faith is possible, but it is important to remember that faith is not necessarily the only element in so-called faith healing. Other magical forces are present in unorthodox methods of healing (Leek 1973:11) and it is possible that more people are healed through the power of suggestion than by faith itself. Suggestion is a great problem for contemporary faith healers. In early Christian times it was easier, because faith was seen to be a sufficient explanation for healing. Today, with the accent on scientific explanations, people and some nurses seek proof and no longer accept the unorthodox methods of faith healing. When the nurse encounters faith healing, it may be helpful to accept that not all laws lend themselves to analytic logic and that some unidentifiable forces, of which faith is a component, can bring about miracles.

Certain researchers hold that a patient's capacity for faith healing is greatly strengthened if trust in, and love and admiration for, the healer exist (Leek 1973:15). The greater the sick person's love for and faith in the healer, the more readily the sick person responds to suggestion. A further requirement for faith healing is the active co-operation of the sick person.

Prayer healing

Prayer healing is a familiar concept in many faiths. Prayer and healing play an important role in the Black independent churches in South Africa. According to Taryor (1976:121), some churches have adopted the name A*l-adura Church of the Lord*, which means 'prayerful people'. This group believes particularly in faith healing and rejects traditional and modern Western medicine. Purification by water is very important to them. The preacher blesses the water and then the holy water is used for healing and for the washing of hands and feet before the place of worship is entered. The group does not believe that the water has any magical power; it simply symbolises the faith in Jesus, who is the Living Water. Because illness is associated with sin, public confession plays an important role in prayer healing (Taryor 1976:121-122).

The prophet

In some religious cults there has been a transition from soothsaying to prophecy. Steegman (1982:13) asserts that the prophets are of Christian origin and that they operate for the most part in Apostolic Zionist churches. The prophets receive their healing power from God and sometimes also from ancestral spirits. Male and female prophets are, as in the case of traditional soothsayers, called to service. The vocation is associated with certain illnesses that can only be healed by other prophets. Then follows a period of training, purification and initiation as a prophet. The prophets *believe* that God has called them through the mediation of ancestral spirits. Training involves sacrifices to God and ancestral spirits, purification rites through immersion in water, emetics and the observation of the activities of other prophets. Prophets perform their work at church healing services, are available for private consultation, and sometimes found their own churches (Steegman 1982:13-14).

According to Steegman (1982:22), the healing practices of prophets correspond in certain respects with those of soothsayers, but the emphasis is different. The female soothsayer derives her power from ancestral spirits, while the prophet receives his power from the Holy Spirit through the mediation of the ancestral spirits.

The word 'Spirit' has different connotations for different population groups and churches. Of importance to health care professionals are those people who identify with the traditional concept of spirit meaning 'wind' and 'coolness'. The belief is that this force regulates the fever condition in illness, which is caused by sorcery and witchcraft. Some churches believe that prophets have been enabled by the power of the Holy Spirit to bring about healing.

For a healing session, the Holy Spirit indicates the colour of the scapular a priest must wear. A Bible, candles and holy water are present at these rites. The prophet questions the sick person, prays, lays hands on and blesses the sick person with a healing staff. The Holy Spirit helps the prophet to prescribe the right medicine. If God has caused the sickness, prayer healing takes place and the sick person is urged to change his/her lifestyle. If evil spirits or the devil has caused the sickness, the sick person is treated with prayers. Sometimes the sick person is given water and sea water - which has been blessed - to drink, to bath in, to steam and to use as an enema. It can also be an ingredient in emetics. Steegman (1982:25) also points out that the Holy Spirit indicates to the prophet how hot or how cold the bathwater should be and how many candles should be placed around the bath. With a view to possible side effects and further treatment at health clinics, it is important for nurses to be aware of the treatment that the prophets prescribe and apply. Enemas and emetics are used to purify the body. Water and milk enemas are prescribed. For emetics the following are used: vinegar, a mixture of sugar and water, or a mixture of vinegar and ash. Ash is an important remedy, because it comes from a fire that has burnt out and cooled down, and therefore has a cooling effect on illness. It is rubbed on the body or sprinkled around the house for protection. Ash is mixed with water and drunk to cool down the condition. If the sick person vomits, this is visible evidence that the illness and the evil spirits have been cast out. Ointments for painful parts of the body are also prescribed and consist of vinegar, Vaseline, methylated spirits, sulphur and petrolatum. Some of the above-mentioned ingredients may be mixed (for example Vaseline) with methylated spirits or with sulphur (Steegman 1982:24-25).

Diverse other healers

Some healers believe in Christ and that their healing ability is received from God. Sometimes ancestral spirits are also invoked. They are instructed to act as healers through dreams and visions.

There are also prayer healers, who hold prayer sessions for the sick during or outside the church service. Then there is the 'secret prayer group', people who heal illnesses through divine powers or the powers of the ancestral spirits. In the latter group the person must move through various stages before he can become a healer. Such a person moves from the position of a sick person to that of a witness; thereafter he/she undergoes a trial period to determine his/her healing ability, then he/she becomes an intercessor and lastly a preacher. The higher the position of the member in the group, the higher the spirit involved in his healing work. In the low ranks the ancestral spirits assist, in the middle ranks angels and apostles are involved, while the spirit of Christ works in the highest rank (Steegman 1982:16).

Treatment by prayer healers includes prayers, the laying on of hands, holy water, ash, steam and immersion in water. Steegman (1982:28) points out that some healing rites take place in both a Christian and a traditional manner. The founder of the church heals in the traditional manner, her assistant heals through prayer and the laying on of hands, while a woman from the church heals with holy water. Here, too, enemas are a favourite treatment and these consist of salt water, castor oil and ash. The healing rites are aimed at purifying the sick person so that he can rid himself of his bile and take over his ancestral spirits. To prepare the sick person for receiving the ancestral spirits, he/she is anointed with a mixture of glycerine or linseed oil and ash. Convulsions and headaches are treated with castor oil (Steegman 1982:28).

Traditional healing

In order to understand traditional healing in South Africa, it is necessary to consider how people experience illness and death. To be in a position to render holistic nursing care, nurses should have an understanding of the patient's culture and religious convictions. Recognition must be given to the patient's view of health, life, illness and death.

View on illness

Church groups and church communities may have an important influence on a black person's conception of illness and adversity. In the Zionist Church, for example, a strong group consciousness exists and illness and adversity are regarded as deriving from outside the group. If someone falls ill, this means that the Zionist codes of conduct have not been adhered to (Steegman 1982:7).

Some black people believe that illness and adversity are caused by sorcery, witchcraft and the vengeance of the ancestors. Others believe that there are natural causes of illness or that God causes illness. Then there are those who believe that God punishes humanity for its sin by bringing about illness and adversity. Steegman (1982:4) has found that Xhosa Christians may believe that their traditional Supreme Being (uQamatha) corresponds with God and that He can bring about adversity. Belief in the ancestral spirits may be prevalent among many black patients. If the descendants forget or do not honour the ancestors, the ancestral spirits may cause illness. Ancestral rites are, for the most part, performed only during times of illness and adversity.

According to West (in Steegman 1982:2), the black urban population may consult the ritual healer for a variety of physical pains, for example stomachache, headache, dizziness, menstrual problems and pimples. The non-physical problems which drive people to ritual healers are numerous and include the following: problems with marriage, work, children, the home, family, housing, love and poverty. In addition to the aforementioned problems, accidents, nightmares, visions and problems with the Holy Spirit may also be mentioned.

Health care professionals must remember that because patients are often uncertain about the true nature of their illness, it is not always possible for the ritual healers to determine the nature of the illness in order to prescribe treatment. The Christian view has also had an influence on the determination of the nature of illness. Some Zionists believe, for example, that spirits who wish to prejudice and destroy prosperity cause illness and adversity. Patients may seek the aid of ritual healers because they have a better understanding and knowledge of their frame of reference than do Western doctors and nurses (Steegman 1982:3).

View on death

In Africa, the traditional viewpoint is that death means the disappearance of a being whose last reality is entirely relative to entities such as his offspring, the community and the world that existed before him and that will continue to exist after him. The true reality does not lie in the individual, but in the above-mentioned entities. According to Staples (1981:127), traditional Africans are, in life, never entirely separated from these entities, and neither do they view death as a total break with these entities. Naturally, the person holding such beliefs knows that it is painful to leave this life with its uncertainties of pleasure and pain, but he/she has always regarded him/herself as an integral part of the endless stream of life. This thought helps him/her to come to terms with death.

Health care professionals must remember that some black people who hold traditional beliefs do not believe that an accident happens by chance. They believe that the variations that occur in nature, such as too much or too little rain, are caused by shortcomings in human conduct and social relationships. Likewise they also believe that the natural and social orders are together responsible for illness and death. Staples (1981:176) asserts that misfortune is personalised. In general it is believed that untimely deaths are caused by witchcraft, sorcery or the influence of an evil spirit. The most important question with which the next of kin of the deceased person are closely concerned is not so much what has become of the evil spirit or whether it will disappear, but who caused the death? In order to determine the origin of the evil spirit, soothsayers are consulted. When the cause of the death has been explained, compensation can be claimed or medicine can be used against witchcraft. The medicine then serves to strengthen the survivors and to ward off further deaths (Staples 1981:176).

The fundamental concepts of the meaning of death, life after death and the nature and destiny of the ancestors have changed. Belief in the ancestors has very little or nothing in common with the classical Western concept of the soul and life after death.

Ela (in Schmidt & Power 1977:35) asserts that the grave represents the invincible in traditional African beliefs; for this reason the cemetery in which the ancestors lie is a holy place. It is at the grave of the ancestors that sacrifices are made and that the ancestors are consulted. The most solemn oaths are sworn on the grave of the ancestors. Nurses must bear in mind that a characteristic of many traditional cultures is that it is taboo to say that someone is dead. It is rather said that a person has gone away, that he/she has left the living or that he/she is no longer with them (Schmidt & Power 1977:36).

The soothsayer

Soothsayers are traditionally women and are called and trained by ancestral spirits to perform services for them. A person who has been called in this way is afflicted with particular symptoms of nervousness, palpitations, fainting fits and confusion, which are then recognised by other soothsayers as evidence of the calling of the ancestral spirits. The soothsayer receives intensive training that can last for one to three years. The training entails the use of certain medicines, the performance of dances that lead to ecstasy, the making of sacrifices, and the interpretation of dreams and the use of emetics. The soothsayer specialises as a soothsayer, herbalist or rite specialist, or she may be active in more than one of these practices. According to Steegman (1982:12), she makes particular use of magical power.

People who are harassed by unfamiliar and incomprehensible events, who lose their job or experience accidents and illness, usually consult the soothsayer. They believe that the soothsayer will find the causes of and the solution to their problems. It is important for nurses to note the three methods that a soothsayer uses to make a diagnosis: questioning, acting on the impulse of the moment and throwing the bones ('dolosse'). Through intensive questioning the soothsayer gets an idea of the causes of the affliction and she then probes the hidden thoughts of the sick person and arrives at a diagnosis (Steegman 1982:19). Nurses, in fact, use a similar method to obtain data in order to make a nursing diagnosis and draw up a nursing-care plan.

To illustrate the ability of the ancestral spirits to determine the causes of the illness, the sick person must beat the ground with a stick while the soothsayer is speaking. If the sick person beats hard, the soothsayer knows that her utterances are being accepted and if the sick person beats softly, her utterances are not acceptable. In this way the soothsayer arrives at a diagnosis. The sick person's friend may accept or reject the utterances on his/her behalf. The soothsayer may jump around, dance, ask questions and shout out her utterances. The second method is where the soothsayer relies on the impulse of the moment. Here she simply listens to the voices of the ancestral spirits to arrive at a diagnosis. The third method is throwing the bones ('dolosse'). The sick person blows on the bones, whereupon the ancestral spirits speak with the spirit of the soothsayer and reveal the diagnosis (Steegman 1982:20).

Where the questioning method is used to make a diagnosis, the sick person must also indicate his/her approval when it comes to the prescription by beating with a stick or clapping his/her hands. Various ritual procedures of healing can now be followed. To drive out evil spirits there is dancing, singing, shouting and a beating of drums around the patient while the soothsayer treats the sick person. Some soothsayers use fresh water, sea water, salt, vinegar, ash, roots and coloured beads to treat the sick person. Prescriptions consist of medicine which must be drunk or rubbed on. Some soothsayers make small cuts on the sick person's body into which the medicine is rubbed. Where the illness is ascribed to sorcery, the soothsayer uses a stick to which the tail of a cow has been attached to point out the guilty person. The diagnosis and treatment by soothsayers is aimed at combating and preventing illness and adversity which have been caused by ancestral spirits, sorcerers and witches (Steegman 1982:21).

The soothsayer may prescribe that sacrifices be made to the ancestors. Daily sacrifices consist of the pouring of beer, or a few grains of snuff. The sacrifices serve as an expression of respect for and deference to the ancestors. Then there is the annual sacrificial ceremony or the making of sacrifices that the soothsayer may prescribe. The sacrifices serve to prevent or protect against ancestral vengeance. The ceremonies, at which family members and the soothsayer are present, take place on Sundays. First the ancestors are prayed to; then the sacrificial animal is slaughtered and the blood is collected. A portion of the blood is cooked and eaten. The meat is cut into pieces without breaking any bones, and is then cooked and eaten. The gall, a portion of the blood, the contents of the reticulum and specific medicines are then buried as a sacrifice to the ancestors (Steegman 1982:22).

The traditional healer

Nurses must bear in mind that the survival of traditional beliefs in urban areas has ensured the survival of the traditional healer. The traditional healer is, in his/her various forms, a respected and valued member of the community. Many people who are dissatisfied with the results of Western medicine will consult a traditional healer.

The modern trend is that some traditional healers like to regard themselves as herbalists. These traditional healers compare their practice to that of a pharmacist (De Ridder 1961:45). In some tribal communities the 'asangomas' ('the inspired ones') will diagnose an illness and then send the person to the *nyanga* ('a herbalist') for medicine. This works in the same way that a patient consults a Western doctor and receives a prescription from the pharmacist. In the urban areas the *nyanga* has also taken over the functions of the *asangoma* - he/she diagnoses the illness and provides the medicine himself or herself (De Ridder 1961:161). Some of the healers concentrate particularly on soothsaying. The healers are always consulted whenever sick people believe that they have been 'bewitched'.

Witchcraft and sorcery

The belief in witchcraft and sorcery is still widespread among many in South Africa and occurs at all levels of the population (Steegman 1982:5). It is important for nurses to know that some people believe that evil spirits cause death, illnesses and disasters. In order to protect people, to pacify ancestral spirits and to overcome evil spirits, various forms of sorcery may be practised (De Ridder 1961:9).

Illness, adversity and all sorts of evils are attributed to forces that are present in the sorcerer and the witch. Witchcraft and sorcery rely on the magical to achieve their objectives. To give rise to misfortune and illness, witches make use of ministering beings. The sorcerer uses rites to cause misfortune and illness in his fellow human beings. Sorcery and witchcraft are connected to jealousy, conflict and competition. According to Staples (1981:152), some black people believe that witches and sorcerers are the primary agents of disruption in the community.

Gray (in Staples 1981:245) asserts that many Christians still believe in witchcraft, but that the reaction to witchcraft has changed drastically. Many Christians who are confronted with witchcraft now resort to prayer and no longer to traditional witchdoctors and soothsayers.

Western and traditional healers in health services

According to Chiwuzie *et al* (1987:240), all medical practices were, to a certain extent, of a traditional nature up to the beginning of the nineteenth century. Traditional medicine deals with all branches of illness and regards health as the necessary balance between physical, psychological, emotional, moral and social well-being. Ancient forms of medicine have magical or religious aspects that have a powerful influence on the human psyche.

In developing countries there is great potential for combining modern and traditional healers in primary health-care teams. If the important status of the traditional healers and the strong influence that they exert over their people are considered, their contribution to improved health services can be of inestimable value.

According to Hoff and Moseko (1986:416), it is in rural communities in particular, where there is an acute shortage of services, that traditional healers can play an important role. Bellakhdar (1989:197), on the other hand, points out that traditional medicine, which has lost some of its original traditional knowledge, tends towards vagueness when it comes to dosage.

Some people view traditional health services only in terms of their irrational and secret aspects, and accordingly reject traditional healers. In South Africa traditional healing is a very important form of health service to many people. The present attempts to have traditional health services officially accepted and to incorporate them in the health system of the country could encourage the positive aspects of traditional healing. This objective attitude in respect of traditional healing could contribute to all facets of the country's potential now being involved in the health services. Bellakhdar (1989:194) believes that developing countries have little hope of extending health cover without making use of traditional healers and medicines.

Nurses must realise that costs, convenience, beliefs and personal values influence patients' choices of health services. Accordingly, some people will prefer to consult traditional healers because these healers are familiar with and respect their psyche, feelings and dignity. Traditional medicine is a practical art that is deeply rooted in local culture, and the relationship between the healer and the sick person is simple and secretive. The scarcity of health services in remote areas of the country also contributes to the fact that traditional healers are favoured. Bellakhdar (1989:195) points out that traditional healers are close to their clients in respect of way of life, social background and language. Convenient access to traditional pharmacist and herbalist stalls is also advantageous to the sick person.

Efforts to have traditional practices incorporated in basic health care should be encouraged, but this inclusion should be considered with circumspection. Any untested assumptions or prejudices in relation to traditional medicine must be addressed, because only then will it be possible to discuss and plan in an impartial manner (Bellakhdar 1989:199).

According to Bellakhdar (1989:197), arriving at a diagnosis in traditional medicine is a complex matter. In addition to the natural causes of illnesses, it often includes supernatural aetiologies, such as spiritual punishment and evil spirits. A tendency therefore exists among traditional healers to ignore direct causes and a clearly defined pathology of illness, which actually form the basis of nosology (the science of description or classification of diseases).

Trained Western health-care professionals have usually been opposed to traditional medicine, asserting that traditional healers do not possess the necessary knowledge of anatomy, physiology, and the like to be able to make accurate prescriptions for medicine. Environment and places of work are not always hygienic and practices are often clouded in secrecy. Ogunbodebe (1991:443) points out that traditional healers should work more hygienically, while Chiwuzie *et al* (1987:240) assert that this allegation is no longer valid.

In a study by Chiwuzie *et al* (1987) of traditional healers it was found that developing countries support these healers because Western-type health systems are unattainable, expensive and without continuity, and they do not meet the people's needs. Every culture has its own peculiarities and socio-cultural aspects are important. Western medical ethics cannot be adapted to a developing country's local beliefs and traditions. Many people think, however, that the rift between Western and traditional systems can be narrowed, and suggest that these two systems be integrated. The success of this integration will depend on the willingness and co-operation of both Western and traditional healers (Chiwuzie *et al* 1987:241).

A project in the form of working groups was launched in 1983 in Swaziland and was attended by nurses and traditional healers. It came to light that traditional healers had a great interest in personal hygiene, safe water and sanitation in houses. According to Hoff and

Moseko (1986:413), the two parties must, with a view to co-operation, reach consensus on the following measures:

- Traditional healers should refer certain patients to clinics.
- Nurses should accept the referrals and respect both the patient and the traditional healer.
- Traditional healers should know the danger signs of eight children's ailments and know how to mix oral rehydration solutions for dehydration.
- Nurses and traditional healers should concentrate on the prevention of illnesses and provide health counselling on balanced nutrition, safe water, personal hygiene, use of toilets and immunisations.

Upvall (1992:32) emphasises the training of traditional healers so that they know when to refer a sick person to a health service and how to prescribe and use medicine. In developing countries modern and traditional health personnel can be combined in a team at the level of primary health care. Traditional healers can make a great contribution to the self-maintenance of health in a community. Nurses and traditional healers should focus on the health objectives that they have in common. Good co-operation in respect of referrals, immunisations and consultation is important. Hoff and Moseko (1986:415) also emphasise the need for communication and a good relationship between nurses and traditional healers in order to ensure referrals to clinics and the continuation of prescribed treatment. Upvall (1992:29) views the nurse as the key to co-operation between Western and traditional health systems.

Nurses should be mindful of the fact that purgatives and enemas, which are a favourite treatment of traditional healers, can lead to further dehydration and even death in young children. For this reason traditional healers should be encouraged to use and prescribe other rehydration solutions. Where traditional healers refer patients to the health services, nurses should find out what traditional medicine a patient is receiving in order to eliminate the possibility of a reaction to Western medicine (Upvall 1992:32-34).

Traditional healers can best be utilised in the community in areas such as psychiatry, health, orthopaedics, gynaecology and idiopathic illnesses. Chiwuzie *et al* (1987:242) recommend that they should be encouraged in these areas. In respect of their utilisation in the orthopaedic field, Ogunbodebe (1991:444) maintains that the traditional healer's ability to reduce fractures should be further investigated. Chiwuzie *et al* (1987:241) found that most doctors who took part in their study were agreed that certain aspects of traditional practices were useful in health services. However, the respondents disapproved of practices such as quackery and witchcraft and insisted that traditional healers should acknowledge their limitations in knowledge and skills and be prepared to refer patients to modern health services in good time.

Even in dentistry, Western practice can be integrated with traditional dentistry. Tooth decay and periodontal disease are a major problem in Africa. Modern dental services focus on the prevention, diagnosis, healing and correction of dental problems. Traditional healers can be trained in routine diagnostic procedures and be encouraged to refer complex cases to dentists.

One of the most effective methods of preventing tooth decay is to remove plaque. In the Western world this is done by means of toothpaste, toothbrushes, toothpicks and dental floss. In Africa a type of chewing stick is often used. Most of the plants that are used as chewing sticks contain fluoride and have an antimicrobic, anticariogenic, anti-inflammatory, antimalarial and haemostatic effect, according to Ogunbodebe (1991:443). In curative dental treatment some traditional healers use a pulp, which is a concentrated solution of certain leaves, tree bark and roots. If the teeth are loose, they are pulled.

The World Health Organization's Regional Committee for Africa has recommended that:

- all traditional healers be registered
- co-operative organisations for traditional healers be promoted
- legal recognition be given to traditional healers on the basis of competence tests
- the degree of medical knowledge of traditional healers be researched
- wherever possible, traditional healers be incorporated in the health team.

The deeply rooted trust the non-Western inhabitant of Africa has in traditional healers should be utilised to the greatest possible advantage in health services.

South Africa has recently approved a law to recognize sangomas. The Traditional Health Practice Act (Act 35 of 2004) was signed during February 2005. This act regulates the activities of traditional healers but bars them from treating fatal diseases such as cancer and HIV/AIDS. This act will create a licensing council for traditional healers (*Government Gazette* 27775 of 11 February 2005).

Concluding remarks

Nurses should remember that health programmes, and therefore also the nursing process itself, should be designed in such a way that they not only cover medical and nursing aspects, but also take the religious needs of patients into account. It is important that consideration be given to the patient's view of his/her own illness and how it should be treated. Be sensitive in the approach to the patient, ensure his/her privacy and uphold the individual's right to self-respect.

Faith healing will *never* be able to replace the enormous advantages of medical science. Leek (1973:17) points out, however, that faith healing can ensure that the motto 'a healthy mind means a healthy body' can be realised.

Traditional African communities believe that illness and adversity are caused by supernatural beings that punish unacceptable behaviour, or by people who make use of witches and sorcerers to prejudice others. As a result of exposure to Christianity, Westernisation and urbanisation, there are now many different explanations for illness and adversity: 'Owing to the Christian faith and the changed circumstances in cities in relation to the traditional society, accents in healing work have changed from traditional to Christian contents' (Schmidt & Power 1977:30). In the case of some healers a general blending of both traditional and Western contents can be observed, while others, in turn, reject traditional contents and subscribe to Christian ones only.

Critical thinking activities

1. Describe the connection between religion and health and between religion and the health services.
2. Explain how the prescriptions of the following religions and faiths influence nursing:
   - Judaism
   - Hinduism
   - Islam
   - Buddhism
   - Christianity
   - Atheism and agnosticism
   - Jehovah's Witnesses.
3. Discuss the major differences between faith healing and traditional healing.
4. How would you bring about co-operation between Western-trained nurses and traditional healers?

* It is not possible to discuss in depth the complexities of all cultures and all religions in this chapter. Please note that, of necessity, this is an overview which expresses the view's of the author.

part 6

Perspectives on the application of ethical theory in health-care

Ethical conflicts are numerous and are encountered every day in nursing practice. Some conflicts clearly challenge core beliefs about what ought to be done. Others have a moral component that may go unrecognised. Although many ethical conflicts can be examined and dealt with thoughtfully over time, others allow little time for reflection. In either case, professionals must make the best decision they can, based on the information and resources available to them at the time.

(Kopala in Chaska 2001:53)

Ethical principles in caring for HIV/AIDS patients

Dirk van der Wal

Outcomes

Studying this chapter will enable you to:

■ substantiate the foundation of moral literacy and moral competence in HIV/AIDS

■ discuss the impact that the biomedical and bioethical approaches to HIV/AIDS treatment have by comparison with a public health approach

■ clarify the phenomenon 'stigmatisation' as it relates to HIV/AIDS: its origin, course and resolution.

■ illuminate issues pertinent to conducting research in the field of HIV/AIDS

■ explain confidentiality as *the* ethical dictum in HIV/AIDS

■ explain the ethics involved in HIV testing

■ justify the ethical principles involved in HIV/AIDS counselling.

Introduction

'We all have AIDS' (Fedor 1992:65). At no point during the development of the HIV/AIDS pandemic have these words been more fitting than at present. This simple statement carries with it an immense moral weight and the appeal it directs at every human being's conscience can only become more pressing until a cure for HIV/AIDS has been found. In the meantime, HIV/AIDS continues to be a source of much ethical controversy. Much of this controversy centres on the following tenets:

■ What is framed as an ethical dilemma may often be a struggle for *fairness* between more and less dominant groups.

■ Ethical principles can be used *ideologically* to sustain structures and keep things the way they are.

■ Unexamined *myths* and ideologies can shape ethical choices and behaviours.

■ Universal ethical standards applied across *contexts* are not adequate

■ Health professionals practise ethics grounded in the reality of HIV/AIDS (Stevens and Hall 1996:39).

Moral literacy and competency in HIV/AIDS

As was indicated in the model of the individual as an ethical and caring agent (Chapter 2), the freedom of the individual to choose, to align conscience with will 'always assumes responsibility and for that reason bears the character of a moral act' (Bauman 1993 cited in Strassberg 2003:171).

Strassberg (2003:172) argues that moral *competence* is shaped by the gradual accumulation of information rather than by exposure to specific ethical codes. Twenty years ago, when health professionals and patients were first confronted with the realities of HIV/AIDS, and all sorts of 'deceitful' assumptions were made about the social environment (homosexual and heterosexual prostitution and drug abuse by injection) that harboured the virus, moral illiteracy and moral incompetence might to some degree have been tolerated and justified. However, for reasons of simple humanity, this should never have happened. Today, more than twenty years later, a large section of the population and many health-care professionals are still illiterate and, consequently, morally incompetent when it comes to HIV/AIDS. The question needs to be asked: how was 'the gradual accumulation of information' on HIV/AIDS obstructed? The problem is multidimensional. Some might argue that the strict bioethical principles of individual autonomy and confidentiality are to be blamed, that more openness about HIV/AIDS might have prevented a situation in which poor moral competency flourishes. Others might argue the problem is one of too much openness: that sex and sexual relationships were 'normalised' (or de-stigmatised) instead of HIV and AIDS. Within the health professions the focus on a biomedical rather than a public and community health approach towards HIV/AIDS is often blamed for the problem of moral illiteracy and incompetence. The biomedical approach, with its emphasis on statistics and technical issues, might well have taken the focus away from the human impact of the disease, that each and every individual, even if not infected, is affected by HIV/AIDS. As Orr and Patient put it, people react neither to abstracts nor to statistics. They respond to the reality that affects them directly (Orr and Patient 2004:14).

Strassberg (2003:172) points out that *moral competence* stems from *moral literacy* that, in turn, is built up from an ever-changing body of cultural knowledge that includes knowledge of religion (religioliteracy), of the social context (socioliteracy), of the environment (ecoliteracy), and of the universe itself (cosmoliteracy). These sources of moral literacy imply a liberal education for health professionals working in the field of HIV/AIDS, an education that mere technical training cannot provide. The individual health professional's moral competence entails familiarity with and an understanding of the full complexity of the cultural knowledge that is the source of moral literacy.

Moral competence manifests itself in specific choices that people make on the basis of moral literacy, in their emotional responses to the information they have accumulated on a given topic, and in their predispositions for actions shaped by both coded information and emotional responses to that information. Strassberg emphatically states: 'The higher the level of moral literacy, the larger pool of resources available to the construction of moral competence' (Strassberg 2003:172). This underscores a basic ethical tenet of all health professions, namely the need to be informed. For the present discussion, to be informed at all times about all issues relating to HIV/AIDS (biomedical, social, religious, political and the like) is an ethical prerequisite for becoming involved with and caring for a person living with HIV/AIDS.

The morally competent health professional will not label HIV/AIDS a disease of gays, drug-users or prostitutes, or as the punishment deserved by those of alternative sexual orientation. When fully morally literate and competent, health professionals will see HIV/AIDS for what it is: a disease among diseases that attacks without regard for sex, gender, age, sexual orientation, social class, race, ethnic origin and level of education (Strassberg 2003:172).

Beliefs and patterns of behaviour rooted in a lack of scientific information, or in misinformation, in 'knowing' things that are not actually true – in *myth*, in other words – can be very powerful (Strassberg 2003:171). This is compounded when lack of scientific knowledge and information become entwined with powerful religious beliefs stemming either from the narrow interpretation of sacred texts and oral traditions or from the deliberate misinterpretation of such texts and traditions. Some people have internalised traditional religious teachings that promote the view that HIV/AIDS is itself sinful, that it is a curse and an expression of the wrath of God (Strassberg 2003:172). This view is found among health professionals too and often leads to emotional barriers in communication. Not only is this judgmental attitude in itself unethical, but also the barrier it establishes creates a divide that fosters *stigmatisation*. In this regard Kelly and Lawrence (1988:160) point out that when the public or sections of the public are alarmed and frightened - and HIV/AIDS is an alarming and frightening phenomenon - misinformation and opinions not grounded in scientific fact can exacerbate hysteria, further foster misinformation, and adversely affect the civil liberties of people and, ultimately, the quality of life of people living with HIV and AIDS (Kelly and Lawrence 1988:160).

Myth, according to the Concise Oxford Dictionary (1982), refers to: 'traditional narratives [usually] involving supernatural or fancied persons etc. and embodying popular ideas on natural and social phenomenon, etc. . . . fictitious person, thing or idea'. Within the parameters of the discussion above, myth, in the context of HIV/AIDS, is the *antithesis* of moral literacy. Previously, in the absence of scientific knowledge, the medical and social community at large believed that any and all of the known means of viral transmission could be in operation in HIV. At present, with an augmented moral literacy base of scientific knowledge, rooms are no longer sprayed with insecticide, touching an HIV positive person is no longer dreaded, and cutlery used by HIV positive persons is not kept separate from others. Science has led to professional measures being taken that are less insulting, less isolating and less marginalising to HIV-positive persons.

At the community level, there are two separate though related areas of HIV and AIDS in which myth is rife: the origin and cause of the disease and the treatment of the disease Woloschack (2003:164). Without going into details on these issues, time and time again news broadcasts report on cases of child molestation and rape in an attempt to cure the HIV and AIDS victim. On the other hand, the argument is often heard that HIV and AIDS are themselves mythical, and merely an attempt to discourage people from having as many children as they want. It is health professionals' and the health-care workers' moral obligation, as members of the community, to identify these misconceptions and myths, and to do what it takes to eradicate these. Precept and example, trust, rapport, being knowledgeable, all of these might assist professionals in combating myth and ignorance.

Theoretical and philosophical foundation of practice

Three distinct, yet interrelated, challenges surround HIV/AIDS, namely: 1) the HI-virus and being HIV-positive; 2) the disease AIDS; and 3) social, cultural, political, and economic responses to HIV/AIDS (Walker and Frank 1997:31). The biomedical nature of HIV/AIDS, which focuses on the disease and the virus *per se*, justifies a biomedical perspective on the pandemic. The bioethical approach, with its strict adherence to the personal autonomy of patients and clients, accompanies this perspective. By way of contrast, the actual means of transmission of the virus shifts the focus of concern to the realm of human behaviour – the field of social interaction and the behavioural sciences. Indeed, the extent of the pandemic warrants a community and public health perspective, framing the whole pandemic within the context of the availability of resources and distributive justice, thus suggesting a more *paternalistic* approach to the pandemic.

The biomedical and bioethical approach

B*ioethics* has emerged in medicine as an ethic designed to counteract the paternalistic authority of physicians and to promote individual autonomy, and its associated concepts of anonymity, informed consent, confidentiality and privacy. This ethic has permeated the whole health-care industry since physicians used to be regarded as the *de jure* representatives of health care notwithstanding the fact that most health care was, and still is, *de facto*, delivered by health care agencies other than medicine proper.

It is argued that within the hospital and the laboratory setting (including the way in which specimens are obtained from humans and the protocols of clinical trial research), the individual finds him/herself in a controlled, and controllable, social setting or culture, cut off from his/her social milieu. In this clinical setting, although everything about the individual patient is valued, the primary concern is of the individual as a source of information for scientific advancement. Understandably, therefore, the individual living with HIV/AIDS often finds him/herself 'alone against the system'. Under these circumstances it is laudable that the medical profession exercises self-control and self-regulation via bioethics, and more pertinently, via patient individuality and autonomy. However, as has been indicated in the tenets underlying this chapter, universal ethical standards that are applied across *contexts* are not adequate or, as Aroskar (1997:135) points out, ethical answers will not be found unless ethical dimensions are first considered.

The approach of public and community health

When the focus is shifted from the strictly clinical (the HI-virus, the symptomatology of HIV/AIDS, clinical trials involving the testing of antiretroviral drugs, the individual's reaction to these drugs, and the like) to the lived experience of being HIV-positive and of having AIDS, it is essentially shifted towards a *population-based* approach that is more in line with the set of values embraced by the public and community health approach. Bayer and Fairchild (2004:475) emphatically state that the high priority given to individual autonomy in, for instance medical research ethics, cannot be assumed to be appropriate for public health. The focus on population-based health requires an ethics of collective health that entails far more extensive limitations on personal autonomy and on civil liberty than would be justified by current bioethics perspectives. A major issue in HIV/AIDS in this regard is *voluntarism* as it figures, amongst other things, in voluntary versus obligatory (paternalistically prescribed) testing. It also involves arguments around disclosure and non-disclosure of individuals' HIV status. However, it does not follow *logically* that public health is insensitive to the importance of protecting individual rights (Bayer and Fairchild 2004:491) such as confidentiality.

Aroskar (1997:135) further states that community health care, and by implication public health, is fraught with ethical dilemmas and reiterates that the ethics of community health care centres around the ethics of prioritising health care delivery to equally needy and deserving groups of people in a resource challenged environment. In addition, the types of communities that exist - structural, emotional and functional communities - each contribute their own special ethical issues with regard to HIV/AIDS. The ethics of this reality entails striking a balance between the alternative models of morality of *individualism* versus *collectivism* and *paternalism* versus *libertarianism*.

Elements of the debate

Public-health activists argue that the biomedical and bioethical approach, and its associated ethic of individual rights, negates the pandemic's extensive social and behavioural ramifications. This has resulted in what is called an epistemological 'obstacle' (Bayer and Fairchild 2004:475), in other word, an impediment in the way that knowledge relating to HIV/AIDS is perceived, the implications of such knowledge, and the social construction of knowledge about HIV/AIDS. From the point of view of people in favour of a public health approach, the biomedical and bioethical approach skews the way in which we conduct research into HIV/AIDS. A community and public health approach has a broader focus on both physical and mental health care and on the variables that affect health directly or indirectly, such as life-style, family and social interactions, and community resources (Aroskar 1997:136). All of the above fit the HIV/AIDS profile well, making community health the preferred model for the majority of people living with HIV/AIDS. Ultimately, a unilateral biomedical and bioethical approach (any unilateral approach for that matter) skews understanding HIV/AIDS. This becomes quite evident in, for instance, the discrepancies in statistics on the prevalence HIV/AIDS in South Africa, coming from sources as different as the World Health Organisation, Statistics SA and the National Department of Health. This is not an idle argument. As Aroskar (1997:136) indicates, not having a complete and up to date database of the community one serves is itself an ethical issue and harbours ethical dilemmas directly relating to distributive justice. Further, the ethical issues already involved in social intervention, in identifying populations that are vulnerable and needing health and nursing care, become that much more intricate if a reliable data base is absent. Ultimately, a pro-biomedical and bioethical distortion of the epistemology of HIV/AIDS can result in a distortion of the caring ethic towards people living with HIV/AIDS. There needs to be a balance between the bio-perspective (biomedicine, bioethics and biology) on the one hand, and the socio-political, cultural and lived experience perspective, on the other hand.

Notwithstanding the HIV/AIDS pandemic's psychosocial and epidemiological character, Bayer and Fairchild (2004:478) insist that, because of the psychosocial and socio-political climate at the beginning of the pandemic, a commitment emerged to treat HIV/AIDS differently from any other epidemic. The biomedical and bioethical doctrine was projected onto the very first individual cases of HIV/AIDS at a time when principles such as individual autonomy and the like were considered the core principles to adhere to. These principles fell well into place when later, as the pandemic developed, certain social and civil measures appeared to be, or were accused of being, coercive and counter-productive since they tended to 'drive people most in need of services away from such service thereby failing to achieve the public health goal of prevention through behavioural change, care and health support' (Bayer and Fairchild 2004:479). This supported the biomedical and bioethical position that no public health policy that violated the rights of individuals could be effective in controlling the spread of HIV (Bayer and Fairchild 2004:478). Even now, this position is supported by the fact that, where other epidemics, though also sexually transmitted, are treatable and curable, HIV/

AIDS is not curable. Widespread public misunderstanding about and sheer moral illiteracy regarding HIV/AIDS still fuel discrimination, stigmatisation and ostracism (Kelly and Lawrence 1988:165). All of these sustain an approach that emphasises individualism, anonymity, non-disclosure of HIV status, voluntarism and the like, as opposed to a paternalistic, epidemiological public health approach.

The dispute between biomedicine and bioethics, on the one hand, and a public and community health approach, on the other, remains unsettled. There is a question about the risk factor involved in voluntary testing and the non-disclosure of HIV-status as opposed to obligatory testing and obligatory disclosure. The problem that emerges relates to the uncertainty of the risk for others. Vulnerability comes into play here. From a public health point of view, it can be argued that society at large becomes vulnerable and that those who are not HIV-infected become potential victims and are victimised by those who are HIV- positive. In other words, everybody else needs to adapt their life styles to 'accommodate' HIV- positive persons who, being members of a minority group, presumably 'just carry on with their lives'.

Returning to the anonymity/vulnerability risk-factor: this concerns the moral weight assigned to the probability and severity of harm that might be done to others when HIV/AIDS is approached from either an individualistic or from a public health approach. No matter how these matters are resolved, they raise issues that are fundamentally different from those posed by behaviours that represent primarily a threat to individuals themselves. According to the public health point of view, it is the *collective* hazard that warrants paternalistic interventions even when the threat posed by any individual may not be very big (Bayer and Fairchild 2004:489). Adherents of the individualistic approach point out that paternalistic decisions of adherents to the public health approach equally bear a risk in the form of severe discrimination, ostracism and stigmatisation. Nonetheless, public health utilitarians insist that '[t]he central commitment to collective well-being requires a much more robust embrace of paternalism - one that goes beyond interventions designed to protect those whose choices are limited by lack of knowledge and understanding . . . because we are morally bound to prevent avoidable suffering and death' (Bayer and Fairchild 2004:491).

Health-care professionals may get caught up in the middle of the bioethics/biomedicine versus public health dispute. To reiterate, this is a dispute in which the ethics of the alternative models of morality of paternalism versus libertarianism and individualism versus collectivism (utilitarianism) need to be resolved. As Bayer and Fairchild point out, the challenge for professionals is to identify those moments and situations when public health paternalism is justified and to articulate a set of principles that preserves a commitment to the realm of free choice (Bayer and Fairchild 2004:492).

The ethics relating to social intervention

A great deal of effort, time and money has been invested in social interventions in the fight against HIV/AIDS. These social interventions, despite their laudable aim, have not gone undisputed. There is the transformation regarding sex education in our schools, the row between HIV/AIDS activist groups and Government's decisions on the antiretroviral comprehensive treatment plan, and the pro-condom campaign. To illustrate the point at issue, namely the ethics of social intervention, the example of the pro-condom campaign will be used. Aroskar (1997:140) reminds us that ethical issues emerge in relation to four aspects of any proposed social intervention, namely goals, targets for change, means, and evaluation.

The **choice of goals** for the proposed social intervention maximises certain values while minimising others (Aroskar 1997:140). With regard to the propagation of condom use in preventing the spread of HIV, it can be argued that although the intervention had a positive goal, the outcome minimised traditional values relating to age and sexual activity as well as sexual traffic in general. Not only have traditional African values been transgressed by this intervention, but also many religious groups are aggrieved and resentful towards the intervention. An underlying argument is that instead of de-stigmatising and normalising HIV/AIDS, permissive sexual intercourse has been 'de-stigmatised' and 'normalised' – that symptomatic measures and treatment are being carried out instead of addressing the underlying social problem of a lack of chastity. Naturally, some would argue that the condom campaign has enlightened the youth and has freed them and others from the bondage of sexual pettiness. Individual health practitioners will have to see how their own moral beliefs fit in with the aims of the campaign.

Defining what **the target for change** in HIV/AIDS is, is extremely problematic. Despite the opinion of a large section of the general public that the target for social intervention in HIV/AIDS should be the 'obscure' culprit groups of gays, prostitutes and intravenous drug users, the fact of the matter is that these groups are today relatively 'unobscure' and it is precisely these groups that have formed active support groups in the fight against HIV/AIDS. The real issue is that HIV/AIDS has become a predominantly heterosexual disease, and so it has become more diffuse in society, thus making it much more difficult to pinpoint a specific target group. Consequently, mass campaigning is the only way to go. The problem is that whether one wants to hear about HIV/AIDS and condoms or not, one has to. With regard to the condom campaign specifically the ethical issue is that the message has spilt over to a section of the community that is not mature enough to deal with the reality of condom usage.

The **means** chosen to implement social interventions is often a source of concern. In the case of television, for example, there is much concern about the apparent double meaning of the message conveyed. There is hardly a television series or full-length film that does not contain content of a sexual nature. Some images shown on national television fall short of being totally explicit and pornographic only because they do not pertinently show whether a condom is actually being used or not. Many music videos contain explicit and suggestive body language that leaves nothing to the imagination. Most alarming to moralists is the fact that these music videos are televised during prime time. So, though the chosen means may assist the mass social intervention campaign, it can also end up refuting or undermining the goals of that intervention. The bottom line from an ethical point of view is to maintain ethical and moral congruency and authenticity, and to refuse to be compromised by anything other than that which one really stands for and believes in.

Evaluating the consequences of the implementation of social intervention is extremely difficult. In a multifaceted phenomenon such as HIV/AIDS, this is even more of a problem because of multiple interventions and confounding variables. There is, however, one point of serious ethical concern and that is the apparent weariness and aloofness people tend to show towards HIV/AIDS. The fact that the term 'HIV/AIDS fatigue' appears more and more in the literature is alarming. Could it be that a large section of the population has become desensitised to HIV/AIDS? If this is so, then a new set of ethical dilemmas and questions needs to be addressed. Whatever the case, the phenomenon merits further investigation and research.

Ethics relating to communities

Within the context of the broad ethical framework within which HIV/AIDS care is rendered, it is important to define what the term *community* implies, as it is more than merely an aggregate of individuals. Aroskar (1997:137) distinguishes between *structural, emotional* and *functional* communities. Each of these communities provides a pertinent view on HIV/AIDS.

A **structural community** refers to an aggregate of people, usually from a geopolitical area (Aroskar 1997:137). In the case of HIV/AIDS the structural community is referred to, in terms of its general geographic distribution, as global, in terms of its pervasiveness as, for instance, sub-Saharan Africa and, in terms of its intensity, as South Africa (or any other country for that matter). When considering a structural community in the light of HIV/AIDS, one has to look at things like policy, legislation, funding and accessibility to health services. As is often the case, what is legal is not necessarily ethical. AIDS activists have brought this dearly to the attention of both the public and the state. Also, by not involving oneself in the ways in which the structural community addresses HIV/AIDS, one might be accused of wanting to keep things the way they are. This may be unethical.

Individuals who have a feeling of belonging, of togetherness, create emotional communities (Aroskar1997: 137). With reference to HIV-positive individuals and patients suffering from AIDS, these individuals may experience a feeling of belonging-ness with other infected and affected individuals. They may belong to sub-cultural groups such as a drug addicts, gays or haemophiliacs, or simply by virtue of being stigmatised, discriminated against and marginalised. These emotional issues demand of the health professional a special sensitivity and understanding. Emotional communities in this instance spell vulnerability, as emotional grouping is often an attempt to ease personal vulnerability. It is not up to health professionals or any other health-care worker to negate these communities.

Aroskar (1997:137) also classifies special-interest groups in the community as *emotional* groups. The most important of these special-interest groups, as far as the caring ethic is concerned, is the buddy system. However, the buddy system should not further alienate and marginalise people living with AIDS. Nonetheless, the health professional must be aware of the human and emotional resources these special-interest groups have to offer and how they can contribute towards alleviating the vulnerability and suffering of people living with AIDS.

A **functional group**, according to Aroskar (1997:137), is 'a group with an identifiable need'. People who are HIV-positive or suffering from AIDS unquestionably have very specific needs over and above those associated with accompanying socio-economic conditions. These needs are similar to the needs of members of vulnerable groups. For HIV/AIDS sufferers, in the sense of their belonging to a functional group, distributive justice is perhaps the most pressing ethical problem.

Confidentiality: *the* ethical dictum in HIV/AIDS

Confidentiality is, for both the biomedical/bioethical and the public health approaches to HIV/AIDS, of critical importance. In HIV/AIDS confidentiality directs a sober appeal to both health practitioners and clients in respect of professional and patient autonomy. *Veracity*, as a professional and civil obligation, is of cardinal importance. The *advocacy* role of the health practitioner often changes from primarily appealing to other health professionals on behalf of the patient to appealing to the patient on behalf of other health professionals and potential patients. Health practitioners often find themselves caught up within the opposing models of egoism versus altruism, of individualism versus collectivism (utilitarianism), and of paternalism versus libertarianism.

In the health-care arena staff and administrators usually set the boundaries for shared secrets (confidentiality) on the basis of bureaucratic and therapeutic requirements (Brown 1993:197). Given the pandemic proportions of HIV/AIDS, the stealth of infection, the behavioural and social dimensions of the disease, and the involvement of community members as allies and colleagues (rather than patients and clients) of the health team, the professional bureaucratic delimitation of the boundaries for confidentiality becomes blurred. Indeed, the bureaucratic basis for setting boundaries - any boundaries for that matter - has been greatly defeated by the democratic approach to HIV/AIDS and the granting of legal empowerment to people living with the disease to decide whether or not to disclose their status or to be tested. In other words, the whole issue of voluntarism versus paternalism is brought to a head.

Given that health care is becoming more specialised and the number of team members increasing, *vis-à-vis* encounters between health professionals are decreasing and communication via documentation increasing. This, together with the sheer numbers of patients, compromises confidentiality (Wilson *et al* 2002: 439). As a consequence ethical management becomes imperative. However, no matter how ethical management is conducted, it is still the individual health professional's integrity that finally counts, and it is at this point that the dynamics of confidentiality, anonymity, disclosure, non-disclosure, and the like, become very intricate.

The secrecy built into voluntarism is perhaps the only real way to secure 'confidentiality'. However, this has ethical implications, as it requires all patients to be treated as potentially HIV-positive. In some circles this is seen, in effect, as labelling all people as being HIV-positive. So the problem of keeping the patient's HIV-status confidential becomes an issue only once the patient has been tested and the result indicates that the patient is indeed HIV-positive. Each citizen, therefore, has the social responsibility to acquaint him/herself with his/ her HIV status should this in any way be compromised. This calls for an exceptionally diffuse and high level of social responsibility. It involves an alignment of all the sources of moral literacy at all levels of society. In the absence of a cure for the disease, this level of moral education and responsibility is the most important ethical quest for health professionals and other health professionals in combating the HIV/AIDS pandemic.

The whole issue of confidentiality, besides the current permissiveness[1] towards individual autonomy and human rights, relates to personal vulnerability, stigmatisation and ostracism. 'While therapeutic interventions always require sensitivity toward client rights to privacy, the stigma associated with AIDS and the stigma that is associated with merely being perceived of as at risk for AIDS, mandates extraordinary diligence in maintaining confidentiality' (Kelly and Lawrence 1988:159). Though not actively breaching confidentiality, the following might raise the suspicions that Kelly and Lawrence (1988:159) warn against: taking the test; visiting a community health clinic regularly; being visited by a community health worker regularly; working with people living with HIV/AIDS; not breastfeeding one's baby according to cultural dictates; taking medication regularly, including vitamins; losing weight for whatever reason; using condoms; and practising celibacy.

[1] *Note to the reader: the word 'permissiveness' is not used pejoratively here.*

In all these instances health practitioners need to take the necessary measures to ensure that patients and clients are not labelled. In spite of this, confidentiality about other aspects and treatment relating to an individual should not be sacrificed in the quest to maintain confidentiality regarding the patient's HIV-status.

However, closely related though disclosure and confidentiality may be, they are not the same thing. Disclosure means 'making known', while confidentiality, as indicated previously, implies 'keeping what has been disclosed secret'. Though a public health perspective supports an epidemiological approach towards managing the HIV/AIDS pandemic, it does not necessarily support breach of confidentiality, nor does it support disclosure to the point of surrender of anonymity. The 'to whom and 'for what purposes' always form the boundaries within which disclosed information should be strictly guarded.

Whatever the ideological perspective on confidentially and disclosure, intricate logistical problems remain. Some of the questions that arise are: how will we determine whether a person is at any given moment HIV-positive or not? Will we take a person's word for it? Will we repeat tests every two weeks or, depending on how much the window period shrinks owing to new ways of testing for antibodies, as often as might be necessary? Who needs to know? If an HIV-positive person continues with risky behaviour that may endanger others, at what point should the individual's autonomy, privacy and anonymity be overruled by the need for others to know and for the greater good of society? What is the health-care professional's position should the deliberate spread of HIV/AIDS be criminalised? The options available are:

- An appeal to the conscience of each and every citizen to act in a socially responsible way. Such responsibility would include the voluntary testing of any individual whose HIV-status is in any way compromised, the voluntary disclosure of HIV-positive individuals to all who need to know about their HIV-status, and the attendant confidentiality. Voluntarism, as freedom of choice, spells responsibility.
- To de-stigmatise and normalise HIV/AIDS completely. Though such a desirable state will not, in principle, overrule the need for professional confidentiality and secrecy, it may decrease the negative effect that accidental disclosure (or 'accidental' breach of confidentiality) may have on the individual. This in turn may promote self-disclosure of the person living with AIDS, reducing threatening situations for others and reducing the ethical dilemma for health professionals of whether or not to breach confidentiality.

Confidentiality relating to sex partners and the need for partner notification (disclosure) are perhaps the most pressing ethical question faced by health professionals in the HIV arena. Wilson *et al* indicate that counselling in this regard should continue throughout the entire therapeutic relationship. This calls for a much closer and more personal relationship between the health professional and the patient than either the bioethical or the public health approach has to offer. When a third party at risk has been identified, patients should be encouraged to disclose their status and the health professional should offer to assist in the process of disclosure (Wilson *et al* 2002: 439). Reasons for not wanting to disclose, such as when the patient's life may be threatened or severe ostracism is feared, must be determined by the health professional and assistance from other public institution must be sought. According to Wilson *et al* (2002:439) '[u]nder these conditions, since the health-care worker's primary duty is to protect the life of the patient, the HIV status should not be disclosed'. Should the health professional decide, in a case where a patient is merely *unwilling* to disclose his or her status to their sex partners, that it is ethically just to disclose a patient's status, these professionals must realise that they may be brought before a court of law to defend their decision. Such disclosure to the patient's sex partner(s) (third party) should be made only after careful consideration, if the third party is: a known and an identified person; is at risk of infection, i.e. it is known that no precautions for safe sex are being taken or that the sexual act is abusive or in any other way inappropriate; is offered testing; and pre- and post-counselling can be given (Wilson *et al* 2002: 439).

In addition, the patient must be informed that the health practitioner will take these steps and that all communications in this regard will be thoroughly documented (Wilson *et al* 2002: 440).

In contrast to a sex partner's right, under certain conditions and circumstances, to know the HIV-status of the patient, family members do not have the right to know the HIV-status of a member of that family (Wilson *et al* 2002:441). Within the broader focus of public health, the advantage of telling the patient's family should be pointed out to the patient. This should preferably be done before the patient develops observable symptoms or full blown AIDS at which point family members may start asking questions, leaving the health professional feeling uncomfortable.

With regard to disclosure and confidentiality **affecting other health-care workers**, the dictum of confidentiality and autonomy demands that precautionary measures be taken during all nursing and medical procedures. Wilson *et al* (2002:442) pertinently indicate that when referring a patient to another member of the health team is required, the HIV-status of the patient may not be disclosed without his/her prior consent. The patient must, however, be informed that not disclosing his/her HIV-status to other relevant health practitioners may jeopardise the quality of his/her future health care. Once they have been informed, all other members of the health team are duty-bound to maintain confidentiality about the patient's HIV status (Wilson *et al* 2002:442).

In the case of confidentiality **relating to medical and health certificates**, occupational health practitioners and other health-care officials should ensure that what appears in such a certificate is 'a description of the illness, disorder or malady in layperson's language' (Wilson *et al* 2002:443). Under no circumstances should this paraphrasing distort the truth, although every attempt should be made not to disclose the true sensitive nature of the patient's condition. Should the employer request more pertinent information, such information may be made available only if the patient consents to it (Wilson *et al* 2002:443).

With regard to confidentiality **relating to occupational injury**, the measures that count in health facilities are also applicable to the industry. Since the HIV-status of all workers is kept confidential, general barrier measures must be in place in respect of injury on duty. It is both a professional and an ethical duty of health professionals in different occupational areas to teach workers about the prevention of transmission of HIV. This is in line with the Occupational Health and Safety Act 85 of 1993 that stipulates that all employers must adopt measures to reduce the risk of HIV transmission in the workplace (Wilson *et al* 2002:445).

The Employment Equity Act 55 of 1998 that prohibits the unfair discrimination against any employee based on his or her HIV status regulates confidentiality relating to employer/employee matters. An employer may conduct pre-employment testing only with the informed consent of the prospective employee. Only if the employee agrees to it, may the results be made available to the employer, who again should treat it with the necessary confidentiality (Wilson *et al* 2002:445).

In the case of **an occupational accident** involving possible exposure of other workers to the body fluids of the injured person, confidentiality is again of paramount importance. Nonetheless, testing the person who is alleged source is a complex issue (Wilson *et al* 2002:447). This should be undertaken only with the informed consent of the patient. If the source patient is unwilling to give consent, it is preferable to do a rapid test on the health worker who has been exposed and to presume the person who is the source to be positive (Wilson *et al* 2002:447). This also applies to other health-care practitioners who may, for instance, sustain a needle prick.

In conclusion, the fact that HIV/AIDS is not a notifiable disease (Wilson *et al* 2002:448) gives credence to confidentiality as the ethical dictum of the disease.

Ethical issues relating to HIV testing and counselling

Cost efficiency contra-indicates wide scale mandatory **HIV testing**. Given the sheer numbers involved, as well as the ethical issues surrounding personal autonomy, it is more effective, safer and less costly to follow the bioethical principle of voluntarism. Health-care professionals should simply maintain effective levels of body fluid precautions as general practice rather than testing all patients entering health-care facilities to determine their HIV status. In the light of the legal empowerment granted to the individual to decide whether or not he or she wants to know his or her HIV status, Wilson *et al* (2002:436) emphatically state that unauthorised HIV testing contradicts the principle of a person's right to freedom and privacy. A person may, therefore, be tested only at his or her own request, or after he or she has given informed consent, or if the test is authorised by legislation or by court order (Wilson *et al* 2004:436).

Informed consent in this instance also implies telling the patient in a neutral, non-coercive way why it might be necessary to have his or her HIV status determined. In this regard the laws that regulate HIV testing must also be considered. Various laws have a bearing on testing and health professionals must determine which legal stipulations are applicable to any specific situation. Furthermore, given the possibility of drug misuse in HIV/AIDS and the possibility of mental incapacitation during the later stages of the disease, health professionals must determine what the patient's mental status is before commencing counselling for informed consent, obtaining informed consent or referring the patient to have blood taken for the test (Wilson *et al* 2002: 436).

According to Bennett and Erin (1999:39), **counselling** has become a catchword in the context of HIV/AIDS. This is mainly due to the fact that the disease is transmittable; that it has a stigma attached to it; and that it is incurable. Moreover, a large part of the management of the pandemic has been placed in the realm of the behavioural sciences. This presents an opportunity to introduce psychological and sociopsychological care into HIV/AIDS care (Bennett and Erin 1997:40).

Counselling in the context of HIV/AIDS should not be seen as therapy (Bennett and Erin 1999:40). The health professionals who involve themselves in HIV/AIDS counselling should be clear about the boundaries of counselling. The instant counselling becomes therapy, or the need for therapy arises, the patient should be referred to the appropriate allied health professional.

Counselling itself involves a number of ethical principles. Besides the four basic ethical principles of patient autonomy (including informed consent and privacy), beneficence, non-maleficence and justice, the following principles must be upheld by the professional counsellor:

- The basic values of the health professional counsellor should include integrity, impartiality and respect for the patient. Health counsellors must ensure their patients' psychosocial and physical safety by maintaining privacy, professional secrecy and patient autonomy. Counselling sessions should thus be kept non-exploitative, implying a commitment to anti-discriminatory and anti-stigmatising practice. It is thus necessary for health counsellors to address their own personal prejudices by way of periodic values clarification sessions and open conversation with peers.
- Confidentiality is a cornerstone of HIV/AIDS counselling as it secures the patient's privacy and autonomy and is essential for the establishment of the trust without which counselling cannot fruitfully proceed.
- The terms and conditions on which counselling is offered must be negotiated with the patient before counselling commences.
- Appropriate boundaries around the counselling relationship must be established and maintained at all times. This is particularly the case when counseling begins to overlap with psychotherapy. (British Association for Counselling and Psychotherapy: http://www.cma.ca)

HIV/AIDS counselling is not a once-off interaction. It covers the full extent of the health professional's relationship with the patient, before and after the blood test, and irrespective of the outcome of the test.

Pre-test counselling must be made available by the health professional counsellor to all patients requesting HIV testing. Such requests must be respected. It is the health counsellor's ethical obligation to trace the patient's risk history and the reasons for wanting the test done; to assess the possibility of the person having been exposed to the HI-virus or, indeed, of having been infected with the virus; to provide the person with information about HIV infection and testing, including the implications of positive, negative and indeterminate test results, as well as the impact the window-period may have; to explore specific ways in which the person can avoid, or reduce, risk behaviour; to identify testing options available, particularly anonymous testing; to discuss the advantages and disadvantages of testing and the potential benefits and harms of being found HIV-positive; to determine whether in fact the person really wants to know his/her HIV-status; to discuss the confidentiality of test results; to consider the strain of waiting for test results and possible reactions to these results; to assess the window-period by identifying the most recent risk event and plan an appropriate time for testing; to obtain and record informed consent; and to arrange for a follow-up appointment, after a predetermined interval, for a face-to-face visit to inform the patient of the test results. (The Canadian Medical Association: http://www.cma.ca)

During **post-test counselling** the health counsellor must be prepared to give the results in person; to assess the patient's understanding of the test result; to encourage the patient to express feelings and reactions; to consider further interventions; and to ascertain whether the person understands the threat of re-infection (The Canadian Medical Association: http://www.cma.ca). According to Wilson *et al* (2002:437), the responsibility for post-test counselling falls on the practitioner who commissioned the test.

In the case of a **negative and indeterminate result** the health professional counsellor must realise that the patient could not have known the result and that he/she has endured a traumatic experience. The health counsellor must discuss the need for repeat testing with the patient should this be necessary; he/she must reiterate the ways in which HIV is transmitted, revisit the topic of risk behaviour and assess the patient's commitment to risk-reducing strategies (The Canadian Medical Association: http://www.cma.ca).

Counselling patients on **a positive result** requires exceptional sensitivity. Here the health professional counsellor must assess the patient's immediate psychological response to being told that he/she is HIV-positive; plan how the patient can overcome adverse psychological reactions; arrange additional psychological and social support services as needed; provide reassurance about the person's immediate safety; arrange for medical follow-up visits; review transmission modes and risk-reduction strategies; and discuss partner notification, if necessary (The Canadian Medical Association: http://www.cma.ca ; Kelly and Lawrence 1988:162).

In addition to the above, other important issues that the health professional counsellor must attend to involve discussing with the patient health, reproductive and treatment issues; reviewing the importance of partner testing and notification, and offering assistance if the patient requires it; and reiterating the patient's right to privacy and confidentiality (The Canadian Medical Association: http://www.cma.ca).

It is important to remember that a significant proportion of persons with AIDS eventually develop neurological symptoms that impede their cognitive functioning (Herman, 1986; Wolcott, 1986a). Even with the present generation of antiretroviral drugs, the health counsellor and patient must anticipate the occurrence of neurological symptoms and consider important decisions relating to treatment, including decisions about life-support maintenance, resuscitation, last will and testament, and consultation with attorneys familiar with health care ethics and law. It is also important for health-care professionals to obtain information from the AIDS patient about who should assist in decision-making if the patient becomes unable to do so. If the patient appoints an individual who has no clear legal standing, such as a non-spouse lover, legal consultation may also be necessary (Kelly and Lawrence 1988:162). The health professional counsellor must thoroughly record all decisions.

With regard to **HIV-testing in children**, children of 14 years and older can independently provide informed consent for an HIV test (Wilson *et al* 2002: 438). These children have the same right to confidentiality as any other patient. However, the child should be strongly advised on the importance of telling parents, caregivers, partners, and the like. On the other hand, children under the age of 14 years can be tested only if their parents or legal guardians have given informed consent (Wilson *et al* 2002: 438).

Access to treatment and care

With regard to general health care, HIV/AIDS raises many ethical issues about basic rights and fair treatment of infected people. Although some people argue that HIV- positive persons acted irresponsibly and that, therefore, some of their rights as citizens are invalidated, the South African Constitution accords every person the right of access to health care, non-discrimination, privacy and confidentiality, and the right to an environment that is not harmful to their health and well-being (Wilson *et al* 2002: 435). Even in the absence of certainty about an individual's HIV-status, emergency treatment may not be withheld from a patient (Wilson *et al* 2002: 436). If any such uncertainty exists, the general rule of treating all patients as potentially HIV- positive should be upheld.

With regard to available antiretroviral drugs, it is unethical to promote these as the only option for 'surviving' the epidemic. Personal responsibility, knowledge and the cultivation of moral literacy and competence among the broader public are still the most important ways of 'surviving' the epidemic. Alternative treatments and nutrition are also viable options (Galloway 2003:20). Antiretroviral treatment is, in any case, expensive and this immediately reintroduces the problem of scarce commodities: in this instance money, human resources and antiretroviral drugs themselves.

Health professionals, especially those in community health settings, have several important professional and ethical obligations with regard to antiretroviral therapy. Some of these are:

- Observing patients for the side-effects of drugs. Health professionals should not minimise side-effects but should also be aware that what are perceived as 'side-effects' may be symptoms of remission into full-blown AIDS, and that the antiretroviral therapy is perhaps ineffective (Galloway 2003:18). When observing the side-effects of antiretroviral drugs, beneficence and non-maleficence feature pertinently. Patient advocacy features pertinently in cases where side-effects are reported to other health-care professionals.

- Checking that patients are adhering to their regimen. By not adhering to a regimen, drug resistant strains of HIV can be cultivated and spread, making even the drug-naïve person resistant (Galloway 2003:18). The side-effects of drugs are often enough motivation for patients to discontinue their treatment. Health professionals should be specifically on the lookout for this. Again, acting on these observations adheres to beneficence and non-maleficence.

- The dispute about the comprehensive treatment plan of antiretroviral drugs. It needs to be noted that, in view of the perception that antiretroviral treatment entails a rather complex regimen, regimens are in fact becoming much simpler (Galloway 2003:20). 'Exaggerating complexity' is unethical and makes patients feel more vulnerable. Not doing so paves the way for equality and fairness in treatment.

- Concerns about poor people who cannot comply with the regimen even if they want to. Here, health professionals must *advocate* for all patients meeting the criteria for inclusion into the antiretroviral comprehensive treatment plan regardless of their socio-economic standing. This does not, however, rule out the fact that certain socio-economic conditions must be favourable, such as nutrition. Here food packages and vegetable gardens are important. Vegetable gardens promote patient autonomy, empowerment and positive self-image. Concern about poor socio-economic conditions also paves the way for distributive justice.

- A pressing problem is that some people, not knowing their status, come into treatment at a very late stage when their CD4+ count has dropped significantly (Galloway 2003:18). In this instance health professionals have the moral obligation to inform and to educate the general public. Especially in deep rural areas with limited mass media coverage, it is health-care professionals and workers who are instrumental in informing the public, without forcing them to have their HIV-status determined. These actions pave the way towards moral literacy and competence as well as towards autonomy.

Stigmatisation

The Concise Oxford Dictionary defines stigma as 'imputation attaching to person's reputation; stain on one's good name'. Stigmatisation goes hand in hand with the concept of *social labelling* (Louw and Edwards 1997:679). The general character of stigmatisation in HIV/AIDS is that those who have contracted HIV should be punished rather than helped (Wang 2000:57). According to Orr and Patient, there are three perceptions underlying stigma as it relates to HIV/AIDS, namely: HIV positive people have only death to look forward to; they will get sick, will need expensive medication, will use scarce resources and will die; in the process, scarce commodities and resources such as food, money, jobs, education will be exploited by these people without their ever reciprocating (Orr and Patient 2004:10).

Brown (1993:196) points out that by merely being HIV-positive, without a single sign or symptom, people may be stigmatised and discriminated against both from within and from without the health-care arena. Assumptions about the way HIV is contracted are enough justification for further recrimination (Brown 1993:196).

Stigmatisation is, however, not restricted to people living with HIV. In the same way that people living with AIDS are stigmatised by members of the community and health professionals, health professionals working with people living with AIDS become stigmatised and isolated because 'they associate with those people'.

For the stigmatised person, stigmatisation harbours shame, poor self-esteem, and the like. The social isolation resulting from stigmatisation is a kind of psychological death experience (Winiarski 1997: 72). Social isolation can create a number of additional psychosocial problems impacting even more negatively on people living with AIDS. Most burdensome is the fact that stigmatisation becomes an obstacle in dealing effectively with the HIV/AIDS pandemic in that, ultimately, it leads to people not accessing resources out of fear of being further stigmatised (Orr and Patient 2004:10).

Stigmatisation is profoundly unethical. The personhood of the person living with AIDS is negated by stigmatisation; autonomy, anonymity, and the like, are completely disregarded. Stigmatisation reverses the principles of *beneficence* and *non-malificence* as it positively contributes towards the stigmatised person's demise. Stigmatisation is directly opposed to *equality* and bears all the features of unjust action. The health professional who is guilty of stigmatisation acts contrary to the principle of patient *advocacy*. Via stigmatisation, the conflict between egoism and altruism is resolved in favour of the self (egoism).

In view of the multidimensional transgression of ethical concepts by stigmatisation, health professionals are expected to be role models for the acceptance and treatment of HIV-infected people and their loved ones, and they are expected to contribute to the appropriate education of the general public. In this regard, the reader is referred to the quotation by Hall that introduces Part 6 of this book. Health-care workers and health professionals need to be knowledgeable about the policies relating to proper conduct, and to work towards reducing denial and stigmatisation, and myths and legends about HIV and AIDS (Wilson *et al* 2002: 435).

Research and HIV/AIDS

The first issue to revisit when considering the research ethics of HIV/AIDS is that of *vulnerable groups*. People living with AIDS are vulnerable, in the first place, because *stigmatisation* relegates them to this position. In the second instance, people living with AIDS, for the larger part, meet all the criteria set for such groups in chapter 12. A guiding rule is that research that can be conducted equally well using people not living with AIDS, should preferably exclude people living with AIDS. It is quite possible that under the interrogating eye of research, individuals' status may become known without them really having intended this to happen.

The ability to be informed and to comprehend what research entails plays an important role in HIV research, particularly in the light of the stage of the disease in which the research participant finds him/herself, as dementia frequently characterises the later stages of the development of AIDS. The way in which the virus was contracted also deserves attention as the participant may be a regular drug user and may not at all times comprehend what is explained to him/her.

The dominant bioethical perspective on HIV/AIDS may skew research in favour of clinical trials and other biomedical research. Though the knowledge obtained via biomedical research has proved valuable in our understanding of HIV/AIDS and has in some circles contributed towards moral literacy and moral competence (Woloschak 2003), people living with AIDS also need to be understood. Their experience of living with HIV/AIDS, of the treatment they are on and how they perceive human caring, need to be investigated. Ultimately, the transformation of moral literacy into moral competence and moral praxis largely depends on the humanisation of scientific knowledge via human understanding, an understanding that can be brought about only by systematically and scientifically investigating lived experiences via well-conducted qualitative research.

Taking into consideration the vulnerability of people living with AIDS, *advocacy* becomes an important ethical concept in HIV/AIDS research. Ethics in general seems to be made more complex when the people involved belong to poverty-stricken and resource-poor communities (Thomas 2002:8). For this reason, principles of research need to be readdressed when conducting research on HIV/AIDS. For instance, when doing research on the lived experience of a person living with AIDS, researchers must possess at least basic skills in HIV/AIDS counselling (Thomas 2002:10). Though counselling *per se* does not constitute therapy, the possibility that an in-depth qualitative research interview might change into therapy is imminent and may even be justified. In the same way it is advisable that the researcher possess therapeutic skills he or she can apply. Elements of existential therapy, such as those underlying *logotherapy*[2], are indicated in this instance. The aim of applying these principles is to integrate the contents of one's own moral literacy into a sententious whole so that moral competence and meaning can be sustained in an attempt to counteract burnout and AIDS *fatigue*.

Reciprocity is a further issue in HIV/AIDS research that takes on quite a different dimension by comparison with other research projects. Reciprocation in HIV and AIDS research is pertinently indicated. People in impoverished communities, for example, often see the researcher as a resource (Thomas 2002:9) and, therefore, researchers should be aware of the resources available in the community in which they conduct research so that participants can be referred to these for help and assistance. Often, community members are not aware of these resources. Within the broader socio-economic milieu, the research must reaffirm that researching the lives of others is a privilege and the vulnerability associated with HIV/AIDS should not be exploited; that assessing and addressing the needs of those being researched should form an integral part of the research design; that both the research process and the outcome of the research should benefit the individuals and the community; and that

[2] *Logotherapy is therapy or healing through meaning.*

a multidisciplinary approach to HIV/AIDS research is an ethical imperative (Thomas 2002:9). These reaffirmations are supported by the four basic ethical principles of autonomy, beneficence, non-maleficence and justice (Thomas 1998:522).

Clinical trails, especially those conducted by large international pharmaceutical companies, can pose serious ethical and legal questions. Thomas (1998:320) cautions that clinical trials have become profitable for international pharmaceutical companies and clinical researchers. They seek to get the work done as quickly as possible with the minimum of impediment. Trials in developing countries apparently offer such opportunities.

The weak link seems to be the absence of, or poorly operating, research ethics committees in the developing countries where clinical trials are done(Thomas 1998:321). In this regard South Africa has made considerable progress with legislation relating to health research ethics committees (see chapter 12). Once again, the health professional, or any other health-care worker, who becomes involved in any drug trial should make sure that a Research Ethics Committee under the jurisdiction of the authorising authority has approved the whole research protocol.

An important point to consider in clinical trails of antiretroviral drugs relates to the way in which participants (patients) will be treated after completion of the trail. In the case of antiretroviral drugs, it is problematic to offer a lifelong supply of the agent/drug undergoing testing and administering these drugs as monotherapy is not advisable (Wilson *et al* 2002:449). Thomas (1998:323-324) indicates that a systematic follow-up should be conducted once clinical trails have been completed. The aim in this instance should be to counteract subminimal treatment of persons who have been involved in HIV clinical trails. The issues of continued access to advanced treatment technologies, equality, the nature of inter-sectoral collaboration and the human rights of the participants, should also be investigated. Del Rio (1998:330) indicates that investigating researchers and companies should guarantee that those communities where drugs have been tested will be given affordable access to newly developed and approved drugs. Any trials in developing countries for testing interventions primarily applicable to developing countries are unethical (Del Rio 1998:330). All health professionals and other health-care workers who are involved in any way in international and local clinical trials should clarify all these issues with the sponsoring firm and the principal researcher.

Finally, in any kind of research, testing for a participant's HIV-status is permitted only with the candidate's free and informed consent (Wilson *et al* 2002:436).

Concluding remarks

In conclusion we can but reiterate that, in accordance with the introductory quotation to Part 6 of this book, for the changes that are requisite for the maintenance of ethics and humanity as these relate to HIV/AIDS, what is needed is a transformation of heart. In essence, the caring ethic needs to be embraced and lived by both health professionals and patients alike.

Critical thinking activities

1. Identify a number of social interventions that have been implemented in the fight against HIV/AIDS. Evaluate these in terms of Aroskar's four critical considerations for any social intervention. In your evaluation give arguments of an ethical nature, illuminating the success/failure of these interventions from different points of view.
2. Construct a conceptual map (diagram) indicating the theoretical and philosophical grounding for ethics in caring for HIV-positive persons. The diagram should indicate the links between the bioethical and public health approaches, social intervention, different 'communities' and at least the four basic ethical principles in health care and nursing.

References

Chapter 1

References

Bandman & Bandman, EL & Bandman, B. 2002. *Nursing Ethics through the Life Span*. 4th Edition. New Jersey: Prentice Hall.

Beauchamp, TL & Childress, JF. 2001. *Principles of Biomedical Ethics*. 5th Edition. New York: Oxford University Press.

Creasia, JL & Parker, B. 1991. *Conceptual Foundations of Professional Nursing Practice*. St Louis: Mosby.

Davis, AJ, Aroskar, MA, Liaschenko, J & Drought, TS. 1997. *Ethical Dilemmas and Nursing Practice*. 4th Edition. Stamford, Connecticut: Appleton & Lange.

Deloughery, GL (ed.). 1991. *Issues and Trends in Nursing*. St Louis: Mosby.

Fowler, MDM & Levine-Ariff, J. 1987. *Ethics at the Bedside*. Philadelphia: J.B. Lippincott.

Husted, GL & Husted, JH. 1995. *Ethical Decisionmaking in Nursing*. 2nd Edition. St Louis: Mosby.

Lindberg, JB, Hunter, ML & Kruszewski, AZ. 1990. *Introduction to Nursing*. Philadelphia: J.B. Lippincott.

McConnell, TC. 1982. *Moral Issues in Health Care. An Introduction to Medical Ethics*. Monterey, California: Wadsworth Health Science Division.

Nolan, RT & Kirkpatrick, FG. 1982. *Living Issues in Ethics*. Belmont, California: Wadsworth Publishing Company.

Rumbold, G. 1993. *Ethics in Nursing Practice*. 2nd Edition. London: Bailliere Tindall.

Steele, SM & Harmon, VM. 1983. *Value Clarification in Nursing*. Norwalk, Connecticut: Appleton Century Crofts.

Thompson, IE Melia, KM & Boyd, KM. 1988. *Nursing Ethics*. 2nd Edition. London: Churchill Livingstone.

Thompson, JE & Thompson, HO. 1990. *Professional Ethics in Nursing*. Malabar, Florida: Krieger Publishing Company.

Thompson, JE & Thompson, HO. 1992. *Bioethical Decisionmaking for Nurses*. Lanham, Maryland: University Press of America.

Tschudin, V. 1993. *Values. A Primer for Nurses*. London: Bailliere Tindall.

Wright, RA. 1987. *The Practice of Ethics: Human Values in Health Care*. New York: McGraw-Hill.

Article

Fowler, MDM. 1989. Ethical decisionmaking in clinical practice. *Nursing Clinics of North America*. Vol. 24 No. 4, December, 955-965.

Chapter 2

References

Bennett-Goleman, T. 2001. *Emotional Alchemy: How your mind can heal your heart*. London: Rider.

Bevis, EO. 1981. Caring: A life force. In: *Caring: An essential human need*; edited by M. Leininger, Thorofare: Charles B Slack, 1981, p. 49-60.

Chinn, PL & Kramer, MK. 2004. *Integrated knowledge development in nursing*. (6th edition). Hong Kong: Mosby.

Dent, NJH. 1984. *The moral psychology of the virtues*. New York: Cambridge University Press.

Dozzy, BM, Keegan L, Guzzetta CE & Kolkmeier, LG. 1995. *Holistic nursing: a handbook for nursing practice*. Gaithersburg: Aspen Publishers

Dugan, AB. 1988. Compadrazgo: a caring phenomenon among urban Latinos and its relationship to health. In *Care, the Essence of Nursing and Health*. (Ed. Leininger, M.) Detroit: Wayne State University Press.

Gadow, S. 1988. Covenant without cure: letting go and holding on in chronic illness. In: *The Ethics of Care and the Ethics of Cure: Synthesis and Chronicity*, edited by J Watson and MA Ray. New York: National League for Nursing

Gaut, DA. 1979. *An Application of the Kerr-soltis Model to the Concept of Caring in Nursing*. London: University Microfilms International.

Gendron, D. 1990. Learning caring behavior in an integrated manner, in *The Caring Imperative in Education*, edited by M Leininger & J Watson. New York: National League for Nursing: 277-286.

Gouws, LA, Louw, DA, Meyer, WF, & Plug, C. 1979. *Psigologie-woordeboek*. Johannesburg: McGraw-Hill.

Heidegger, M 1996. *Being and Time*. Translated by J. Stambough. Albany: University of New York Press.

Klimek, M. 1990. Virtue, ethics and care: developing the personal dimension of caring in nursing education. In: *The caring Imperative in Education* edited by M Leininger and J Watson, New York: National League for Nursing

Lindberg, JB, Hunter, ML, & Kruszewski, AZ. 1990. *Introduction to Nursing. Concepts, Issues and Opportunities*. Philadelphia: Lippincott Company.

Mautner, T. 2000. *The Penguin Dictionary of Philosophy*. London: Penguin Publishers

Moccia, P. 1990. Deciding to care: a way to knowledge, in *The Caring Imperative in Education*, edited by M Leininger & J Watson. National League for Nursing: New York: 207-216.

Moral Regeneration Movement in South Africa http://www.search.gov.za/info/newresults.jsp/ Accessed 16 Dec 2004).

Noddings, N. 1984. *Caring: a feminine approach to ethics and moral education*. Los Angeles: University of California Press.

Peterson, G. 1982. *Conscience and Caring*. Philadelphia: Fortress Press.

Steiner, G. 1989. *Martin Heidegger*. Chicago: University Press.

Stevenson, JS & Tripp-Reimer T. 1990. *Knowledge about care and caring*. Kansas City: American Academy of Nursing.

The Consice Oxford Dictionary. 1984. Oxford:Clarendon Press.

Tillich, P. 1952. *The Courage to Be*. Welwyn: Nisbet.

Van der Wal, DM. 1996. Caring in Nursing Education. Unpublished master's dissertation. Department of Advanced Nursing Science. University of South Africa.

Van der Wal, DM. 2000. The maintenance of a caring concern by the caregiver. Unpublished doctoral thesis. Department of Advanced Nursing Science. University of South Africa.

Watson, J. 1985. *Nursing: Human Science and Human Care. A Theory of Nursing*. National League for Nursing: New York.

Watson, J. 1999. *Postmodern Nursing and Beyond*. New York: Churchill Livingston.

Articles

Carper, BA. 1978. Fundamental patterns of knowing. *Advances in Nursing Science*, 1(1):13-23.

Carper, BA. 1979. The ethics of caring. *Advances in Nursing Science*, 1(3):11-19.

Dunlop, MJ. 1986. Is a science of caring possible? *Journal of Advanced Nursing*, 11(4):661-670.

Forrest, D. 1989. The experience of caring. *Journal of Advanced Nursing*, 14(10):815-823.

Forsyth, GL. 1979. Exploration of empathy in nurse-client interaction. *Advances in Nursing Science*, 1(2):53-61.

Fry, ST. 1988. The ethics of caring: Can it survive in nursing? *Nursing Outlook*, 36(1):48.

Goddard, NC. 1995. 'Spirituality as integrative energy': a philosophical analysis as requisite precursor to holistic nursing practice. *Journal of Advanced Nursing*, 22 (4):808-815.

Griffin, AP. 1980. Philosophy and nursing. *Journal of Advanced Nursing*, 5(3):261-272.

Harrison, LL. 1990. Maintaining the ethic of caring in nursing. *Journal of Advanced Nursing*, 15(2):125-127.

Kekes, J. 1986. The informed will and the meaning of life. *Philosophy and Phenomenological Research*, 67(1):75-90.

Massey, RF. 1991. Social Conscience in logotherapy. *The International Forum for Logotherapy*, 14(1):32-35.

Schiltz M. 1996. Intentionality: a program for study. *The Journal of Mind-Body Health*, 12(3):31-32.

Chapter 3

References

Beauchamp, TL & Childress, JF. 2001. *Principles of Biomedical Ethics*. 5th Edition. New York: Oxford University Press.

Beauchamp, TL & Walters, L. 1978. *Contemporary Issues in Bioethics*. Belmont, California: Wadsworth Publishing Company.

Creasia, JL & Parker, B. 1991. *Conceptual Foundations of Nursing Practice*. St Louis: Mosby.

Curtin, L & Flaherty, MJ. 1982. *Nursing Ethics. Theories and Pragmatics*. Englewood Cliffs: Prentice-Hall.

Davis, AJ, Aroskar, MA, Liaschenko, J & Drought, TS. 1997. *Ethical Dilemmas and Nursing Practice*. 4th Edition. Stamford, Connecticut: Appleton & Lange.

Deloughery, GL (ed.). 1991. *Issues and Trends in Nursing*. St Louis: Mosby.

Fowler, MDM & Levine-Ariff, J. 1987. *Ethics at the Bedside*. Philadelphia: J.B. Lippincott.

Francoeur, RT. 1983. *Biomedical Ethics. A Guide to Decisionmaking*. New York: John Wiley & Sons.

Husted, GL & Husted, JH. 1995. *Ethical Decisionmaking in Nursing*. 2nd Edition. St Louis: Mosby.

Kozier, B, Erb, G & Blais, K. 1992. *Concepts and Issues in Nursing Practice*. 2nd Edition. Redwood City, California: Addison Wesley Nursing.

Lindberg, JB, Hunter, ML & Kruszewski, ZA. 1990. *Introduction to Nursing*. Philadelphia: J.B. Lippincott.

Loewy, EH. 1989. *Textbook of Medical Ethics*. New York: Plenum Medical Book Company.

McConnell, TC. 1982 *Moral Issues in Health Care*. Monterey, California: Wadsworth Health Science Division.

Oermann, MH. 1991. *Professional Nursing Practice*. New York: J.B. Lippincott.

Rumbold, G. 1993. *Ethics in Nursing Practice*. 2nd Edition. London: Bailliere Tindall.

Thompson, IE, Melia, KM & Boyd, KM. 1988. *Nursing Ethics*. 2nd Edition. London. Churchill Livingstone.

Thompson, JE & Thompson, HO. 1990. *Professional ethics in Nursing*. Malabar, Florida: Krieger Publishing Company.

Thompson, JB & Thompson, HO. 1992. *Bioethlcal Decisionmaking for Nurses*. Lanham, Maryland: University Press of America.

Veatch, RM & Fry, ST. 1987. Case *Studies in Nursing Ethics*. New York: J.B. Lippincott.

Wright, RA. 1987. *The practice of Ethics. Human Values in Health Care*. New York: McGraw Hill.

Articles

Fowler, MDM. 1989. Ethical decisionmaking in clinical practice. *Nursing Clinics of North America*. Vol. 24 No. 4, December, 955-965.

Gibson, CH. 1993. Underpinnings of ethical reasoning in nursing. *Journal of Advanced Nursing*. Vol. 18,2003-2007.

Hoyer, PJ, Booth, D, Spelman, MR & Richardson, CE. 1991. Clinical cheating and moral development. *Nursing Outlook*. Vol. 39, No. 4, 170-173

Smith, JB. 1989. Ethical issues raised by new treatment options. *The American Journal of Maternal Child Nursing*. Vol. 14, May/June, 183-187.

Chapter 4

References

Bandman & Bandman, EL & Bandman, B. 2002. *Nursing Ethics through the Life Span*. 4th Edition. New Jersey: Prentice Hall.

Beauchamp, TL & Childress, JF. 1979. *Principles of Biomedical Ethics*. 2nd Edition. New York: Oxford University Press.

Beauchamp, TL & Childress, JF. 2001. *Principles of Biomedical Ethics*. 5th Edition. New York: Oxford University Press.

Bruce, JAC .1988. *Privacy and Confidentiality of Health Care Information*. 2nd Edition. American Hospital Association: American Hospital Publishing, Inc.

Burkhardt, MA & Nathaniel, AK. 2002. *Ethics and Issues in Contemporary Nursing.* 2nd Edition. United States: Delmar.

Davis, AJ, Aroscar, MA, Liaschenno, J & Drought, TS. 1997 *Ethical Dilemas and Nursing Practice.* Stamford, Connecticut: Appleton & Lange.

Deloughery, GL. 1995. *Issues and Trends in Nursing.* 2nd Edition. St Louis: Mosby.

McHale, JV. 1993. *Medical Confidentiality and Privilege.* London: Routledge.

Neethling, J, Potgieter, JM & Visser, PJ. 1999. *Law of Delict.* 3rd Edition. Durban: Butterworths.

Oermann, MH. 1991. *Professional Nursing Practice. A Conceptual Approach.* Philadelphia: J.B. Lippincott.

Quinn, CA & Smith, MD. 1987. *The Professional Commitment: Issues and Ethics in Nursing.* Philadelphia: Saunders.

Rumbold, G. 1993. *Ethics in Nursing Practice.* 2nd Edition. London: Bailliere Tindall.

Searle, C & Pera, S. 1992. *Professional Practice: A South African Nursing Perspective.* 2nd Edition. Durban: Butterworths.

Strauss, SA. 1992. *Legal Handbook for Nurses and Health Personnel.* 7th Edition. Cape Town: King Edward VII Trust.

Strauss, SA & Maré, MC. 2001. *Medical Law.* L.C.R. 404 U. Pretoria: University of South Africa.

Tschudin, V. 1992. *Ethics in Nursing. The Caring Relationship.* 2nd Edition. Oxford: Butterworth-Heinemann.

Tschudin, V. 1993. *Ethics. Nurses and Patients.* London: Scutari Press.

Veatch, RM. 1989. *Cross Cultural Perspectives in Medical Ethics: Readings.* Boston: Jones & Bartlett.

Wright, RA. 1987. *The Practice of Ethics. Human Values in Health Care.* New York: McGraw-Hill.

Articles

Curran, M & Curran, K. 1991. The ethics of information. JONA. Vol. 21 No. 1, January, 47-49.

High, DM. 1989. Truth-telling, confidentiality and the dying patient: New dilemmas for the nurse. *Nursing Forum.* Vol. 24 No. 1, 5-10.

Lee, S. 1987. Do you want to know a secret? *Nursing Rimes.* Vol. 83 No. 49, 24-31

Martin, J. 1993. Lying to patients: Can it ever be justified? *Nursing Standard.* Vol. 7 No. 18, January, 29-31.

Melia, K. 1988. To tell or not to tell. Nursing Times. Vol. 84 No. 30, 37-39.

Milholland, OK. 1994. Privacy and confidentiality of patient information. Challenges for nursing. JONA. Vol. 24 No 2, February, 19-24.

Chapter 5

References

Bernzweig, EP. 1990. *The Nurse's Liability for Malpractice.* 5th Edition. St Louis: Mosby.

Catalano, JT. 1991. *Ethical and Legal Aspects of Nursing.* Springhouse, Pennsylvania: Springhouse Notes.

Cheadle, MH; Davis, DM & Haysom, NRL. 2002. *South African Constitutional Law: The Bill of Rights.* Durban: Butterworths.

Claassen, NJB & Verschoor, T. 1992. *Medical Negligence in South Africa.* Pretoria: Digma Publications.

De Waal, J; Currie, I & Erasmus, G. 2001. *The Bill of Rights Handbook.* 4th Edition. Cape Town: Juta.

Fenner, KM. 1980. *Ethics and Law in Nursing.* New York: D van Nostrand Company.

Fiesta, J. 1988. *The Law and Liability: A Guide for Nurses.* 2nd Edition. New York: Delmar Publishers.

Hemelt, MD & Mackert, ME. 1982. *Dynamics of Law in Nursing and Health Care.* 2nd Edition. Reston, Virginia: Prentice-Hall.

Kleyn, D & Viljoen, F. 2002. *Beginner's Guide for Law Students.* 3rd edition. Cape Town: Juta.

Mahoney, KE & Mahoney, P. 1993. *Human Rights in the Twenty-First Century: A Global Challenge.* Dordrecht: Kluwer Academic Publishers.

Strauss, SA. 1991. *Doctor, Patient and the Law. A Selection of Practical Issues.* 3rd Revised edition. Pretoria: Van Schaik.

Verschoor, T, Jansen, RM, Fick, GA & Viljoen, DJ. 1995. *Nursing and the Law.* Cape Town: Juta.

A National Health Plan for South Africa. 1994. Prepared by the African National Congress, Johannesburg. May.

Articles

Strydom, HA. 1994. The private domain and the Bill of Rights. Paper delivered at the course on Human Rights Litigation, University of the Orange Free State, May-August.

Van der Vyver, JD. 1994. General principles of the Declaration of Fundamental Rights. Notes prepared for the course on Human Rights Litigation, University of the Orange Free State, May-August.

The Reconstruction and Development Programme: A policy framework. 1994. Prepared by the African National Congress. Johannesburg: Umanyano Publications.

Chapter 6

References

Bandman, EL & Bandman, B. 1990. *Nursing Ethics Through the Life Span.* 2nd Edition. Norwalk: Appleton & Lange.

Curtin, L & Flaherty, MJ. 1982. *Nursing Ethics. Theories and Pragmatics.* Englewood Cliffs: Prentice Hall.

Duxbury, J. 2000. *Difficult patients.* Oxford: Butterworth-Heinemann.

Guido, GW. 2001. *Legal and ethical issues in nursing.* 3rd edition. New Jersey: Prentice Hall.

Haynes, L, Boese, T & Butcher, H. 2004. *Nursing in contemporary society. Issues, trends and transition to practice.* New Jersey: Pearson Prentice Hall.

Hudak, CM, Gallo, BM & Morton, PG. 1998. *Critical care nursing. A holistic approach.* 7th edition. Philadelphia: Lippincott.

McCloskey, JC & Grace, HK (eds.). 1990. *Current Issues in Nursing.* 3rd Edition. St Louis: Mosby.

Muyskens, JL. 1982. *Moral Problems in Nursing. A Philosophical Investigation.* Totowa, New Jersey: Rowman & Littlefield.

Oermann, MH. 1997. *Professional Nursing Practice.* Stamford, CT: Appleton & Lange.

Pence, T & Cantrall, J. 1990. *Ethics in Nursing: An Anthology.* New York: National League for Nursing.

Searle, C. 2000. *Professional Practice: A South African Nursing Perspective.* 4th Edition. Kwa Zulu-Natal: Heinemann.

Tadd, GV. 1998. *Ethics and values for care workers.* Oxford:Blackwell Science.

Thompson, JE & Thompson, HO. 1990. *Professional Ethics in Nursing.* Malabar, Florida: Krieger Publishing Company.

Thompson, JE & Thompson, HO. 1992. *Bioethical decision making for nurses.* Lanham;University Press of America.

Tschudin, V. 1992. *Ethics in Nursing. The Caring Relationship.* 2nd Edition. Oxford: Butterworth-Heinemann.

Tschudin, V (ed). 1993. *Ethics, Nurses and Patients.* London: Scutari Press.

Tschudin, V. 1999. *Nurses matter. Reclaiming our professional identity.* Hampshire: Macmillan

Articles

Asworth, P. 2000. Nurse-doctor relationships: conflict, competition or collaboration. *Intensive and Critical Care Nursing.* Vol 16. 127-128.

Baker, C & Diekelmann, N. 1994. Connecting conversations of caring: Recalling the narrative to clinical practice. *Nursing Outlook.* Vol. 42 No. 2, March/April, 65-70.

Blue, I & Fitzgerald, M. 2002. Interprofessional relations: case studies of working relationships between registered nurses and general practitioners in rural Australia. *Journal of Clinical Nursing.* Vol 11. 314-321.

Castledine, G. 2004. The importance of the nurse-patient relationship. *British Journal of Nursing.* Vol 13. No 4. 231.

Davidhizar, R & Dowd, S. 2001. How to get along with doctors and other health professionals. *The Journal of Practical Nursing*. Spring. 12-15.

Davidhizar, R & Dowd, S. 2003. The doctor-nurse relationship. *The Journal of Practical Nursing*. Vol. 53 No 4. 9-12.

Germain, CP. 1992. Cultural care: A bridge between sickness, illness, and disease. *Holistic Nursing Practice*. Vol. 6 No. 3, 1-9.

Jones, RAP. 1994. Nurse-physician collaboration: A descriptive study. *Holistic Nursing Practice*. Vol. 8 No. 3, April, 38-53.

Marck, P. 1990. Therapeutic reciprocity: A caring phenomenon. *Advances in Nursing Science*. Vol. 13 No. 1, 49-59.

Murphy, K & Macleod Clark, J. 1993. Nurses' experiences of caring for ethnic-minority clients. *Journal of Advanced Nursing*. Vol. 18 No. 3, 442-450.

Olsen, DP. 1993. Populations vulnerable to the ethics of caring. *Journal of Advanced Nursing*. Vol. 18 No. 11, 1696-1700.

Oosthuizen, MJ. 2002. Die realiteit van transkulturele verpleging: 'n etiese perspektief. *Health SA/Gesondheid*. Vol 7 No. 2, 3-13.

Pike, AW. 1991. Moral outrage and moral discourse in nurse-physician collaboration. *Journal of Professional Nursing*. Vol. 7 No. 6, November-December, 351-363

Ramos, MC. 1992. The nurse-patient relationship: Theme and variations. *Journal of Advanced Nursing*. Vol. 17 No. 4, 496-506.

Snelgrove, S & Hughes, D. 2000. Interprofessional relations between doctors and nurses: perspectives from South Wales. *Journal of Advanced Nursing*. Vol 31. No 3. 661-667.

Snowdon, AW & Rajacich, D. 1993. The challenge of accountability in nursing. *Nursing Forum*. Vol. 28 No. 1, 5-11.

Taylor, C, Lillis, C & LeMone, P. 2001. *Fundamentals of Nursing*. 4th edition. Philadelphia: Lippincott.

Thorne, SE & Robinson, CA. 1988. Reciprocal trust in health care relationships. *Journal of Advanced Nursing*. Vol. 13 No. 1, 782-789.

Trnobranski, PH. 1994. Nurse-patient negotiation: Assumption or reality? *Journal of Advanced Nursing*. Vol. 19 No. 4, 733-737.

Yuen, FKH. 1986. The nurse-client relationship: a mutual learning experience. *Journal of Advanced Nursing*. Vol. 11 No. 1, 529-533.

Chapter 7

References

Bezuidenhout, MC, Garbers, CJ & Potgieter, S. 1998. *Managing for healthy labour relations. A practical guide for health services in Southern Africa*. Van Schaik: Pretoria.

Curtis, MBJ. 1981. *Ethics in nursing*. New York: Oxford University Press.

Du Toit, D, Woolfrey, D, Murphy, J, Godfrey, S, Bosh, D & Christie, S. 2000. *Labour relations law. A comprehensive guide*. 3rd Edition.

Frith, L (Ed). 1996. *Ethics and Midwifery. Issues in contemporary practice*. Oxford: Butterworth-Heinemann.

Fry, ST. 1993. *Ethics in Nursing Practice: A guide to ethical decision making*. Switzerland: ICN.

Grogan, J. 2003. *Workplace Law*. 7th Edition. Juta Law: Lansdowne

Hall, JK. 2002. *Law & ethics for Clinicians*. Jackhall Books: Texas, USA.

INTERNATIONAL COUNCIL OF NURSES 1999. Position paper: Strike Policy. ICN: Geneva.

INTERNATIONAL COUNCIL OF NURSING (ICN) 1999. Press release ICN/PR/99 No. 21. ICN: Geneva.

Jameton, A. 1984. *Nursing practice: the ethical issues*. Englewood Cliffs, NJ Prentice Hall.

South Africa 1966. Unemployment Insurance Act (Act 30 of 1966). Pretoria: Government Printer.

South Africa 1978. Nursing Act (Act 50 of 1978). Pretoria: Government Printer.

South Africa 1993. Occupational Health and Safety Act (Act 85 of 1993). Pretoria: Government Printer.

South Africa 1993. Compensation for Occupational Injuries and Diseases Act (Act 130 of 1993). Pretoria: Government Printer.

South Africa 1995. Labour Relations Act (LRA) (Act 66 of 1995). Pretoria: Government Printer.

South Africa 1996. Constitution of the Republic of South Africa, 1996. Pretoria: Government Printer.

South Africa 1997. Employment Equity Act (Act 55 of 1998). Pretoria: Government Printer.

South Africa 1997. Administrative Justice Act (Act 3 of 2000). Pretoria: Government Printer.

South Africa 1997. Promotion of Equality and Prevention of Unfair Discrimination Act (Act 4 of 2000). Pretoria: Government Printer.

South Africa 2000. Promotion of Access to Information Act (Act 2 of 2000). Pretoria. Government Printer.

South Africa 2003. National Health Act (Act 61 of 2003). Pretoria. Government Printer.

Steinman-Marais, S. 2002. Workplace violence in the health sector. *Country Case Study: South Africa* An international research project commissioned by the INTERNATIONAL LABOUR ORGANISATION, INTERNATIONAL COUNCIL FOR NURSES, WORLD HEALTH ORGANISATION, AND PUBLIC SERVICES INTERNATIONAL.

Thompson, IE, Melia, KM & Boyd, KM. 1988. *Nursing ethics*. 2nd Edition. New York: Churchill Livingstone.

Thompson, JE & Thompson, HO. 1990. *Professional ethics in nursing*. Malabar, Florida: Krieger Publishing Company.

Webster, GC & Bayliss, F. 2000. *Moral residue*. (In: Rubin SB, Zoloth L eds. Margin of error. The ethics of mistakes in the practice of medicine. Hagerstown, MD. University Publishing).

Xaba, J & Phillips, P. 2002. Nurse immigration. Durban: TURP.

Articles

CLarke, J & O'Neill, CS. 2001. How the Irish Times portrayed Irish nursing during the 1999 strike. *Nursing Ethics* 8(4): 350 – 59.

Corley, MC. 2002. Nurse Moral distress: a proposed theory and research agenda. *Nursing Ethics*, 9(6) 636 – 650.

Geyer, N Ethics & Law : Moonlighting.Nursing Update March 2001: 30-31

Jameton, A. 1993. *Dilemmas of moral distress: moral responsibility and nursing practice*. Clinical Issues Perinat Women's Health Nurse 4: 542 – 51.

Killen, AR. 2002. Stories from the operating room: moral dilemmas for nurses. *Nursing Ethics* 9(4): 405 – 415.

Macdonald, C. 2002. Nurse autonomy as relational. *Nursing Ethics*, 9(2): 194 – 201.

Muula, AS & PHIRI, A. 2003. Health workers' strike in Blantyre, Malawi. *Nursing Ethics*, 10(2): 208 – 14.

Redman, KR & FRY, ST. 2000. Nurses' ethical conflicts: What is really known about them? *Nursing Ethics* 7(4): 360 – 66.

Woods, M. 2001. Balancing rights and duties in 'Life and Death' decision making involving children: A role for nurses? *Nursing Ethics*, 8(5):

Chapter 8

References

Burnard, P & Chapman, CM. 1993 *Professional and Ethical Issues in Nursing. The Code of Professional Conduct*. 2nd Edition. London: Scutari Press.

Curtin, L & Flaherty, MJ. 1982. *Nursing Ethics. Theories and Pragmatics*. Englewood Cliffs: Prentice-Hall.

Curtis, MBJ. 1981. *Ethics in Nursing*. New York: Oxford Universtiy Press.

Davis, AJ & Aroskar, MA, Liaschenka, J & Draught, TS. 1997. *Ethical Dilemmas and Nursing Practice*. 4th Edition. Stamford: Appleton & Lange.

Deloughery, GL (ed). 1991. *Issues and Trends in Nursing*. St Louis: Mosby.

Grippando, GM & Mitchell, PR. 1989. *Nursing Perspectives and Issues*. 4th Edition. New York: Dlemar.

Harron, F, Bumside, J & Beauchamp, T. 1983. *Health and Human Values. A Guide to Making Your Own Decisions*. New Haven: Yale University Press.

Husted, GL & Husted, JH. 1991. *Ethical Decisionmaking in Nursing*. St Louis: Mosby.

INTERNATIONAL COUNCIL OF NURSING (ICN) 2004b: ICN Fact Sheet. Nurse: Patient ratios. Retrieved from http://www.icn.ch/matters mptratio.htm on 31/12/2004.

INTERNATIONAL COUNCIL OF NURSING (ICN) 2004b: ICN Fact sheet on Nursing Matters: Nurses and Overtime. Retrieved from http://www.icn.ch/matters overtime.htm on 31/12/2004.

INTERNATIONAL COUNCIL OF NURSING (ICN) 2004b: ICN Fact sheet on Nursing Matters: ICN on occupational stress and the threat to worker health. Retrieved from http://www.icn.ch/matters stress.htm on 31/12/2004.

Murschison, I, Nichols, TS & Hanson, R. 1982. *Legal Accountability in the Nursing Process*. St Louis: Mosby.

Pence, T & Cantrall, J. 1990. *Ethics in Nursing: An Anthology*. New York: National League for Nursing.

Rumbold, G. 1986. *Ethics in Nursing Practice*. London: Bailliere Tindall.

Rumbold, G. 1989. *Ethics in Nursing Practice*. London: Bailliere Tindall.

Rumbold, G. 1993. *Ethics in Nursing Practice*. 2nd Edition. London: Bailliere Tindall.

Searle, C. 1987. *Ethos of Nursing and Midwifery*. *A General Perspective*. Durban: Butterworths.

Searle, C & Pera, S. 1992. *Professional Practice*. A *South African Nursing Perspective*. 2nd Edition. Durban: Butterworths.

South African Nurses' Association 1986: *Desirable Conditions of Service for Nursing Personnel*. Pretoria: SANA.

Strauss, SA. 1992. *Legal Handbook for Nursing and Health Personnel*. 7th Edition. Cape Town: King Edward VII Trust.

Steinman-Marais S. 2002: Workplace violence in the health sector. *Country Case Study: South Africa* An international research project commissioned by the INTERNATIONAL LABOUR ORGANISATION, INTERNATIONAL COUNCIL FOR NURSES, WORLD HEALTH ORGANISATION, AND PUBLIC SERVICES INTERNATIONAL.

Thompson, JE, Melia, KM & Boyd, KM. 1988. *Nursing Ethics*. 2nd Edition. New York: Churchill Livingstone.

Tschudin, V (ed.). 1993. *Ethics. Nurses and Patients*. London: Scutari Press.

Wright, RA 1987. *The Practice of Ethics: Human Values in Health Care*. New York: McGraw-Hill.

Articles

Fokus op gesondheidsorg: 2004. Bylae tot *Finansies en Tegniek*. 6-10 September, 35-44.

Goodlad, J. 1987. Hepatitis B and nursing in the UK. *Report from the Wembley Conference*. London: Royal College of Nursing.

International Council of Nurses. 1987. International portable health record: The patient's right to know. *Position Statements*. Geneva: ICN.

Kleinman, I. 1986. Force feeding: The physician's dilemma. *Canadian Journal of Psychiatry*. Vol. 31 No. 4, 313-316.

Miller, WP. 1986. The hunger-striking prisoner. *Journal of Prison & Jail Health*.. Vol. 6 No. 1, 40-61.

Pettifor, JL. 1985. Patient rights, professional ethics and situational dilemmas in mental health services. Canada's *Mental Health*. Vol. 33 No. 3, September, 20-23.

Taylor, M & Ryan, H. 1988. Fanaticism, political suicide and terrorism. *Terrorism*. Vol. 11, No. 2, 91-111.

Wilson, DR. 1985. Patients' rights and ethics committee, Douglas Hospital Center. Canada's *Mental Health*. Vol. 33 No. 3, September, 24-27.

Chapter 9

References

Bandman, EL & Bandman, B. 2002. *Nursing ethics through the life span*. 4th Edition. Upper Saddle River, NJ:Prentice Hall.

Bartter, K (ed.). 2001. *Ethical issues in advanced nursing practice*. Oxford: Butterworth-Heinemann.

Burkhardt, MA & Nathaniel, AK. 2002. *Ethics and issues in contemporary nursing*. 2nd Edition. Albany, NY: Delmar.

Charo, RA. 2002. And baby makes three – or four, or five, or six: redefining the family after the reprotech revolution, in *Legal and ethical issues in human reproduction*, edited by B. Steinbock, Burlington: Dartmouth: 215-237.

Devine, RJ. 2000. *Good care, painful choices. Medical ethics for ordinary people.* 2nd Edition. New York: Paulist Press.

Dooley, D, McCarthy, J, Garanis-Papadatos, T & Dalla-Vorgia, P. 2003. *Ethics of new reproductive technologies.* New York: Berghahn.

Fremgen, BF. 2002. *Medical law and ethics.* Upper Saddle River, N.J. Prentice Hall.

Frith, L & Draper, H (eds.). 2004. *Ethics and midwifery. Issues in contemporary practices.* 2nd Edition. Edinburg: Elsevier.

Gastmans, C (ed.). 2002. *Between technology and humanity. The impact of technology on health care ethics.* Leuven, Belgium: Leuven University Press.

Gupta, S. 1990. Psychosocial development in a genetic male surgically reassigned as a female at birth. *American Journal of Psychotherapy.* Vol XLIV, No 2, 283–289.

Hafez, ESE & Semm, K. (eds.). 1982. *Instrumental insemination.* Den Haag: Martinus Nijhof.

Hull, RT. (ed). 1990. *Ethical issues in the new reproductive technologies.* California: Wadsworth.

Rae, SB. 1996. *Brave new families. Biblical ethics and reproductive technologies.* Michigan: Baker Books.

Searle, C & Pera, S. 1992. *Professional Practice: A South African Nursing Perspective.* 2nd Edition. Durban. Butterworths.

South Africa. 1996. Choice on Termination of Pregnancy Act, 92 of 1996. Pretoria: Government Printers.

Spradley, BW & Allender, JA (eds.). 1997. *Readings in community health nursing.* 5th Edition. Philadelphia: Lippincott.

Strauss, SA & Maré, MC. 2001. *Medical Law.* Only study guide for LCR404-U. Pretoria: Unisa.

Tancredi, LR & Weisstub, DN. 1986. Technology assessment: its role in forensic psychiatry and the case of chemical castration. *International Journal of Law and Psychiatry.* Vol 8 No3, 257–271.

Articles

Aley, P & Mitchell, E. 1991. Preventing cot death. The role of the nurse. *New Zealand Nursing Journal.* July, 22-24.

Bar-Joseph, H & Tzuriel, D. 1990. Suicidal tendencies and ego identity in adolescence. *Adolescence.* Vol. XXV No. 97, 215-223.

Brooks-Gunn, J & Furstenburg, JR. 1990. Coming of age in the era of AIDS: Puberty, sexuality and contraception. *The Milbank Quarterly.* Vol. 68, Suppl. 1, 59-84.

Carr, EK, Friedman, T, Lannon, B & Sharp, PC. 1990. The study of psychological factors in couples receiving artificial insemination by donor: A discussion of methodological difficulties. *Journal of Advanced Nursing.* Vol. 15, 906-910.

Czechowicz, D. 1988. Adolescent alcohol and drug abuse and its consequences—an overview. *American Journal of Drug Alcohol Abuse.* Vol. 14 No. 2, 189-197.

Ehlers, VJ. 2003. Adolescent mothers' knowledge and perceptions of contraceptives in Tswane, South Africa. *Health SA Gesondheid,* (8) 1:13-25.

Heywood, A. 1991. Immaculate conception? *Nursing Times.* Vol. 87 No. 22, 62-63.

Lundqvist, A, Nilstun, T & Dykes, A. 2003. Neonatal end-of-life care in Sweden. *Nursing in Critical Care,* 8 (5): 197-202.

Marmaduke, A & Bell, SK. 1989. *In vitro* fertilization and embryo transfer dilemmas. Nursing Forum. Vol. XXIV No. 3/4, 24-28.

Mogotlane, S. 1993. Teenage pregnancy: An unresolved issue. *Curationis.* Vol. 16 No. 1, 11-14.

Ndaki, K. 2004. Risky business. SA youth and HIV/AIDS. *AIDS Bulletin,* Vol. 13. No. 2, 52-53.

Ogden, J. 1993. Getting it wrong. *Nursing Times.* Vol. 89 No. 16, 18.

Oosthuizen, MJ. 1993. Kan ons toetree by kindermishandeling? *Nursing RSA Verpleging.* Vol. 8. No. 11/12, 20, 44-46.

Poggenpoel, M, Myburgh, CPH & Gmeiner, AC. 1998. One voice regarding the legislation of abortion: nurses who experience discomfort. *Curationis,* 21(3): 2-7.

Pretorius, R. 1987. Surrogaat-moederskap: Implikasies in die Suid-Afrikaanse regstelsel. *De Rebus*. June, 270-278.

Redelinghuys, IF & Mazarakis, E. 1994. Kindermishandeling – identifikasie en aanmelding. *Nursing RSA Verpleging*. Vol. 9 No. 4, 10-13.

Schoeman, MN. 1990. Sexuality education among black South African teenagers: What can reasonably be expected? Curationis. Vol. 13 No. 3/4, 13-18.

Setiloane, CWM. 1990. Contraceptive use amongst urban and rural youths in South Africa—a comparative study. Curationis. Vol. 13 No. 3/4, 44-48.

Simbayi, LC, Chauveau, J & Shisana, O. 2004. Behavioral responses of South African youth to the HIV/AIDS epidemic: a nationwide survey. AIDS Care, Vol. 16, No 5, 605-618.

Strydom, G. 1993. Contraceptives for teenagers—an ethical issue. *Nursing RSA Verpleging*. Vol. 8 No. 8, 29-32.

Townshend, P. 1990. A challenge for neonatal nurses. Nursing Times. Vol. 86 No. 26, 38-41.

White, GL, Murdock, RT, Richardson, GE, Ellis, GD & Schmidt, LJ. 1990. Development of a tool to assess suicide risk factors in urban adolescents. *Adolescence*. Vol. XXV No. 99, 655-666.

Chapter 10

References

Burkhardt, MA & Nathaniel, AK. 2002. *Ethics and issues in contemporary nursing*. 2nd Edition. Albany, NY: Delmar.

Butler, RN & Jasmin, C (eds). 2000. *Longevity and quality of life. Opportunities and challenges*. New York: Kluwer Academic/Plenum Publishers.

Cohen, MH. 2003. *Future medicine. Ethical dilemmas, regulatory challenges, and therapeutic pathways to health care and healing in human transformation*. Michigan: University of Mitchigan Press.

Devine, RJ. 2000. *Good care, painful choices. Medical ethics for ordinary people*. 2nd Edition. New York: Paulist.

Fremgen, BF. 2002. *Medical law and ethics*. Upper Saddle River, New Jersey: Prentice Hall.

Galanti, G. 2004. *Caring for patients from different cultures*. 3rd Edition. Philadelphia: University of Pennsylvania.

Gastmans, C (ed.). 2002. *Between technology and humanity. The impact of technology on health care ethics*. Leuven, Belgium: Leuven University.

Hall, MA, Bobinski, MA & Orentlicher, D. 2003. *Health care law and ethics*. 6th Edition. New York: Aspen.

Lindberg, JB, Hunter, ML & Kruszewski, AZ. 1998. *Introduction to nursing concepts, issues and opportunities*. 3rd Edition. Philadelphia: Lippincott.

Monagle, JF & Thomasma, DC. 1994. *Health care ethics. Critical issues*. Gaithersburg, Maryland: Aspen.

Nattrass, N. 2004. *The moral economy of AIDS in South Africa*. Cambridge, UK: Cambridge University Press.

Searle, C & Pera, S. 1992. *Professional Practice: A South African Nursing Perspective*. 2nd Edition. Durban: Butterworths.

Smith, D. 1996. *Life and morality. Contemporary medico-moral issues*. Dublin: Gill & MacMillan.

Spradley, BW & Allender, JA (eds.). 1997. *Readings in community health nursing*. 5th Edition. Philadelphia: Lippincott.

Strauss, SA & Maré, MC. 2001. *Medical law*. Only study guide for LCR 404-U. Pretoria: Unisa.

Articles

Bachman, MO & Booysen, FLR. 2004. Relationships between HIV/AIDS, income and expenditure over time in deprived South African households. AIDS Care. Vol. 16, No 7:817-826.

Bohn, DK. 1990. Domestic violence and pregnancy. Implications for practice. *Journal of Nurse-Midwifery*. Vol. 35 No. 2, 86-98.

Bradshaw, D, Groenewald, P, Laubscher, R, Nannan, N, Nojilana, B, Norman, R, Pieterse, D & Schneider, M. 2003. Initial estimates from the South African National Burden of Disease Study, 2000. AIDS Bulletin. Vol. 12 No 2:22-27.

Chong, JML. 1990. Social assessment of transsexuals who apply for sex reassignment therapy. *Social Work in Health Care*. Vol. 14 No. 3, 87-104.

Davis, AJ, Davidson, B, Hirschfield, M, Lauri, S, Lin, JY, Norberg, A, Phillips, L, Pitman, E, Shen, CH, Van der Laan, R, Zhangh, HL & Ziv, L. 1993. An international perspective of active euthanasia: Attitudes of nurses in seven countries. *International Journal of Nursing Studies*. Vol. 30 No. 4, 301-310.

Edwards, S. 1990. Battered women who kill. *New Law Journal*. Vol. 140 No. 6474, 1380-1381, 1392.

Fry, ST. 1991. Are new proposals to increase organ donations ethical? *Nursing Outlook*. Vol. 39 No. 4, 192.

Grassly, NC, Lewis, JJ/C, Mahy, M, Walker, N & Timaeus, IM. 2004. Comparison of household-survey estimates with projections of mortality and orphan numbers in sub-Saharan Africa in the era of HIV/AIDS. 2004. *Population Studies*. Vol. 58, No. 2:207-217.

Groenewald, MM. 1993. Vigs: Die etiese implikasies. *Nursing RSA Verpleging*. Vol. 8 No. 7, 22-23.

Jenkins, T. 2002. *The health care of the aged : some ethical issues : Part 1 Update*, 18(3):67.

Kalichman, SC & Simbayi, L. 2004. Traditional beliefs about the cause of AIDS and AIDS-related stigma in South Africa. *AIDS Care*. Vol. 16, No. 5:572-580.

Kuhse, H & Singer, P. 1993. Voluntary euthanasia and the nurse: An Australian survey. *International Journal of Nursing Studies*. Vol. 30 No. 4, 311-322.

Miteff, L. 2001. *Palliative care ethics : autonomy in aged care*. Australian Nursing Journal, 9(6):1-4.

Orr, N & Patient, D. 2004. Stigma. Beliefs cause behaviour. *AIDS Bulletin*. Vol. 1, No. 13:10-14.

Pang, SM. 2003. *Medical techonology, end-of-life care and nursing ethics*. Nursing Ethics, 10(3):236-237.

Parker, B & Ulrich, Y. 1990. A protocol of safety: Research on abuse of women. *Nursing Research*. Vol 39 No. 4, 248-250.

Ringerman, ES & Koniak-Griffin, D. 1992. A re-examination of euthanasia: Issues raised by Final Exit. *Nursing Forum*. Vol. 27 No. 4, 5-8, 34.

Waterhouse, J & Metcalfe, M. 1991. Attitudes toward nurses discussing sexual concerns with patients. *Journal of Advanced Nursing*. Vol. 16, 1048-1054.

WHO says failure to deliver AIDS medicines is a global emergency. Global AIDS emergency requires urgent response – no more business as usual. 2004. *AIDS Bulletin*.Vol. 13 No. 1:24-25.

Wilkes, L, White, K & Tolley, N. 1993. Euthanasia: A comparison of the lived experience of Chinese and Australian palliative care nurses. *Journal of Advanced Nursing*. Vol. 18, 95-102.

Chapter 11

References

Donaldson, T, Werhane, PH & Cording, M. 2002. *Ethical issues in business. A philosophical approach*. 7th edition. New Jersey: Prentice Hall.

Groenewald, MM. 2001. *Contemporary issues in health services*. Only Study Guide for HMA305-D. Pretoria:University of South Africa.

Swansburg, RC & Swansburg, RJ. 2002. *Introduction to management and leadership for nurse managers*. 3rd edition. Massachusetts;Jones and Bartlett Publishers.

Tappen, RM. 2001. *Nursing leadership and management. Concepts and practice*. 4th edition. Philadelphia: F.A. Davis Company.

Articles

George S. May International Company. 2004(a). *More guides to acting ethically*. Retrieved from http:/ /ethics.georgemay.com/14/htm on 2004-11-19.

George S. May International Company. 2004(b). *Business ethics takes on more importance as business scandals make headlines*. Retrieved from http://ethics.georgemay.com/6/htm on 2004-11-19.

Geyer, N. 2004. Re-marketing the nursing profession. *Nursing Update*. 28(3): 34-37.

Llewellyn, S, Eden, R & Lay, C. 1999. Financial and professional incentives in health care. Comparing the UK and Canadian experiences. *The International Journal of Public Sector Management*. Vol.12 No.1, 6-16.

Shindul-Rothschild, J, Berry, D & Long-Middleton, E. 1996. Where have all the nurses gone? Final results of our patient care survey. *American Journal of Nursing*. 96(11):25-39.

Schlegelmilch, BB & Houston JE. 1989. Corporate codes of ethics in large UK companies: an empirical investigation of use, content and attitudes. *European Journal of Marketing*. Vol 23. No. 6. 7-24. Retrieved from http://miranda.emeraldinsight.com/vl=3894655/cl=49/nw=1 on 2004-11-18.

Von Baeyer, C. 2004. Our Code of Ethics: A shared vision, high principles and some good housekeeping. Retrieved from http://www.workplaceethics.ca/work.html on 2004-11-19.

Von Baeyer, C. 2004. What's workplace ethics? Retrieved from http://www.workplaceethics.ca/work.html on 2004-11-19.

Wells, B & Spinks, N. 1996(a). Ethics must be communicated from the top down. *Career development International* Vol 1. No 7. 28-30.

Wells, B & Spinks, N. 1996(b). The context of ethics in the health care industry. *Health Manpower Management*. Vol. 22, No. 1, 21-29.

Chapter 12
References

Ashcroft, R. 2002. An ethical perspective – nursing research. In: *Nursing Law and Ethics* (2nd edition) edited by J Tingle and A Gibbs. Oxford: Blackwell. pp.278-286.

Bandman, EL and Bandman, B. 1995. *Critical Thinking in Nursing*. (2nd ed.) Norwalk: Appleton & Lange.

Brink, HI. 2001. *Fundamentals of Research Methodology for Health Care Professionals*. Landowne: JUTA.

Burns, N and Grove, SK. 2001. *The Practice of Nursing Research.: Conduct, Critque and Utilization* (4th edition). Philadelphia: Saunders.

De Villiers, L and Van der Wal, DM. 2004. Researching cultural issues in health care. In: *Cultural Issues in Health and Health Care*, edited by A Tjale and L de Villiers. Lansdowne:Juta. pp:255-265).

De Vos, AS (Ed.). 2002. *Research at Grassroots* (2nd edition).Pretoria: Van Schaik

Eysenbach, G. 2000. Report of a case of cyberplagiarism - and reflections on detecting and preventing academic misconduct using the Internet. *Journal of Medical Internet Research*. Http//:www.jmir.org/2001/1/e4/ . . . Accessed 18 December 2004.)\

Fox, M. 2002. Clinical research and patient. The legal perspective. In: *Nursing Law and Ethics* (2nd edition) edited by J Tingle and A Gibbs. Oxford: Blackwell. pp.252-276.

Garbers, JG (Ed.). 1996. *Effective Research in the Human Sciences*. Pretoria: Van Schaik.

Krüger, JS, Lubbe, GJA and Steyn, HC. 1996. *The Human Search for Meaning: A Multireligious Introduction to the religions of Humankind*. Hatfield: Via Afrika.

Kuhse, H and Singer, P. 1999. *Bioethics: an anthology*. Oxford: Blackwell.

Latimer, J (Ed.). 2003. *Advanced Qualitative Research for Nursing*. Oxford: Blackwell.

Mautner, T. 2000. *The Penguin Dictionary of Philosophy*. London: Penguin Publishers

Muller, M. 2001. *Nursing Dynamics* (3rd edition). Sandow: Heinemann.

Siegler, M. 1999. ethics committees: Decisions by bureaucracy. In: *Bioethics: an anthology*, edited by Kuhse, H and Singer, P Oxford: Blackwell. pp. 583-586.

Streubert Speziale, JH and Carpenter, DR. 2004. *Qualitative Research in Nursing: Advancing the Humanistic Imperative* (3rd edition). New York: Lippencott.

Articles

Garattini, S, Bertele, V and Li-Bassi, L. 2003. How can research ethics committees protect patient better? *British Medical Journal*, 326(7400):1199-1201

Tschudin, V. 2001. European experiences of Ethics Committees. *Nursing Ethics*, 8(2):142-151.

Internet website references

- South African Medical Research Council (MRC). Guidelines on Ethics for Medical Research: General Principles: www.sahealthinfo.org/ethics/ethicsbook1.pdf (Accessed 10 November 2004)

- Helsinki Declaration: http://www.wma.net/e/policy/pdf/17c.pdf Accessed 18 December 2004.
- South African Medical Council http://www.sahealthinfo.org/ethics/ethicsbook1.pdf (Accessed 18 December 2004)
- National Health Act (Act 61 of 2003) http://www.doh.gov.za/docs/index.html (Accessed 18 December 2004)
- Patient Rights Charter: http://www.doh.gov.za/docs/legislation/patientsright/chartere.html (Accessed 18 December 2004)
- Health Research Policy in South Africa 2001: http://www.doh.gov.za/search/index.html (Accessed 18 December 2004)
- Guidelines for Good Practice in the Conduct of Clinical Trials in Human Participants in South Africa. http://www.doh.gov.za/docs/index.html (Accessed 18 December 2004)
- University of Alberta, http://www.library.ualberta.ca/guides/plagiarism/terminology/index.cfm Accessed 17 December 2004).

Chapter 13

References

Andrews, MM & Boyle, JS. 1999. *Transcultural concepts in nursing care.* 3rd edition. Philadelphia:Lippincott

Brink, PJ. 1990. *Transcultural Nursing.* A *Book of Readings.* Illinois: Waveland Press Inc.

Burkhardt, MA & Nathaniel, AK. 2002. *Ethics and issues in contemporary nursing.* 2nd edition. Albany NY: Delmar.

Giger, JN & Davidhizar, R. 2004. *Transcultural Nursing. Assessment and Intervention.* 4th edition. St Louis: Mosby.

Haynes, L, Boese, T & Butcher, H. 2004. *Nursing in contemporary society. Issues , trends and transition to practice.* New Jersey: Pearson Prentice Hall.

Henderson, G & Primeaux, M. 1981. *Transcultural Health Care.* Menlo Park: Addison-Wesley Publishing Company.

Lindeman, CA & McAthie, M. 1999. *Fundamentals of contemporary nursing practice.* Philadelphia: W.B. Saunders Company.

McCloskey, JC & Grace, HK (eds.). 1990. *Current Issues in Nursing.* 3rd Edition. St Louis: Mosby.

Oermann, MH. 1997. *Professional Nursing Practice.* Stamford, CT: Appleton & Lange.

Sullivan, EJ. 1999. *Creating nursing's future. Issues, opportunities and challenges.* St Louis: Mosby

Tjale, AA & De Villiers, L. 2004. *Cultural issues in health care*: A *Resource book for Southern Africa.* Cape Town: Juta.

Articles

Eliason, MJ. 1993. Ethics in transcultural nursing care. *Nursing Outlook.* Vol 41 No. 5, 225-228.

Lynam, MJ. 1992. towards the goal of providing culturally sensitive care: principles upon which to build nursing curricula. *Journal of Advanced Nursing.* Vol.17, 149-157.

Chapter 14

References

Beaver, RP, Bergman, J, Langley, MS, Metz, W, Romarheim, A, Walls, A, Withycombe, R & Wootten, RWF. 1982. *The World's Religions.* Malaysia: Struik Christian books (Pty) Ltd.

Burnard, P & Chapman, CM. 1993. *Professional and Ethical Issues in Nursing. The Code of Professional Conduct.* 2nd Edition. London: Scutari Press.

Davis, AJ & Aroska, MA & Draught, TS. 1997. *Ethical dilemmas and nursing practice.* 4th Edition. Stamford,Connecticut: Appleton & Lange.

De Ridder, JC. 1961. *The Personality of the Urban African in South Africa.* London: Routledge & Kegan Paul.

Dolan, JA. 1978. *Nursing in Society. A Historical Perspective*. Philadelphia: Saunders.

Dreyer, M, Hattingh, S & Lock, M. 1993. *Fundamental Aspects in Community Health Nursing*. Halfway House: Southern Book Publishers.

Giger, JN & Davidhizar, RE. 1999. *Transcultural nursing assessment and intervention*. 3rd Edition. St Louis: Mosby.

Gruss, EG. 1975. *We Left Jehovah's Witnesses—A Non-prophet Organisation*. United States of America: Presbyterian and Reformed Publishing Co.

Helman, CG. 1990. *Culture, Health and Illness. An Introduction for Health Professionals*. 2nd Edition. London: Wright.

Hewat, EGK. 1967. *Meeting Jehovah's Witnesses*. Edinburgh: The Saint Andrew Press.

Holden, P & Littlewood, J (eds.). 1991. *Anthropology and Nursing*. London: Routledge.

Holy Bible – Good News Edition. 1988. Goodwood, Cape: National Book Printers.

Larue, GA. 1985. *Euthanasia and Religion: A Survey of the Attitudes of World Religions to the Right to Die*. Los Angeles: The Hemlock Society.

Leek, S. 1973. *The Story of Faith Healing*. New York: MacMillan.

McGilloway, O & Myco, F. 1985. *Nursing and Spiritual Care*. San Francisco: Harper & Row.

Rosner, F. 1986. The Jewish patient in a non-Jewish hospital. *Journal of Religion and Health*. Vol. 25 No. 4, Winter, 316-324.

Schmidt, H & Power, D (ed.). 1977. *Liturgy and Cultural Religious Traditions*. New York: The Seabury Press.

Searle, C. 1965. *The History of the Development of Nursing in South Africa 1652-1960*. Pretoria: SANA.

Sherr, L (ed.). 1989. *Death, Dying and Bereavement*. Oxford: Blackwell Scientific Publications.

Taryor, LNK. 1976. *Impact of the African Tradition on Christianity in Africa Through the Independent Church Movements*. Ann Arbor: University of Microfilms International.

Articles

Bellakhdar, J. 1989. A new look at traditional medicine in Morocco. *World Health Forum*. Vol. 10, 193-199.

Brock, G. 1990. Ritual and vulnerability. *Journal of Religion and Health*. Vol. 29 No. 4, Winter, 285-294.

Chiwuzie, J, Ukoli, F, Okojic, O, Isak, E and Esiator, I. 1987. Traditional practitioners are here to stay. *World Health* Forum. Vol. 8, 240-244.

Cox, JL. 1989. Karma and redemption: A religious approach to family violence. *Journal of Religion and Health*. Vol. 28 No. 1, Spring, 16-24.

Edwards, KL. 1987. Exploratory study of black psychological health. *Journal of Religion and Health*. Vol. 26 No. 1, Spring, 73-79.

Glueck, N. 1988. Religion and health: A theological reflection. *Journal of Religion and Health*. Vol. 27 No. 2, Summer, 109-117.

Hodgson, K. 1989. A responsive service: Health education for Asians with diabetes. *The Professional Nurse*. Vol. 5 No. 3, December, 129-130, 132-133.

Hoff, W & Maseko, DN. 1986. Nurses and traditional healers join hands. *World Health* Forum. Vol. 7, 412-415.

Koekemoer, PJT. 1989. Genadedood en die teologie. *Vroue Hervormer* supplement to *Die Hervormer*. No. 107, October.

Lecso, PA. 1986. Euthanasia: A Buddhist perspective. *Journal of Religion and Health*. Vol. 25 No. 1, Spring, 51-57.

Ogunbodebe, E. 1991. Dental care: The role of traditional healers. *World Health* Forum. Vol. 12, 443-444.

Ontwaak. 1990. Bloedverkope is 'n reusebedryf. Vol. 52 No. 20, 22 October, 1-30.

Government Gazette 27775. SA Government Printer, 11 February 2005.

Staples, RL. 1981. Christianity and the cult of the ancestors: Belief and ritual among the Bantu-speaking peoples of South Africa. Doctoral dissertation. New Jersey: Princeton.

Steegman, HJ. 1982. Rituele genesing onder die Bantoesprekende stedelike bevolking van Suid-Afrika. Submission for BA Hons Ethnology. Pretoria: University of South Africa.

Upvall, MJ. 1992. Nursing perceptions of collaboration with indigenous healers in Swaziland. *International Journal of Nursing Studies*. Vol. 29. No. 1, 27-36.

Vanderpool, HY & Jeffrey, SL. 1990. Religion and medicine: How are they related? *Journal of Religion and Health*. Vol. 29 No. 1, Spring, 9-17.

Chapter 15

References

Aroskar, MA. 1997. Ethical issues in Community Health Nursing. In: *Readings in Community Health Nursing*, edited by BW Spradley and JA Allender (5th edition). New York: Lippencott. pp.135-143.

Bauman, Z. 1993. Intimations of postmodernity. London:Routledge.

Havenga Coetzer, P. 2003. *Viktor Frankl's Avenues to Meaning: A compendium of Concepts, Phrases & Terms in Logotheapy*. Benmore: PattiHavengaCoetzer.

Kelly, JA and Lawrence, JS. 1988. *The AIDS Health Crisis: Psychological and Social Interventions*. Ney York: Plenum Press.

Louw, DA and Edwards, DJA. 1997. *Psychology: An Introduction for Students in South Africa*. 2nd Ed. Johannesburg: Heinemann

Mbigi, L and Maree, J. 1995. *Ubuntu: The Spirit of African Transformation Management*. Johannesburg: Sigma Press.

Walker, MB and Frank, L. 1997. HIV/AIDS: an imperative for a new paradigm for caring. In: *Readings in Community Health Nursing*, edited by BW Spradley and JA Allender 5th Ed. New York: Lippencott. pp.30-38.

Wilson, D, Naidoo, S, Bekker, L-G, Cotton, M and Maartens, M. 2002. *Handbook of HIV Medicine*. Cape Town: Oxford University Press.

Winiarski, MG. 1997. HIV *mental health for the 21st century*. New York: New York University Press.

Articles

Bayer, R and Fairchild, AL. 2004. The genesis of public health ethics. *Bioethics*, 18(6):473-492.

Brown, KH. 1993. Descriptive and normative ethics: class, context and confidentiality for mothers with HIV. *Social Science & Medicine*, 36(3):195-202.

Del Rio, C. 1998. Is ethical research feasible in developed and developing countries? *Bioethics*, 12(4):328-330.

Edwards, SJL, Ashcroft, R and Kirchin, S. 2004. Research ethics committees: differences and moral judgment. *Bioethics*, 18(5):408-427.

Fedor, M. 1992. AIDS: advocacy and activism. *Nursing and Health Care*, 13(2):65.

Galloway, MR. 2003. ART – promises, experience and pitfalls. AIDS *Bulleting*, 12(2):18-20.

Orr, N and Patient, D. 2004. Stigma: beliefs cause behaviour. AIDS *Bulletin*, 13(1):10-14.

Stevens, PE and Hall, JM. 1997. An occupational transmission of HIV: collision of ethical worlds in nursing practice. *Advances in Nursing Science*, 19(1):38-50.

Strassberg, BA. 2003. "The plague of bood": HIV/AIDS and the ethics of the global health-care challenge. *Zygon*, 38(1):169-183.

Thomas, K. 2002. Ethics and HIV research. AIDS Bulletin, 11(1):8-10.

Thomas, J. 1998. Ethical challenges of HIV clinical trails in developing countries. Bioethics, 12(4):320-327.

Wang, Y. 2000. A strategy of clinical tolerance for prevention of HIV and AIDS in China. *Journal of Medicine and Philosophy*, 25(1):18-61.

Woloschak, GE. 2003. HIV: how sciences shaped the ethics. *Zygon*, 38(1):163-167.

Internet sites

The Canadian Medical Association Counselling Guidelines for HIV Testing. (http://www.hivpositive.com/f-TestingHIV/CanadaGuidelines/checklis.htm (Accessed 16 February 2005) British Association for Counselling and Psychotherapy. (http://www.emintel.com/code.htm (Accessed 16 February 2005).

Index

abnormalities, congenital, newborn infants
118-9
abortion 116-8
and Sterilisation Act 116
abuse
children 119-20
women 128-9
access to treatment and care, HIV/AIDS 214-6
accountability 53-4
and responsibility 54
nurse-patient relationship 73-4
research 148
Acquired Immune Deficiency Syndrome
(AIDS) *see also* HIV/AIDS
adolescents 121-2
adults 126-7
act-deontologism 31
act-utilitarianism 30
active euthanasia 137
Jewish view 179
Christian view 183
administrative accountability 5
Administrative Justice Act 83
adolescents, nursing care for 120-3
advanced directives 138
advocacy 51-2, 208, 216-7
affective skill 21
aging, nursing care for the 130-4
agnosticism 188
alcohol, adolescents 122
allocation of resources 35, 143
alternative nursing science 13
analytical ethics 7
ancestral spirits 192-3
anonymity, research 154-5
antenatal care 115
antiretroviral treatment 126, 214-5, 218
apathy 16-7
'armchair caring' 16-7
artificial
insemination 111-2
nutrition and hydration 135
asangoma 194
assault 64
atheism 188
attitudes 8
culture shock 172
attribution, research 159
autonomy

and nurse as employee 84-5
health-care research 149, 152, 154
principle of 32-3, 43
respect for 46-7

Basic Conditions of Employment Act (BCEA)
84-6, 90-1
beliefs 8
culture shock 172
beneficence, principle of 33-5, 43-4, 216
bill of rights 59, 61-3
bioethical
approach, HIV/AIDS 203-4, 205-6
decision-making model 42
bioethics (biomedical ethics) 6, 150
Births, Marriages and Deaths Registration
Act 125
brain-damaged patients and consent 49
breach of service contract 86-7
Buddhism 186-8
view of illness 187
view of dying 187-8

care, access to, HIV/AIDS 214-5
caring 4, 4-17
and nursing ethics 6
'armchair' 16-7
as ethical principle 12
definition 15-7
ethic 11-22
Gilligan's theory of moral development 40-1
'pseudo' 16-7
variants of 16-7
words associated with 16
castration 126
certificates, medical and health, HIV/AIDS
211
cessation of treatment 100
child abuse 119-20
Child Care Act 48, 114, 119
children
and consent 49
HIV tests 214
Children's Status Act 111, 114-5
Choice of Termination of Pregnancy Act 61,
116-7
Christianity 182-3
view of illness 182-3
view of dying 183

citation 159
civil
  liability 65
  rights 60
claim 98
clinical trails 218
code
  nursing 6
  of ethics 6
  of practice for medical practitioners 111
  organisational 144-5
cognitive skill 21
collaborative relationships 79
collective bargaining 92
collegial relationships 79-80
common
  knowledge 160
  law 64
  morality 5
communication
  culture shock 171
  intercultural 168, 169-70, 173
  of research findings 162
communities and HIV/AIDS 208
community
  health approach, HIV/AIDS 204-6
  the elderly in the 132-4
Compensation for Occupational Injuries and
  Diseases Act 84
competence 21
  moral, in HIV/AIDS 201-3
  research 158-62
computerisation and confidentiality 50-1
confidentiality 36-7, 50-2
  and privacy of patient information 50-1
  and the law 50
  computerisation and 50-1
  health-care research 154
  HIV/AIDS 208-12
  problems of 102-3
  right to 102-3
  violation of 103
conflict
  ethical, in bureaucratic environment 91-2
  of loyalties 91
congenital abnormalities, newborn infants
  118-9
conscience 17-20
consent
  informed 47-9
  legal validity of 47-8
  right to refuse 48-9
consequentialism 29-30

Constitution of the Republic of South Africa
  83, 84, 214
context for caring 13
contraception 115
contracts, employment 85-7
controlling paradigm 12-14
conventional level, moral development 38-9
copyright 159
cosmoliteracy 202
cost benefit analysis principle 34
cot death 119
counselling, HIV 212-4
crimen injuria 64-5
culpable homicide 64
cultural
  differences 74-5, 167-73
  forces, transcultural nursing 175-97
  imposition 170-1
  orientation, own 173
  traditions and nursing 177-97
culturally congruous care 172-3
culture
  -sensitive care, obstacles to 168-71
shock 171-2
cure paradigm 12-4
curing 12-5
cyberplagiarism 159

data
  analysis and interpretation 161
  collection 161
death 136-7
  Buddhist view 187
  Christian view 183
  Hindu view 186
  Islamic view 181-2
  Jehovah's Witnesses' view 184
  Jewish view 179-80
  traditional healers' view 192
decision-making
  ethical principles in 46-55
  ethical theory and 27-45
models and process 41-4
moral 37-44
Democratic Nursing Organisation of South
  Africa (DENOSA) 92, 117
deontology 30-2
descriptive ethics 7
dietary practices
  Judaism 178
  Islam 180
differences, labour 92
difficult patients 74

dignity of participants, research 151
dilemma, ethical, research 147
disclosure, HIV/AIDS status 208-12
discrimination, prevention of 83
disputes, labour 92
dissimilar values 9
distorting truth 52
distress, moral 88-9
doctor-nurse relationship 78-80
drug addiction, adolescents 122
due process 83
duties of nurses 104
dying 136-7

ecoliteracy 202
economic-ethical issues 129-30
egoism 29-30
elderly, nursing care for the 130-4
embryo transfer 113-4
emotional
communities 208
  skill 21
employees
  health care industry 143
  rights of 105
employing authorities and nurses 84-92
employment contracts 85-7
Employment Equity Act 83
essential services 93-5
ethical
  agent, individual as 17-22
  business practices in health care
  organisations 141-2
  concepts, application for research 151-62
  conflict in bureaucratic environment 91-2
  decisions in the workplace 141
  dilemma in research 147-8
  intention of research 147
  issues in health care organisations 145-6
  liability, nurses 65-8
  mediators, nurses as 89-90
  principles 32-5
        application for research 151-62
        in decision-making 46-55
        in HIV/AIDS care 201-18
        in professional-patient
  relationships 46-55
  theories 27-32
        application for research 151-62
  theory and decision-making 27-45
ethics
  analytical 7
  clearance 155

committee 44
descriptive 7
foundation of 4-6
in nursing practice 3-4
in research 147-62
management 140-6
nature and scope 6-7
normative 7
organisational 140-1
sources of, for research 150-1
ethnocentrism 74, 168, 170-1
euthanasia 34, 61, 64, 137-8
  adults 128
  Buddhist view 188
  Christian view 183
  Hindu view 186
  Islamic view 182
  Jehovah's Witnesses' view 184
  Jewish view 179
  neonatal 119
  traditional healers' view 192
experience 18-20

fairness, HIV/AIDS 201
faith healing 189
family planning 115
family-member
  -nurse relationships 75-6
  older person as 131-2
fidelity 36, 43-4
fieldworker 147
first-generation human rights 60
formal
ethical decision-making model 43-4
law 64
formalist theories 31
foundation of ethics 4-6
freedom, patient's 43
functional group 208

Gilligan's theory of moral development 40-1
grievances 92
Grundnorm 61
habits, culture shock 172
healing 12-5
  spiritual 188-91
  traditional 191-4
health certificates, HIV/AIDS 211
hermaphrodite 125
Hinduism 184-6
view of illness 185
  view of dying 186
HIV counselling and testing 212-4

HIV/AIDS 126-7, 201-18
/STD Strategic Plan for South Africa 126
holistic patient care, transcultural nursing 168-73
homosexual transsexualism 125
horizontal application, Bill of Rights 59, 61
human rights 59-63
as patient rights 98-103
as rights of nurses 105
violation of 63
Human Tissue Act 114
humanism, secular 188
Husted's formal ethical decision making model 43-4

ideology, HIV/AIDS 201
illness
Buddhist view 187
Christian view 182-3
Hindu view 185
Islamic view 180-1
Jehovah's Witnesses' view 184
Jewish view 178-9
traditional healers' view 191
immoral patients 169
in vitro fertilisation 113-4
indeterminate result, HIV test 214
individual as ethical agent 17-22
infants, newborn 118-9
infertility 111-5
information
patient, privacy 50-1
right to 100-1
technology and confidentiality 50-1
withholding of 101-2
informed consent 47-9
HIV/AIDS research 218
research 152-3
infringement 160
institution, research 154-7
institutional care, the elderly 133-4
instrumental relativism 38
intellect 21
intentions, ethical research 147
intentionality 18
intuition 18, 20
investors, health-care industry 142-3
Islam 180-2
view of illness 180-1
view of dying 181-2
isolation, culture shock 172

Jehovah's Witnesses 183-4
view of illness 184
view of dying 184
Jewish dietary laws 178
Judaism 178-80
view of illness 178-9
view of dying 179-80
justice
and legislation 83-4
principle of 35

knowledge 18, 21-2
culturally congruous care 172-3
right to 100-1
Kohlberg's hierarchy of moral development 38-40

Labour Relations Act 84
language differences 170
law, classification of 64-5
legal
accountability 53
liability of nurse 63-8
rights of nurses 105-6
validity of consent 47-8
legalisation of patient rights 103
legislation 83-4
liability, legal, of nurse 63-8
limited consequentialism 30
literacy, moral, in HIV/AIDS 201-3
literature review, research 159
long-term care, the elderly 133-4
longevity revolution 130-1
low birth-mass neonates 118

management
ethics 140-6
of resources 143-4
role in ethical business practices 141-2
meaning 18, 20
mechanical differences, culture shock 171-2
medical certificates HIV/AIDS 211
mentally handicapped and consent 49
moonlighting 90-1
mercy killing *see* euthanasia
moral
accountability 53
action guides, decision-making 28
competency 201-3
decision-making 37-44
development 37-44
distress 88-9
implications of nursing children 119-20

judgements, nature of 29
literacy in HIV/AIDS 201-3
obligation to do research 149
patients 169
philosophy 4
reasoning 37-44
rights of nurses 106
rules 36-7
values 5
morality 5
motherhood, surrogate 114-5
multicultural nursing 168-73
  religious and cultural forces 175-79
murder 64
mutual
  respect for values and beliefs 73
  trust 73
myths, HIV/AIDS 201, 203
National Health Act 82, 103, 111
negative result HIV test 214
negligence 65-8
negotiation, nurse-patient relationship 73
neonatal euthanasia 119
neonates 118-9
newborn infants 118-9
non-coercive disclaimer 153
non-consequentialism 30-2
non-maleficence, principle of 33-5, 216
non-moral action guides, decision-making 28
non-verbal communication 169-70
normative ethics 7
norms 5
notification of sex partners, HIV/AIDS 210-1
nurse
  and trade unions 92-6
  as ethical mediator 89-90
  autonomy and 46
  -doctor relationships 78-80
  -employer relationships 84-92
  -family member relationship 75-6
  -nurse relationships 76-7
  -patient agreement 43
  -patient relationship 46-55, 70-5
rights of 103-7
  role of in consent 49
nursing practice
  ethics in 3-5
  values in 7-10
nyanga 194

objectivity 29
Occupational Health and Safety Act (OHSA)
  83, 84, 211

occupational injury, HIV/AIDS 211-2
option to withdraw statement 153
organ transplantation 136
organisational
  code of ethics 144-5
ethics 140-1
ostracism, HIV/AIDS 209
own cultural orientation 173
ownership of records 88

paediatrics care 118-20
painless death *see* euthanasia
palliative care 134-6
paraphrasing 160
participation in health-care research 148-9
participants, research 147
passive euthanasia 137, 183
paternalism, principle of 34
patient
  access to information 51
autonomy 47
brain-damaged, and consent 49
difficult 74, 169
freedom of 43
information, privacy of 50-1
moral and immoral 169
nurse- agreement 43
-nurse relationships 46-55, 70-5
perspective of 173
  rights of 97-103
  role in health-care industry 143
  self-determination 46
  unpopular 74, 169
permission in research 152, 154
perspective of patient 173
pilot study, research 160
plagiarism 159
political rights 60
population-based approach to HIV/AIDS 204
positive result, HIV test 214
post-conventional level, moral development
  39-40
post-test counselling, HIV 213
practical model for moral decision-making
  42-3
prayer healing 189-91
preconventional level, moral development 38
prejudice 169-71
premature neonates 118
pre-test counselling, HIV 213
prevention of evil 33
privacy 36-7, 43-4
  research 154

right to 102-3
private law 64-5
privilege 98
  therapeutic 48
privileges, nurses' rights as 104
professional
  accountability 53
  liability 65-8
  morality 5
  patient relationships 46-55
  rights 105-6
Promotion of Equality and Prevention of
  Unfair Discrimination Act 83
promotion of good 33
prophet, healing 189-90
'pseudo-caring' 16-7
psychological contract 86
psychomotor skill 21
public
  health approach to HIV/AIDS 204-6
  law 64

quality of life
  of the elderly 133
  principle 34

racism 171
reason 18, 20
reciprocity
HIV/AIDS research 217-8
therapeutic 72-3
records, ownership of 88
recruiting, research 160
referencing 160
refusal
of consent, right to 48-9
  of treatment, right to 137
relationships
  between nurses 76-7
  nurse-doctor 78-80
  nurse-employer 84-92
  nurse-family members 75-6
  nurse-patient 46-55, 70-5
  nurse-trade unions 92-6
trusting 80
relativism 29
religioliteracy 202
religion
  and health, connection 176
  and health service 176-7
religious
  forces, transcultural nursing 175-97
  traditions and nursing 177-97

reproductive
  care 111-5
  technology 111-5
research
ethics 147-162
  HIV/AIDS 216-8
Research Ethics Committee 155-7
researcher 147
  competence 158-82
  scientific integrity 157
resources
  allocation of 35, 143
  management of 143-4
respondents, research 147
responsibilities of nurses 104
responsibility
  and accountability 54
  of nurse in consent 49
retirement 132-3
right
  to die 137
  to refuse consent 48-9
rights
  bill of 59, 61-3
  human 59-63
  of patients 97-103
  of nurses 103-7
role of nurse in consent 49
rule
of deontology 31-2
  -utilitarianism 30

sampling, research 160
sanctity of life principle 34
scientific integrity 157
second-generation human rights 60
secular humanism 188
sedation, palliative care 135-6
self respect of participants, research 125-6
sex
-change surgery 125-6
partners, confidentiality 210-1
sexism 171
sexual
  activity, adolescents 120
  activity, adults 125
  freedom 124
skills 18, 21-2
  communication 173
  for culturally congruous care 172-3
social
intervention, HIV/AIDS 206
  responsibility programmes 144

socio-economic rights 60
socioliteracy 202
soothsayer 192-3
sorcery 194
South African
Bill of Rights 59, 61-3
    Democratic Nurses Union (SADNU) 92
    Nursing Council (SANC) 83
special rights of nurses 105
spiritual healing 188-91
spirituality 18
stakeholders, health-care industry 142-3
statutory law 64
stereotyping 74, 168
sterilisation 115
stigmatisation, HIV/AIDS 127, 203, 209, 216
stressors, culture shock 171-2
strikes 92-6
structural community 208
subjectivity 29
subjects, research 147
surrogate motherhood 114-5

technology, culture shock 171-2
teenage
    pregnancy 120-1
    suicide 122
teleology 29-30
termination of contract 86-7
testing, HIV 212-4
therapeutic
    privilege 48
    reciprocity 72-3
third-generation human rights 61
Thompson and Thompson's bioethical
    decision-making model 42
Thompson, Melia and Boyd's practical mode
    for moral decision-making 42-3
trade unions 92-6
traditional
    healer 193-4
    healing 191-4
    medical-natural science-human context 13
    practices and Western medicine 194-7
transcultural nursing 168-73, 175-97
transpersonal caring-healing model 22
transplantation, organ 136
transsexualism 125
transvestite transsexualism 125

treatment
    access to HIV/AIDS214-5
    cessation of 100
refusal to receive 100, 137
right to 99
trusting relationships 80
truth
    distortion of 52
    in research 161
    -telling 52-3, 101
    withholding of 52, 101

unconscious patient and consent 49
unpopular patients 74, 169
utilitarianism 30

validity, legal, of consent 47-8
values 5, 8
and beliefs, respect for 73
in nursing practice 7-10
variants of caring 16-7
veracity 36, 43-4, 52-3
    HIV/AIDS 208
    research 152
verbal communication 169-70
vertical application, Bill of Rights 59, 61
violation of human rights 63
violence, workplace 87-8
virtue 21
voluntarism, HIV/AIDS 204, 209
voluntary refusal of treatment 137
vulnerability
    HIV/AIDS 209, 216
    research 148-50

Western medicine and traditional healers
    194-7
will orientation 17-9
witchcraft 194
withholding
    information 101
    truth 52
words associated with caring 16
working conditions 87-90
workplace violence 87-8

Xhosa Christians 191

Zionist Church 191